FABrithwood

Endocrinology
Specialist Handbook

Endocrinology Specialist Handbook

Stephen Robinson
Department of Endocrinology and Metabolic Medicine
Imperial College School of Medicine
St Mary's Hospital
London, UK

Karim Meeran
Department of Endocrinology and Metabolic Medicine
Imperial College School of Medicine
Hammersmith and Charing Cross Hospitals
London, UK

MARTIN DUNITZ

© 2002 Martin Dunitz Ltd, a member of the Taylor & Francis group

First published in the United Kingdom in 2002 by
Martin Dunitz Ltd,
The Livery House,
7–9 Pratt Street,
London NW1 0AE

Tel.:   +44 (0) 20 7482 2202
Fax.:   +44 (0) 20 7267 0159
E-mail: info@dunitz.co.uk
Website: http://www.dunitz.co.uk

A CIP record for this book is available from the British Library.

ISBN 1-84184-158-7

Distributed in the USA by
Fulfilment Center
Taylor & Francis
10650 Tobben Drive
Independence, KY 41051, USA
Toll Free Tel.: +1 800 634 7064
E-mail: taylorandfrancis@thomsonlearning.com

Distributed in Canada by
Taylor & Francis
74 Rolark Drive
Scarborough, Ontario M1R 4G2, Canada
Toll Free Tel.: +1 877 226 2237
E-mail: tal_fran@istar.ca

Distributed in the rest of the world by
Thomson Publishing Services
Cheriton House
North Way
Andover, Hampshire SP10 5BE, UK
Tel.: +44 (0)1264 332424
E-mail: salesorder.tandf@thomsonpublishingservices.co.uk

Composition by EXPO Holdings, Malaysia

Printed and bound in Singapore by Kyodo Printing Co (S'pore) Pte Ltd

Contents

Foreword

Too often medicine retreats into the realms of molecular biology and the *raison d'être* of doctors is forgotten — to make a diagnosis, to devise a treatment plan and, simplistically, to make patients feel better or, indeed, occasionally to cure them. Endocrinology often falls into this trap: there is a kind of magic to molecules, and the molecular and genetic basis of many endocrine disorders have been beautifully explored in minute detail. The large textbooks of endocrinology seem at times to contain little else. This is intellectually stimulating, but we still have to treat patients.

This handbook focuses specifically on the latter. It is an invaluable guide for the doctor in training to the diagnosis and treatment of all the common endocrine disorders. It is based, wherever possible, on evidence rather than anecdote and is logical in its approach and format. It should be invaluable for the intending endocrinologist, particularly when set against the bewildering array of minutiae that could have been included. At first sight, it may seem odd to include dyslipidaemias, however these are often referred to the endocrinologist/diabetologist and certainly trainees in these specialties need to be familiar with them.

I commend this volume to trainees and to consultants requiring an *aide-mémoire* and look forward to the parallel volume in diabetes.

Sir George Alberti
Professor of Medicine

Preface

This book has been written for the specialist registrar, but we hope it will also be useful for the consultant and SHO. It concentrates on day-to-day management issues; much of the physiology which allows us to understand best practice has been left out on purpose, in order to achieve a small, compact volume which can easily be carried in the pocket rather than sit on a shelf.

Much of endocrinology is best practice. Seldom in endocrinology do we find large placebo-controlled randomised trials with endpoint outcomes. Our practice is often dictated by anecdotal evidence, or trials using surrogate markers, or common sense based on physiological understanding of the principles. Undoubtedly, some experts will disagree with some of the management in this book, but even when there are clear outcome data for a condition, there is still no unanimity on management.

Endocrinology is an enticing subject. It spans the entire field of medicine – from the physiology of cortisol and cortisone to the anatomy of the pituitary *fossa*; from the pharmacology of somatostatin analogues to cytology of thyroid nodules. In clinical practice we can offer a treatment, and indeed a cure, of many conditions, through to the more subtle new answers of persuading patients about the benefits of preventive therapy, finally to epidemiological practice and decisions on screening programmes. We do not have so much clear evidence-based practice of our *alter ego*, the diabetologist. We attempt to follow sensible practice both in terms of the science and physiology of the situation but also the merits of treating a condition in an individual patient.

There may be some differences between the endocrinologist and the diabetologist, however, both have to work in a multidisciplinary area. The thyroid clinic will rely upon the skills of a surgeon, the technical know-how of the cytologist and the oncologist, in addition to the ability of the ultrasonographer. The pituitary service will include a neurologist and neuro-ophthalmologist, a surgeon, a radiotherapist and a neuro-radiologist. The endocrinologist will attempt to put these services into a complete, rounded practice addressing all aspects of patient care. We have attempted to review the roles of the specialities around endocrinology.

At the end of each chapter there is a reading list, this is not intended to be an extensive reference list, but rather suggest review articles which give evidence supporting or disagreeing with the practice suggested in that chapter. Many specialist registrars would read *Clinical Endocrinology* and the *Journal of Clinical Endocrinology and Metabolism*. Both journals give review and best clinical practice articles, in addition to original scientific papers.

The appendix includes the common endocrine investigations and how to perform them. Some centres may have different protocols and different normal ranges, and one needs to check first. There are also some useful addresses of patient and professional organisations.

Stephen Robinson
Karim Meeran

Contributors

Stephen G Ball
The Medical School
University of Newcastle upon
    Tyne
Framlington Place
Newcastle upon Tyne
NE2 4HH, UK

Pierre-Marc Gilles Bouloux
Centre for Neuroendocrinology
Royal Free Hospital
Pond Street
London
NW3 2QG, UK

Nicola A Bridges
Chelsea and Westminster
    Hospital
369 Fulham Road
London
SW10 9NH, UK

Helen C Cocks
88 Montagu Avenue
Godforth
Newcastle-upon-Tyne, UK

Juliet E Compston
University of Cambridge
    School of Clinical Medicine
Department of Medicine Box
    157
Addenbrooke's Hospital
Hills Road
Cambridge
CB2 2QQ, UK

Jayne A Franklyn
Division of Medical Sciences
Queen Elizabeth Hospital
Edgbaston
Birmingham
B15 2TH, UK

Dimitrous Goulis
Department of Metabolic
    Medicine
Imperial College School of
    Medicine
St Mary's Hospital
Praed Street
London
W2 1NY, UK

Ashley Grossman
Department of Endocrinology
King George V Block
St Bartholomew's Hospital
London
EC1A 7BE, UK

David Heath
Department of Endocrinology
Selly Oak Hospital
Raddlebarn Road
Selly Oak
Birmingham
B29 6JD, UK

Paul J Jenkins
Department of Endocrinology
King George V Block
St Bartholomew's Hospital
London
EC1A 7BE, UK

Desmond G Johnston
Department of Endocrinology
  and Metabolic Medicine
Imperial College School of
  Medicine
St Mary's Hospital
Praed Street
London
W2 1NY, UK

Tara M Kearney
Department of Endocrinology
  and Metabolic Medicine
Imperial College School of
  Medicine
St Mary's Hospital
Praed Street
London
W2 1NY, UK

Michael F Laker
Department of Clinical
  Biochemistry
Royal Victoria Infirmary
Newcastle-upon-Tyne
NE2 4HH, UK

John H Lazarus
Department of Medicine
University of Wales College of
  Medicine
University Hospital of Wales
Heath Park
Cardiff
CF4 4XN, UK

Miles J Levy
Endocrine Unit
Imperial College School of
  Medicine
Hammersmith Hospital
Du Cane Road
London
W12 0NN, UK

Catherine A Lissett
Department of Endocrinology
Christie Hospital
Wilmslow Road
Withington
Manchester
M20 4BX, UK

Callum Livingstone
Royal Surrey County Hospital
Guildford
Surrey
GU2 7XX, UK

Anne Marie McLaughlin
Department of Investigative
  Endocrinology
St Vincent's University
  Hospital
Elm Park
Dublin 4
Ireland

Karim Meeran
Department of Endocrinology
  and Metabolic Medicine
Imperial College School of
  Medicine
Hammersmith and Charing
  Cross Hospitals
Du Cane Road
London
W12 0NN, UK

John DC Newell-Price
Endocrine Unit
Division of Clinical Sciences
University of Sheffield
Northern General Hospital
Sheffield
S5 7AU, UK

Kofi Obuobie
Department of Medicine
University of Wales College of
    Medicine
University Hospital of Wales
Heath Park
Cardiff
CF4 4XN, UK

Jean O'Connell
Department of Investigative
    Medicine
St Vincent's University Hospital
Elm Park
Dublin 4
Ireland

Donal O'Shea
Department of Investigative
    Medicine
St Vincent's University
    Hospital
Elm Park
Dublin 4
Ireland

Adam CJ Robinson
Department of Diabetes &
    Endocrinology
Diabetes Centre
Oldham Royal Hospital
Rochdale Road
Oldham
OL1 2JH, UK

Stephen Robinson
Department of Metabolic
    Medicine
Imperial College School of
    Medicine
St Mary's Hospital
Praed Street
London
W2 1NY, UK

Andrew Rodin
Department of Endocrinology
    and General Medicine
St Helier Hospital
Wrythe Lane
Carshalton
Surrey
SM5 1AA, UK

Stephen M Shalet
Department of Endocrinology
Christie Hospital
Wilmslow Road
Withington
Manchester
M20 4BX, UK

Ayesha Siddiqi
Department of Endocrinology
King George V Block
St Bartholomew's Hospital
London
EC1A 7BE, UK

Shahrad Taheri
Endocrine Unit
Imperial College School of
    Medicine
Hammersmith Hospital
Du Cane Road
London
W12 0NN, UK

Rajesh V Thakker
May Professor of Medicine
The Oxford University Institute
   of Musculoskeletal Sciences
Botnar Research Centre
Nuffield Department of
   Clinical Medicine
Nuffield Orthopaedic Centre
Headington
Oxford
OX3 7LD, UK

Anthony D Toft
The Royal Infirmary of
   Edinburgh
1 Lauriston Place
Edinburgh
EH3 9YW, UK

Shahid T Wahid
Department of Diabetes &
   Endocrinology
Diabetes Centre
Oldham Royal Hospital
Rochdale Road
Oldham
OL1 2JH, UK

Diana F Wood
Department of Endocrinology
King George V Block
St Bartholomew's Hospital
London
EC1A 7BE, UK

List of abbreviations

ACA	adrenal cortex autoantibodies
ACTH	adrenocorticotrophic hormone
AD	androgen deficiency
ADH	antidiuretic hormone
ALT	alanine aminotransferase
ANCA	antineutropihil cytoplasmic autoantibody
ANP	atrial natriuretc peptide
ApoA-II	apolipoprotein A-II
ApoB	apolipoprotein B
APUD	amine precursor uptake and decarboxylation
AQPs	aquaporins
ATD	antithyroid drug
BIPSS	bilateral inferior petrosal sinus sampling (BIPSS)
BMD	bone mineral density
BMI	body mass index
CAH	congenital adrenal hyperplasia
CBG	corticosteroid-binding globulin
CCF	congestive cardiac failure
CCK	cholecystokinin
CK	creatine kinase
COC	combined oral contraceptives
COMT	catecholamine-O-methyl transferase
CRE	cAMP response element
CREB	cAMP response binding protein
CRH	corticotrophin-releasing hormone
CT	computed tomography
DDAVP	desmopressin
DHEAS	dehydroepiandrosterone sulphate
DHT	dihydrotestosterone
DOPA	dihydroxyphenylalanine
DTC	differentiated thyroid cancer
DXA	dual energy X-ray absorptiometry
FBH	familial benign hypercalcaemia
FH	familial hypercholesterolaemia
FHA	functional hypothalamic amenorrhoea
FHH	familial hypocalciuric hypercalcaemia

FNAC	fine needle aspiration cytology
GABA	γ-aminobutyric acid
GGT	γ-glutamyl transferase
GH	growth hormone
GH	growth hormone gene
GHRH	growth hormone releasing hormone
GHRH-R	GHRH receptor
GIP	glucose-dependent insulinotropic polypeptides
GLP-1	glucagon-like peptide-1
GLP-2	glucagon-like peptide-2
GnRH	gonadotrophin-releasing hormone
GRF	growth hormone releasing factor
hCG	human chorionic gonadotrophin
hCS	human chorionic somatotrophin
hMG	human menopausal gonadotrophin
HDDST	high-dose dexamethasone-suppression test
HDL	high-density lipoprotein
hGH-N	gene for pituitary GH
hGH-V	gene for placental GH
HMGCoA	3-hydroxy-3-methylglutaryl coenzyme A
HPA	hypothalamic–pituitary–adrenal
HPT	hypothalamic–pituitary–testicular
IFG	impaired fasting glucose
IGF-1	insulin-like growth factor-1
IGFBP	insulin-like growth factor binding protein; e.g. IGFBP-3
IGT	impaired glucose tolerance
IHD	ischaemic heart disease
IHH	idiopathic hypogonadotrophic hypogonadism
INR	international normalised ratio
ITT	insulin tolerance test
IVC	inferior vena cava
JGA	juxta glomerular apparatus
LDL	low-density lipoprotein
LDDST	low-dose dexamethasone-suppression test
LFT	liver function test
LOH	loss of heterozygosity
Lp(a)	lipoprotein(a)
LPL	lipoprotein lipase
MCV	mean cell volume
MEN	multiple endocrine neoplasia
MIBG	meta-iodobenzylguanidine
MRI	magnetic resonance imaging

MSH	melanocyte-stimulating hormone
NP	neurophysin
NPY	neuropeptide Y
NSAIDS	nonsteroidal anti-inflammatory drugs
OGTT	oral glucose tolerance test
OCP	oral contraceptive pill
PAC	plasma aldosterone concentration
PAI-1	plasminogen activator inhibitor 1
PCOS	polycystic ovary syndrome
PGA	polyglandular autoimmune syndrome
PHA	primary hyperaldosteronism
PNMT	phenylethanolamine N-methyl transferase
POMC	pro-opiomelanocortin
PP	pancreatic polypeptide
PRA	plasma renin activity
PRL	prolactin
PSA	prostate-specific antigen
PTH	parathyroid hormone
PTHrp	parathyroid hormone-related protein
PUO	pyrexia of unknown origin
PVN	paraventricular nuclei
R–A	renin–angiotensin (system)
RIA	radio immuno assay
SCC	side chain clearage
SCRT	stereotactic conformal radiotherapy
SERM	selective oestrogen receptor modulator
SHBG	sex hormone-binding globulin
SIADH	syndrome of inappropriate antidiuretic hormone
SON	supraoptic nuclei
SSCP	single-strand conformation polymorphism analysis
SSRIs	serotonin reuptake inhibitors
T_3	triiodothyronine
T_4	thyroxine
TBI	total body irradiation
TENS	transcutaneous electrical nerve stimulation
TIBC	total iron binding capacity
TRAb	TSH-receptor antibody
TRH	thyrotrophin-releasing hormone
TRIGS	triglycerides
TRT	testosterone replacement therapy
TSH	thyroid-stimulating hormone
TSHR-Ab	thyroid-stimulating hormone receptor antibodies

UFC	urinary free cortisol
ULN	upper limit of normal
USS	ultrasound
VHL	von Hippel-Lindau syndrome
VIP	vasoactive intestinal peptide
VP	vasopressin

Pituitary Adenomas

Tara M Kearney and Desmond G Johnston

Introduction

Tumours arising from the pituitary gland may present to the endocrinologist, neurologist or ophthalmologist, but are increasingly discovered incidentally while imaging the brain for other reasons. The differentiation from hypothalamic tumours may be extremely difficult and is sometimes possible only following surgery.

Epidemiology

Pituitary adenomas constitute 10% of all intracranial tumours. The prevalence is ~200/million and the incidence ~15/million/year. At post-mortem, occult pituitary tumours are found in 11–23% of unselected adult cases. In clinical practice, 70% of pituitary tumours present between 30 and 50 years; only 3–7% occur in patients under 20 years old. An equal sex distribution is observed, except for microprolactinomas, which are 20 times more common in women.

Aetiology

Pituitary adenomas may be primary or secondary. Primary pituitary tumours are usually sporadic, but can be inherited, e.g. as part of the MEN1 syndrome (multiple endocrine neoplasia type 1). This is a syndrome comprising hyperplasia or neoplasia of the anterior pituitary, pancreas or parathyroid glands, which is inherited in an autosomal dominant fashion.

Rarely, pituitary tumours may be secondary in the sense that they arise following a prolonged period of hyperplasia. This may be seen with ectopic hormone secretion, e.g. ectopic secretion of growth hormone releasing hormone (GHRH) from carcinoma of the pancreas, lung or gastrointestinal tract, leading to somatotroph hyperplasia and subsequent adenoma formation. Loss of negative feedback may be important in some instances and may contribute to the development of adrenocorticotrophic hormone (ACTH)-secreting pituitary adenomas following bilateral adrenalectomy for Cushing's disease (Nelson's syndrome).

Pathogenesis

Several studies have demonstrated that some pituitary tumours are monoclonal, suggesting an underlying genetic defect. There are two main mechanisms.

Oncogenes

Oncogene expression may lead to phosphorylation of intracellular growth factors promoting cell proliferation, altering signal transmission by GTPases or altering DNA transcription. Some growth hormone (GH)-secreting tumours have somatic mutations in the G-protein, which normally inhibit GTPases, resulting in elevated cAMP levels in one-third of such tumours.

Tumour suppressor genes

Tumour suppressor genes exert their influence in a recessive manner; hence, the tumour suppressor genes on both chromosomes must be mutated before suppression of proliferation is lifted. MEN1 tumours may show a mutation of a tumour suppressor gene localised to chromosome 11q13. The same defect has been found in up to 20% of sporadic tumours.

Classification

Pituitary tumours can be classified according to size, function, cell composition, staining characteristics and degree of invasion. An overview is given in Table 1.1.

Table 1.1 Overview of pituitary tumours

Tumour type	Hormone secreted	Per cent adenoma	Cellular composition	Staining characteristics	Macroadenomas (%)[a]	Invasion (%)[a]
Functional	Prolactin	30–40	Lactotroph	Acidophilic	40 F, 90 M	50
	GH	2–17	Somatotroph	Acidophilic	90	60
	ACTH	2–10	Corticotroph	Basophilic	11	60
	TSH	<1	Thyrotroph	Basophilic	~100	50
	Multiple	15	Mixed	Variable	70	50
Non-functional	α-subunit	7–15	Gonadotroph	Chromophobic	~100	21
	Nil	10–20	Primitive	Chromophobic	~100	40

F = female, M = male; ACTH = adrenocorticotrophic hormone; GH = growth hormone; TSH = thyroid-stimulating hormone.
[a] At diagnosis.

Size

Microadenomas are defined as tumours less than 10 mm in diameter on imaging, and commonly include prolactinomas in women and ACTH-secreting tumours. *Macroadenomas* are defined as tumours greater than 1 cm in diameter, and include most other tumours, particularly non-functioning tumours. Some investigators recognise an intermediate category of *mesoadenoma* (tumours 10–20 mm).

Functioning/non-functioning

Functioning tumours secrete hormones to produce a clinically recognisable syndrome, such as prolactinomas, Cushing's disease, acromegaly and, rarely, thyroid-stimulating hormone (TSH)- or gonadotrophin-secreting tumours (secretion of biologically active gonadotrophins, unlike α-subunit secretion, is rare). Details of these tumours can be found in other chapters. Functional tumours account for ~75% of all pituitary tumours which present clinically.

   Non-functioning tumours do not secrete hormones, or secrete hormones without clinical sequelae. These are further classified, as described in Table 1.2. Non-functioning tumours account for ~25% of all pituitary tumours.

Cellular composition

Pituitary adenomas may also be described according to the cell of origin and include corticotrophs, lactotrophs, thyrotrophs, somatotrophs, gonadotrophs, null cells and oncocytes.

Staining characteristics

The ability of pituitary tumours to stain with haematoxylin and eosin (H&E) produced an early classification of pituitary tumours which is still widely employed in initial reports following surgery. Tumours that stain poorly are referred to as chromophobe adenomas, and include non-functioning tumours. Tumours staining well are referred to as chromophilic and are further divided into those that stain in acid conditions (mainly prolactinomas and somatotrophic adenomas) and those that stain in basic conditions (thyrotrophic, corticotrophic and gonadotrophic adenomas).

Table 1.2 Characteristics of non-functioning tumours

Non-functioning tumour	Histological characteristics	Staining characteristics
Null cell	Primitive cells, mitochondria deplete	Sparse staining for FSH, LH, α-subunit
Oncocytomas	Primitive cells, filled with mitochondria	Sparse staining for FSH, LH, α-subunit
Silent corticotrophs type 1	Identical to basophilic adenomas, but little ACTH secretion	Most cells stain for ACTH
Silent corticotrophs type 2	Smaller secretory granules than typical basophilic adenomas	Most cells stain for ACTH
Silent corticotrophs type 3	Similar to glycoprotein-secreting adenomas; chromophobic	Few cells stain for ACTH or POMC

ACTH = adrenocorticotrophic hormone; FSH = follicle-stimulating hormone; LH = luteinising hormone; POMC = pro-opiomelanocorticotrophin.

Extent of invasion

A further classification system is that based on invasion of surrounding tissue: Hardy's classification (Table 1.3).

Clinical Features

Patients may present with symptoms relating to the pituitary mass, endocrine insufficiency or clinical syndrome arising from hormone hypersecretion.

Table 1.3 Hardy's classification of pituitary tumour invasion

Grade	Finding
0	Normal sella turcica
I	Focal changes seen, confined to the sella
II	Macroadenoma with sella enlargement
III	Macroadenoma with focal sella destruction
IV	Extensive sella destruction with erosion of the skull base

Features related to a pituitary mass

Symptoms related to a pituitary mass are usually found in cases of macroadenomas, and are therefore most commonly seen in non-functioning tumours, acromegaly and, in men, prolactinomas. The most common symptoms are headache and visual field defects. Symptoms of raised intracranial pressure, cranial nerve palsies and cerebrospinal fluid (CSF) rhinorrhoea are less commonly observed. These symptoms are described in Table 1.4. Rarely, microadenomas may also cause such symptoms.

Features related to hypopituitarism

Compression or replacement of functional pituitary tissue leads to the sequential loss of follicle-stimulating hormone (FSH), luteinising hormone (LH), GH, TSH and then ACTH. The early loss of gonadotrophins, combined with hyperprolactinaemia which

Table 1.4   Clinical features of a pituitary mass

Symptoms/signs of pituitary mass	Frequency observed	Characteristic features
Headache	50–72% macros	Worse in the morning, on straining and coughing
Visual field defect	50–60% macros	Classically a bitemporal hemianopia, but any abnormality can be seen
Symptoms of raised ICP	5%	Headache, nausea, vomiting, hypothalamic dysfunction, i.e. hyperphagia, dysthermia
Cranial nerve palsies	Uncommon	Ophthalmoplegia (CN III, VI), facial pain, optic atrophy, papilloedema
CSF rhinorrhoea	Rare	Nasal discharge (positive for glucose on dipstick)
Pituitary apoplexy	Rare	Sudden headache, meningism, visual loss, visual field deficit and hypopituitarism. Signs of ↑ICP. Patient may be moribund

CN = cranial nerve; CSF = cerebrospinal fluid; ICP = intracranial pressure.

often coexists, results in amenorrhoea, which may lead to the earlier detection of pituitary tumours in women compared with men. Men tend to present later with macroadenomas, as the early symptoms of failing sexual function may deter patients from seeking help. The symptoms related to hypopituitarism are discussed in Chapter 2, but are briefly summarised in Table 1.5.

Features related to endocrine oversecretion

The clinical syndromes produced by oversecretion of GH, ACTH, prolactin (PRL) and TSH are discussed in separate chapters. Hyperprolactinaemia may result from compression of the pituitary stalk by any form of pituitary or hypothalamic tumour. This occurs as a result of the loss of the inhibitory action of dopamine, which is released from the hypothalamus and passes to the pituitary via the neurohypophyseal vein. The hyperprolactinaemia that results is usually modest (< 3000 mU/l). Prolactin levels greater than 5000 mU/l would suggest the presence of a prolactinoma rather than stalk compression.

Table 1.5   Clinical features of pituitary insufficiency

Deficient hormone	Incidence[a]	Symptoms and signs
LH, FSH	45% women	Amenorrhoea, infertility, breast and vaginal atrophy
	40% men	Reduced libido, impotence, reduced shaving, lethargy
GH	80%	Lethargy, weakness, obesity, low mood, fatiguability, thin skin, reduced sweating
TSH	20–30%	Apathy, dry hair, pallor, bradycardia, hypothermia, weight gain
ACTH	20–30%	Weight loss, pallor, postural hypotension, hyponatraemia
Panhypopituitarism	10%	As above, may be moribund

ACTH = adrenocorticotrophic hormone; FSH = follicle-stimulating hormone; GH = growth hormone; LH = luteinising hormone; TSH = thyroid-stimulatiing hormone.
[a] In macroadenoma.

Investigations

The aim of the investigations is to assess endocrine function, pituitary size and neuro-ophthalmic complications.

Assessment of endocrine function

The assessment of endocrine function may incorporate tests to establish endocrine deficiency and oversecretion. Basal and dynamic pituitary function tests are often required. In general, stimulation tests are required to demonstrate endocrine deficiency and can be found in detail in Chapter 2. In cases of suspected endocrine oversecretion, suppression tests are usually required and are detailed in the relevant chapters. A summary of the tests that may be required can be found in Tables 1.6 and 1.7.

Assessment of pituitary size

A high-resolution magnetic resonance imaging (MRI) scan is the imaging technique of choice, as it allows high-resolution imaging with assessment of the optic chiasm and surrounding structures. MRI scanning also permits visualisation without the need for X-irradiation, of importance especially in patients requiring further imaging following treatment. No imaging technique can differentiate functioning from non-functioning tumours. An empty sella is seen in 4% of normal volunteers. Skull X-rays may show ballooning of the sella, with bony erosions, but have been superseded by MRI scans. When MRI imaging is available, computed tomography (CT) scans are usually reserved for emergency use and for patients with pacemakers, claustrophobia or other contraindications to MRI scanning.

Neuro-ophthalmic assessment

Compression of the optic chiasm by a pituitary mass may threaten vision, and hence a thorough neuro-ophthalmic assessment is required. This involves the assessment of external eye muscle movements, visual acuity, visual fields and fundoscopy, and should preferably be performed in conjunction with an ophthalmologist.

Table 1.6   Tests of endocrine Insufficiency

Deficient hormone	Basal tests	Dynamic stimulation test
Prolactin	Low prolactin	None usually employed (TRH, domperidone, IST)
FSH / LH	Low / normal FSH/LH Low testosterone/oestrogen or clinical evidence of oestrogen deficiency	LH releasing hormone (LHRH) test is rarely employed
TSH	Low/normal ???TSH, low ?FT_4 or total T_4	Thyroid hormone releasing hormone test is rarely employed
ACTH	Low plasma cortisol, ACTH Possible low plasma sodium	Cortisol levels on stimulation test, i.e. IST, glucagon test, short tetracosactrin test (30-min value)
GH	Low IGF-1 and random GH unreliable	GH < 6 mU/l on stimulation test, i.e. IST, glucagon test
AVP	Urine output > 3 litres/day. Low urine osmolality with raised plasma osmolality	Water deprivation test

ACTH = adrenocorticotrophic hormone; AVP = arginine vasopressin; FSH = follicle-stimulating hormone; FT4 = free thyroxine; GH = growth hormone; IST = insulin stress test; IGF-1 insulin-like growth factor-1; LH = luteinising hormone; T4 = thyroxine; TRH = thyrotrophin-releasing hormone; TSH = thyroid-stimulatiing hormone.

Treatment

Pituitary tumours may be managed medically, surgically or with radiotherapy. In some cases, all three treatment modalities will be required.

Medical therapy

Medical therapy may be indicated for several reasons, including the following.

Table 1.7 Tests of endocrine oversecretion

Excess hormone	Basal tests	Dynamic suppression test
Prolactin	Random prolactin level	None employed
FSH / LH	↑ FSH, LH, sex hormone	None employed
TSH	↑ TSH, Free T_3, T_4	None employed
ACTH	↑ Urinary free cortisol, ↑ ACTH in 50%	Dexamethasone suppression test (low-dose, 2 mg/day for 48 hours)
GH	↑ IGF-1, GH	Oral glucose tolerance test
AVP	Hyponatraemia, plasma and urine osmolalities	None employed

ACTH = adrenocorticotrophic hormone; AVP = arginine vasopressin; FSH = follicle-stimulating hormone; GH = growth hormone; IGF-1 = insulin-like growth factor-1; LH = luteinising hormone; T_3 = triiodothyronine; T_4 = thyroxine; TSH = thyroid-stimulatiing hormone.

Control of symptoms

Medical therapy may be used to decrease the hormone production in pituitary tumours secreting excessive amounts of hormone. Examples of this include the use of dopamine agonists to reduce prolactin secretion or metyrapone to reduce cortisol production. Such treatment may be used prior to surgery or may be the treatment of choice for the long term. A brief summary of the drugs currently available to reduce excessive hormone secretion and the effect achieved is outlined in Table 1.8. More detailed descriptions can be found in the relevant chapters.

Reduction of tumour size (debulking)

In some cases, medical therapies can also cause shrinkage of the pituitary tumour. Dopamine agonists are associated with a significant decrease in the size of prolactinomas in 80% of cases, and are thus the treatment of choice. Rarely, dopamine agonists may also reduce the size of GH-secreting tumours, but surgery is usually required to achieve a satisfactory result. Somatostatin analogues cause a (usually small) reduction in tumour size in acromegaly. Concerns regarding the GH-receptor antagonist, pegvisomant, leading to tumour enlargement, have not been

Table 1.8.   Medical treatment of endocrine oversecretion

Drug group	Examples	Used in	Success (%) in ↓ secretion	Success (%) in ↓ tumour size
Dopamine agonists	Bromocriptine Cabergoline Quinagolide	Prolactinomas Acromegaly FSHomas Non-functioning	90 15 10 Not applicable	80 5 0 <10
Somatostatin analogues	Octreotide Lanreotide	Acromegaly TSHomas	55 15	50 Nil
11β-hydroxylase inhibitor	Metyrapone	Cushing's disease	>50%	Nil
Cytochrome P450 inhibitor	Ketoconazole Etomidate	Cushing's disease	>50%	Nil

borne out but longer-term data on large numbers of patients are awaited.

Replacement of endocrine deficiencies

Pituitary tumours, or their treatment, are commonly associated with endocrine insufficiencies. Medical replacement therapy is required. Further details of this can be found in Chapter 2.

Surgical therapy

Indications

Surgery is generally indicated for macroadenomas, except for macroprolactinomas, which usually respond to dopamine agonists. Surgery is also indicated in cases where medical therapy has failed to control the oversecretion of hormones, either by a micro- or macroadenoma. This is commonly the case with Cushing's disease. In the rare case of pituitary apoplexy, surgical intervention may be required as an emergency for prevention of permanent blindness or other neurological deficit.

Preoperative assessment

Attempts should be made preoperatively to delineate the size (and function if possible) of the pituitary tumour. Visual fields should be formally assessed and recorded. In cases of endocrine insufficiency, satisfactory replacement should preferably be achieved prior to surgery. This is particularly important in the case of ACTH deficiency, where surgery without adequate steroid cover would be hazardous. Where endocrine oversecretion has been documented, attempts may be made to suppress hormonal production. This may be of benefit in Cushing's disease, where the general health of the patient and tissue healing can be improved by medical control prior to surgery.

Consent

During consent, it is necessary to advise the patient that a small amount of fat may be taken from the thigh to 'plug' the hole left by breaching the floor of the fossa, that a nose pack will be required for 24 hours and that a headache may be experienced postoperatively. Some centres administer antibiotics for 5 days to reduce meningitis and sinus thrombosis. Patients should also be advised that pituitary function might deteriorate as a result of the surgery.

Choice of surgical approach

The size of the sinuses, the size and position of the tumour and direction of extrasellar extension will govern the surgical approach. Most (96%) of adenomectomies are now performed trans-sphenoidally and only 4% by craniotomy. Some advantages and disadvantages of the surgical approach are described in Box 1.1.

Success rates of surgery

Surgical success can be measured in terms of preservation or achievement of normal endocrine function and effect on pituitary size. Outcome is dependent on the initial tumour size and, to some extent, on the experience of the surgeon; optimal published results are recorded in Table 1.9. The long-term outcome in terms of hypersecretion is generally considerably less favourable than the values quoted for recurrence of tumour mass (see individual chapters).

Complications

Infection, thrombosis or haemorrhage may complicate pituitary surgery as with most other surgery. Complications specific to trans-sphenoidal pituitary surgery include a CSF leak (reduced by

Box 1.1 Trans-sphenoidal hypophysectomy

Advantages of trans-sphenoidal approach:
Brain undisturbed, thus less confusion and epilepsy. No scars or blood transfusions, well tolerated. Better decompression, thus quicker visual recovery and preservation of pituitary tissue. If the tumour recurs, it tends to extend into the sinuses, rather than intracranially

Disadvantages of trans-sphenoidal approach:
Restricted field of view, optic nerve is not visualised, cerebrospinal fluid (CSF) rhinorrhea, incomplete removal of large tumours

Contraindications of trans-sphenoidal approach:
If at operation tumour appears very tough then it may be prudent to take a biopsy and abandon the operation; otherwise, removal is traumatic and CSF leak is likely

packing the sphenoid sinus at operation), nasal morbidity (reduced by displacing rather than removing the nasal septum), visual disturbance, pituitary insufficiency and diabetes insipidus. In one series of patients with preoperative visual disturbance, visual acuity improved in 87% of cases, was unchanged in 9% and worsened in 4%. Following resection of a macroprolactinoma, transient diabetes insipidus is observed in almost 25%

Table 1.9 Surgical success rates

Tumour type	Immediate cure of oversecretion	10-year mass recurrence rates
Acromegaly	82% micro/mesoadenoma 37% macroadenoma	8%
Prolactinoma	73% mesoadenoma 40% macroadenoma	24%
Cushing's disease	91%	8%
Nelson's syndrome	60%	17%
Non-functioning tumours	Not applicable	16%

of cases, and is permanent in approximately 2%. Similar post-operative diabetes insipidus rates are probably observed with other pituitary surgery. The degree of endocrine function loss is dependent upon the degree of pituitary resection required.

Radiotherapy

Indications

Radiotherapy is indicated where the pituitary tumour has been incompletely excised. It may occasionally be used as a primary treatment to reduce tumour bulk and secretion where surgery is not feasible or would be hazardous.

Success rates of radiotherapy

The effectiveness of radiotherapy is dependent upon the nature and size of the pituitary tumour. Reduction in pituitary mass of 40–60% is achieved with most tumours, which is usually sustained. Radiotherapy is more successful in smaller tumours. The onset is slow, with maximal effects observed at 2 years, but effects continue up to 15–20 years later.

Indications

In non-functioning tumours, radiotherapy after trans-cranial surgery increases the 10-year recurrence-free survival from 9% to 79%. When used following trans-sphenoidal surgery, this figure is closer to 93%. Thus, most patients with non-functioning macroadenomas now receive radiotherapy as a routine post surgery. In GH-secreting tumours, radiotherapy is reserved for those cases where an adequate biochemical response (GH levels of less than 5 mU/l during an oral glucose tolerance test) has not been achieved with surgery alone and where residual tumour tissue is visible on imaging. Microprolactinomas rarely require surgery or radiotherapy (generally reserved for those intolerant of dopamine agonist treatment). Most macroprolactinomas can be satisfactorily managed with dopamine agonists. Surgery is indicated for those macroprolactinomas unresponsive to medical therapy, and most centres advocate the use of radiotherapy post-operatively. Patients with Cushing's disease frequently require both surgery and radiotherapy, as biochemical cure may not achieved with surgery alone (see Chapter 5).

Advantages and disadvantages of radiotherapy

Radiotherapy is noninvasive and can be performed in an outpatient setting. It can be of use when surgery is contraindicated on grounds of general ill health. However, it is nonselective and will damage normal pituitary tissue as well as the adenoma. A high incidence of hypopituitarism is therefore observed in the years following treatment. The slow onset means that alternative, shorter-term therapies are required for more immediate effect.

Side effects and complications of radiotherapy

Short-term side effects include nausea, vomiting, skin irritation and hair loss, although these are uncommon. Visual impairment, secondary to damage to the vascular supply to the optic nerve, occurs in 12.5% of people who receive > 220 cGy per day. The risk is increased as the daily and total dose increases. Typically, patients receive 45–50 Gy in total, given over 4–5 weeks in 20–25 fractions. Hypopituitarism may result from hypothalamic or pituitary damage. The development of hypopituitarism increases with fractional and total dose, and incidence increases with time. The GH axis appears to be most sensitive, followed by the sequential loss of gonadotrophins, ACTH and TSH. The effect of radiotherapy on endocrine function is shown in Table 1.10. Second tumours, e.g. meningiomas, have been described following radiotherapy, although it is unclear as to whether this is a direct consequence of the treatment or not. There is also evidence to suggest that the incidence of cerebrovascular accidents is four-fold higher in the next 10 years compared with control subjects. The role of radiotherapy is an area of intensive debate.

Newer forms of pituitary irradiation

The results described above were derived from treatment using conventional fractionated external beam radiotherapy in which

Table 1.10   The effect of radiotherapy on pituitary function

New endocrine deficiencies 5 years post radiotherapy	Radiotherapy alone	Surgery and radiotherapy
Hypogonadism	47%	70%
Hypoadrenalism	30%	54%
Hypothyroidism	16%	38%

radiation is delivered to the tumour and entire fossa with a 1–2 cm margin. The radiation field arrangement leads to relatively high doses being applied to regions in the frontal and temporal lobes. Stereotactic radiosurgery, using either a cobalt unit (gamma knife) or a modified linear accelerator, delivers small localised spheres of irradiation. The gamma-knife technique permits single fraction therapy, but as high single doses of irradiation cause damage to the adjacent central nervous system (CNS), it is suitable only for small intrasellar tumours 0.5–1 cm away from the optic structures. For most tumours, linear accelerator stereotactic irradiation permits the treatment fields to conform to the individual's tumour shape. This combination of conformal therapy and sterotactic localisation with focused radiation (stereotactic conformal radiotherapy, SCRT) is administered by conventional fractionation to diminish the risks of damage to adjacent nervous structures. Early results with SCRT have suggested tumour control similar to that obtained with conventional external beam radiotherapy. SCRT has the theoretical advantage of reducing damage to adjacent structures, but long-term prospective studies are required to confirm its efficacy.

Follow-up

Patients undergoing surgery for pituitary tumours should be reassessed 6–12 weeks postoperatively. This should include an MRI of the pituitary fossa, basal and dynamic tests of the anterior and posterior pituitary where appropriate and a neuro-ophthalmic review. This may be repeated after 6 months, then annually thereafter. Education of the patients to enable them to cope with intercurrent illness – (especially regarding management of their glucocorticoid and DDAVP (desmopressin) replacement) – is mandatory. When the pituitary mass is stable, an MRI need only be performed every 3 years. Long-term follow-up in specialist centres is desirable for most patients.

Other Pituitary Masses

Incidentalomas

Incidentalomas are pituitary lesions found in patients being evaluated with MRI or CT for other reasons, with no symptoms or signs of pituitary disease. They are found in approximately 10% of

Table 1.11   Management of incidentalomas

Category	Action
History & examination	• Symptoms and signs of hypersecretion of hormones and local pressure symptoms should be sought. Family history is important.
Investigation	• Basal blood tests, such as IGF-1, PRL, TSH, FSH, LH, testosterone, T_4 should be checked, as well as routine blood tests (blood count, creatinine and electrolytes, fasting glucose and lipids) • 24-hour urine free cortisol and urine volume • Dynamic tests as indicated • Neuro-ophthalmic assessment if a macroadenoma
Treatment	• Microadenomas – nil necessary, if nonsecretory • Macroadenomas – drugs, surgery or radiotherapy if indicated clinically
Follow-up	• Microadenomas – assessment at 1 year, then 2-yearly • Macroadenomas – assess at 6 months, then as above
Long-term outcome	• In one study of untreated microadenomas without endocrine dysfunction, after 22 months: pituitary size remained unchanged in 70%, increased in 20% and decreased in 10%; endocrine function remained normal in 93% and 7% developed some dysfunction

FSH = follicle-stimulating hormone;
IGF-1 = insulin-like growth factor-1;
LH = luteinising hormone;
PRL = prolactin;
T4 = thyroxine;
TSH = thyroid-stimulating hormone.

people undergoing imaging for other reasons. Management of incidentalomas is given in Table 1.11.

Pituitary carcinomas

These tumours are rare and are difficult to differentiate from adenomas on histology. The presence of distant metastasis is necessary for the diagnosis to be made. Spread most commonly occurs via the CSF to the spine, but also to bone, liver, kidney, lymph nodes and heart. These tumours may be of insidious onset, with no local invasion and benign histology at diagnosis, leading to the hypothesis that carcinomas may arise from adenomas. However, there is little evidence for this. Carcinomas are usually endocrinologically active, with PRL, GH, ACTH and TSH secretion described.

Lymphocytic hypophysitis

Lymphocytic hypophysitis affects mainly young women. It typically presents in the last trimester of pregnancy or during the early period during delivery. The presentation may be with local pressure symptoms or symptoms from hypopituitarism (which is the rule at some stage). MRI scans typically show an isointense, diffusely enlarged gland. The diagnosis is usually made following surgery.

Pituitary metastases

These are uncommon, but occur in patients with melanomas or breast cancer.

Other pathological conditions

Rarely, pituitary adenomas may be confused with pathology other than hypothalamic tumours. Occasional confusing conditions are granulomatous disease, pituitary abscesses, germinomas within the sellar, parasellar meningiomas, optic nerve gliomas and carotid arterial aneurysms.

Physiological changes

Pituitary size increases throughout childhood, peaking in adolescence, then shrinking in adulthood. Women have larger pituitary glands than men, with 53% of all females aged 11–20 years demonstrating upper convexity of the gland, and in 25% the pituitary may appear almost spherical. The pituitary also increases in convexity and size in pregnancy, in proportion to gestation, to as much as 136% of normal. This begins to revert 6 days postpartum, reaching pre-pregnancy size 1 week to 6 months later, independent of lactation.

Further Reading

Brada M, Rajan B, Traish D *et al*. The long term efficacy of conservative surgery and radiotherapy in the control of pituitary adenoma. *Clin Endocrinol* 1993;**38**:571–8.

Ciric I, Mikael M, Stafford T, Lawson L, Garces R. Transsphenoidal microsurgery of pituitary microadenomas with long term follow up results. *J Neurosurg* 1983;**59**:395–401.

Clayton RN, Stewart PM, Shalet SM, Wass JA. Pituitary surgery for acromegaly – Should be done by specialists? *BMJ* 1999;**319**:588–9.

Elster AD. Modern imaging of the pituitary. *Radiology* 1993;**187**:1–14.

Klibanski A, Zervas NT. Diagnosis and management of hormone secreting pituitary tumours. *N Engl J Med* 1991;**324**:822–31.

Melmed S (ed). *The Pituitary*. Cambs, Mass: Blackwell Science Inc., 1995.

Plowman PN. Pituitary adenoma radiotherapy – when, who and how. *Clin Endocrinol* 1999;**51**:265–71.

2

Hypopituitarism

Catherine A Lissett and Stephen M Shalet

Introduction

Incidence

Hypopituitarism is the deficiency of one or more pituitary hormones. It is relatively rare, with an incidence in adulthood of eight to ten new cases per million. It is, however, seen commonly in endocrine practice and, importantly, is associated with increased morbidity and mortality. Clinical manifestations are influenced by the aetiology, severity and rate of onset of pituitary hormone deficiency.

Mortality

There is now overwhelming evidence that hypopituitary patients have an excess mortality compared with the normal population. The first study to demonstrate this was from Göteborg, Sweden. Of 333 subjects diagnosed as having partial or complete hypopituitarism between 1956 and 1987, 104 died during follow-up, representing a 1.8-fold higher mortality than the normal population. Patients with acromegaly and Cushing's disease were excluded, as these patients are known to have higher mortality. The principal cause of the two-fold increase in mortality in both men and women was vascular disease. Deaths from malignancy were lower than expected in men but not in women. Neither the type nor degree of pituitary insufficiency influenced the excess mortality.

Two other studies, one from the UK and the other from Lund, Sweden, confirmed that hypopituitary patients have excess mortality, ranging from 1.75- to 2.2-fold greater than the normal population. Again, vascular disease was responsible for the majority of excess deaths, although this figure was not statistically significant in the UK cohort.

Pathological correlates

In adults with hypopituitarism:

- ↑ atherosclerosis
- ↓ aortic distensibility.

Possible causative factors

- Growth hormone (GH) deficiency secondary to adverse changes in:
  - body composition
  - endothelial function
  - lipid profile
  - fibrinogen level
  - insulin sensitivity
  - plasminogen activator inhibitor levels.
- Long-standing over-substitution with corticosteroids: adverse changes in body composition
  - ↑ insulin resistance.
- Failure to replace or under-replacement with sex steroids.

Causes

The causes of hypopituitarism are varied (Table 2.1). In adulthood, however, the most common cause is a pituitary adenoma and/or treatment with pituitary surgery or radiotherapy.

Table 2.1　Causes of hypopituitarism

Pituitary and parapituitary tumours
Radiotherapy
Surgery
Trauma, including perinatal
Infarction, including apoplexy and Sheehan's syndrome
Infiltration, including sarcoidosis, Langerhans' cell histiocytosis, haemochromatosis
Lymphocytic hypophysitis
Infection, including tuberculosis
Genetic/embryological disorders
Idiopathic

Pituitary and hypothalamic mass lesions

- Pituitary adenomas account for the vast majority of pituitary mass lesions although secondary tumours do occur, with metastasis to the pituitary gland reported from carcinomas of the breast, lung, colon and prostate.
- Pituitary microadenomas (< 1 cm) are surprisingly common, being found in between 1.5 and 27% of patients at autopsy; these tumours are very rarely, if at all, associated with hypopituitarism.
- Macroadenomas (> 1 cm) are less common, but are more frequently associated with pituitary hormone deficiencies; some 30% of patients with pituitary macroadenomas have one or more anterior pituitary hormone deficiencies. Evidence suggests the causative mechanism of hypopituitarism in these patients is compression of the portal vessels in the pituitary stalk, either secondary to the expanding tumour mass directly, or to raised intrasellar pressure.
- Craniopharyngiomas are the third most common intracranial tumour and account for the majority of parapituitary tumours. They are thought to arise from Rathke's pouch and may be cystic or solid, commonly showing calcification: 50% occur in children under 15 years. The diagnosis is usually precipitated by visual problems and headaches, although most patients show features of hypopituitarism at presentation.
- Derangement of central endocrine regulation also occurs with other parapituitary space-occupying lesions such as chondromas, chordomas, suprasellar meningiomas, astrocytomas of the optic nerve and primary tumours of the third ventricle.

Pituitary surgery

- Hypopituitarism is a common consequence of pituitary surgery.
- The incidence and degree of hypopituitarism depends on a number of factors, including:
  1. the size of the original tumour
  2. the degree of infiltration
  3. the experience of the surgeon.
- Prompt postoperative assessment of pituitary function should be performed and the patient warned of a possible deterioration of pituitary function postoperatively. However, a decline in pituitary function postoperatively is not universal. Paradoxically, surgery for non-functioning pituitary adenomas may be associated with a significant recovery of pituitary function. In those patients in

whom recovery of pituitary function occurs, the process begins immediately after surgery.

The type of preoperative endocrine deficiency is related to postoperative endocrine recovery. Preoperative thyroid-stimulating hormone (TSH), adrenocorticotrophic hormone (ACTH), gonadotrophin and GH deficiency were associated with endocrine recovery in 57, 38, 32 and 15% of patients, respectively. Prognostic indicators for recovery were smaller tumours and less severe hypopituitarism before the operation. The pituitary hormone least likely to recover was GH; this may reflect the fact that severe deficiency of GH was more common preoperatively than for other pituitary hormones.

Radiotherapy

- Hypopituitarism may follow treatment with external radiation when the hypothalamic–pituitary axis lies within the fields of radiation.
- Hypopituitarism has been described in patients who received radiation therapy for nasopharyngeal carcinoma, tumours of the pituitary gland or nearby structures and primary brain tumours, as well as in children who underwent prophylactic cranial irradiation for acute lymphoblastic leukaemia or total body irradiation (TBI) for a variety of tumours and other diseases.
- The radiobiological impact of an irradiation schedule is dependent on:
  1. total dose
  2. number of fractions
  3. duration of treatment.
- The same total dose given in fewer fractions over a shorter time is likely to cause a greater incidence of pituitary hormone deficiency than if the schedule is spread over a longer time interval with a greater number of fractions.
- After lower radiation doses, isolated GH deficiency ensues, while higher doses may produce panhypopituitarism (Figure 2.1)
- Radiation dose also determines the speed of onset of hormonal deficiency. The greater the radiation dose, the earlier GH deficiency will occur after treatment, so that between 2 and 5 years after irradiation 100% of children receiving > 30 Gy (over 3 weeks) to the hypothalamic–pituitary axis showed subnormal GH responses to an insulin tolerance test (ITT) whereas 35% of those receiving < 30 Gy (over 3 weeks) still show a normal GH response (Figure 2.2).

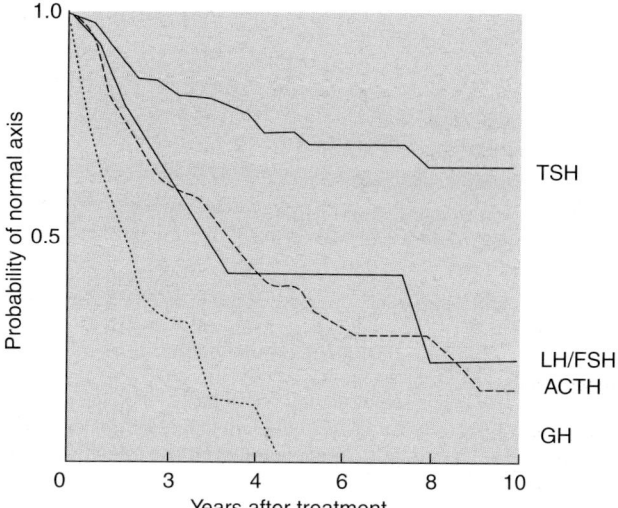

Figure 2.1 Life-table analysis indicating probabilities of initially normal hypothalamic–pituitary–target gland axes remaining normal after radiotherapy (3750–4250 cGy).

Growth hormone (GH) secretion is the most sensitive of the anterior pituitary hormones to the effects of external radiotherapy and thyroid-stimulating hormone (TSH) secretion the most resistant. In two-thirds of patients, gonadotrophin deficiency develops before adrenocorticotrophic hormone (ACTH) deficiency and vice versa in the remaining one-third. LH/FSH = luteinising hormone/follicle-stimulating hormone.

- Paradoxically, while high doses of cranial irradiation may render a child gonadotrophin-deficient, lesser doses of irradiation may be associated with early puberty. The mechanism for early puberty after irradiation is likely to be related to disinhibition of cortical influences on the hypothalamus.

With increased longevity of survival, follow-up of patients irradiated for tumours of the brain and surrounding structures will need to focus less on the possibility of tumour recurrence and more on the delayed effects of therapy, including the endocrine effects.

Genetic causes

Genetic or familial causes of hypopituitarism are rare but, over recent years, study of these conditions and their diverse pathophysiological

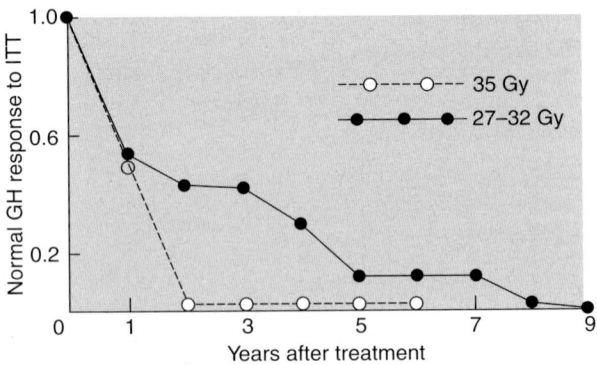

Figure 2.2. The incidence of growth hormone (GH) deficiency in children receiving 27–32 Gy or 35 Gy of cranial irradiation for a brain tumour in relation to time from irradiation (DXT). The speed at which individual pituitary hormone deficits develop is dose-dependent: the higher the radiation dose, the earlier growth hormone (GH) deficiency occurs. ITT = insulin tolerance test.

mechanisms has increased the understanding of anterior pituitary gland development and gene regulation in normal and disease states.

Isolated GH deficiency

Two broad types of genetic defect have been identified which cause isolated GH deficiency. These are mutations of the GH gene and of the growth hormone releasing hormone (GHRH) receptor gene.

- Four mendelian disorders of GH deficiency have been identified to date: two with autosomal recessive inheritance and an autosomal dominant as well as an X-linked form.
- The human *GH* gene is located on chromosome 17 in a cluster of five genes: *hGH-N* encodes the gene for pituitary GH, *hGH-V* encodes the gene for placental GH and three genes for human chorionic somatotrophin (hCS). Children with gene mutations or deletions of *hGH-N* present with severe short stature and, in males, microgenitalia. They have the characteristic phenotypic features of GH deficiency.
- The gene encoding the GHRH receptor (GHRH-R) is expressed in pituitary somatotroph cells and belongs to a family of G

protein coupled receptors. A mutation in this gene has been identified in a number of kindreds, resulting in a severely truncated receptor lacking the seven membrane spanning domains.

GnRH deficiency

Isolated gonadotrophin-releasing hormone (GnRH) deficiency is a genetic defect characterised by a functional deficit in hypothalamic GnRH production or secretion.

- Patients with accompanying anosmia or hyposmia are referred to as having *Kallmann's syndrome* whereas those without other associated abnormalities are described as having *idiopathic hypogonadotrophic hypogonadism* (IHH).
- The hypogonadotrophic state results from deficient hypothalamic secretion of GnRH and may be explained by a defect in the migration of GnRH neurones from their origin in the olfactory placode to the hypothalamus, whereas anosmia is due to agenesis of the olfactory bulbs.
- Whether IHH and Kallmann's syndrome represent a spectrum of manifestations of GnRH deficiency remains controversial. X-linked (*Kal 1* gene), autosomal recessive and autosomal dominant patterns of inheritance have been described.

ACTH/TSH deficiency

Isolated deficiencies of TSH or ACTH are very rare; however, in a number of cases a genetic abnormality has been described or proposed. Mutations of the coding region of the TSH β-subunit gene resulting in TSH deficiency have been identified in a number of different families. Whereas a genetic basis for ACTH deficiency has not yet been elucidated, kindred studies suggest that abnormalities of the CRH gene may result in this rare phenomenon.

Transcription factor defects (Table 2.2)

Pit-1, PROP1 and HESX1 and have all been associated with hypopituitarism.

Other causes of hypopituitarism

1. *Post-traumatic* dysfunction of the hypothalamic–pituitary axis is uncommon, but well described. In particular, the pituitary stalk may be severed in deceleration injuries, leading to diabetes

Table 2.2   Transcription factor defects associated with multiple pituitary hormone deficits

Transcription factor	Pituitary hormone deficiencies	Pituitary size	Inheritance
Pit-1	GH, PRL and TSH	Normal or small	Dominant and recessive
PROP1	GH, PRL, TSH, FSH and LH (sometimes ACTH occurs later)	Normal or hyperplastic	Recessive
HESX1	Variable (GH, TSH, ACTH, FSH, LH and ADH) in association with midline brain abnormalities and optic nerve hypoplasia	Hypoplastic	Sporadic and autosomal recessive

ACTH = adrenocorticotrophic hormone, ADH = antidiuretic hormone, FSH = follicle-stimulating hormone, GH = growth hormone, LH = luteinising hormone, PRL = prolactin, TSH = thyroid-stimulating hormone.

insipidus. Isolated pituitary hormone deficiencies, particularly GH (1 in 3000–6000 live births) or gonadotrophin deficiency, have also been attributed to trauma, including *perinatal trauma*.

2.   *Pituitary apoplexy* is the abrupt destruction of pituitary tissue, resulting from infarction or haemorrhage into the pituitary, usually into an underlying pituitary tumour. Severe headache accompanies a variable degree of visual loss and/or cranial nerve palsies. The consequent pituitary hormone deficiencies may develop rapidly.

3.   In *Sheehan's syndrome,* pituitary infarction occurs secondary to severe postpartum haemorrhage and ensuing circulatory failure. The pituitary may double or treble in volume in a normal pregnancy; a relatively small fall in blood pressure may precipitate pituitary infarction. Once common, this complication is now mainly confined to areas where obstetric services are less well developed.

4.   *Granulomatous diseases* including sarcoidosis, tuberculosis and Langerhans cell histiocytosis can affect the hypothalamic–pituitary axis and cause hypopituitarism, including diabetes insipidus. Diabetes insipidus complicates sarcoidosis rarely

(1%). It is more common, however, in Langerhans cell histiocytosis, with 15% of childhood cases developing diabetes insipidus, but may also occur in patients presenting in adulthood. Diabetes insipidus may be masked by cortisol deficiency (cortisol is needed for free water excretion).

5. *Lymphocytic hypophysitis*
   - This is an immune-mediated diffuse infiltration of the anterior pituitary with lymphocytes and plasma cells.
   - It occurs predominantly in women and is often first evident in pregnancy or after delivery.
   - The classical presentation is peripartum hypopituitarism, often with a pituitary mass and visual failure. Secondary adrenal failure is an almost universal feature which when undiagnosed has proven fatal.
   - The headaches of this condition do not appear to be related to dural stretching and are worse than the size of the pituitary would seem to predict.
   - At an early stage the pituitary gland is enlarged and cannot be distinguished from a pituitary tumour by computed tomography (CT) or magnetic resonance imaging (MRI) scanning, while in the latter stages the gland may atrophy, leaving an empty sella. Exclusion of a surgically remediable problem such as pituitary apoplexy is essential.
   - Lymphocytic hypophysitis is more common in patients with another autoimmune endocrine disease. Cytosolic autoantigens against the pituitary can be demonstrated in some cases, but are also present in patients who were hypopituitary secondary to other causes and in normal patients; thus, the definitive diagnosis of this condition remains difficult without pituitary biopsy.
   - Spontaneous resolution of both the mass and the hypopituitarism have been reported and, in some cases, neurosurgical intervention has led to irreversible pituitary failure. Therefore, conservative management is appropriate in the majority of patients.

6. Lastly, *iron overload states*, i.e. haemochromatosis and patients with β-thalassaemia receiving frequent blood transfusions, are associated with pituitary hyposecretion secondary to siderosis and a reduction of pituitary cell number. The gonadotrophs are particularly vulnerable to this mode of damage; however, as affected patients live longer due to improved medical care, other pituitary hormone deficits, including GH and ACTH deficiency,

are becoming more common. Iron overload may affect other endocrine organs such as the gonads; primary and secondary failure can exist.

Clinical Features

Clinical features of hypopituitarism are outlined in Table 2.3.

- The clinical features of hypopituitarism are determined principally by the *degree, type,* and *speed of onset* of the pituitary hormone deficiency.
- Local pressure effects and/or hormonal hypersecretion can, however, complicate the clinical picture.

In many forms of hypopituitarism, i.e. secondary to a pituitary adenoma and following irradiation, a characteristic evolution of pituitary failure is apparent: typically, secretion of GH fails first, followed by luteinising hormone (LH), follicle-stimulating hormone (FSH) and, finally, by failure of ACTH and TSH secretion. However, the endocrine deficiency may occur in any order.

$$GH \rightarrow LH/FSH \rightarrow ACTH \rightarrow TSH$$

Table 2.3   Clinical features of hypopituitarism

Hormone deficiency	Symptoms and signs
GH	Short stature in children, abnormal body composition, increased fracture rate, reduced well-being and exercise capacity
Gonadotrophins	In men: poor libido/impotence, infertility, small soft testes, reduced facial/body hair In women: amenorrhoea/oligomenorrhoea dyspareunia, infertility, breast atrophy
TSH	Growth retardation in children, decrease in energy, constipation, sensitivity to cold, dry skin, weight gain
ACTH	Weakness, tiredness, pallor, hypoglycaemia
Prolactin	Failure of lactation
ADH	Polyuria, polydipsia, nocturia and hypotension

ACTH = adrenocorticotrophic hormone, ADH = antidiuretic hormone, GH = growth hormone, TSH = thyroid-stimulating hormone.

- Prolactin deficiency is rare, except as a component of Sheehan's syndrome. Hyperprolactinaemia is much more common, either secondary to interference with the secretion or delivery of dopamine to the pituitary, thereby releasing the normal lactotrophs from tonic inhibition, or because of hypersecretion from a prolactinoma.
- Diabetes insipidus is not generally a feature of pituitary disease, and the presence of diabetes insipidus usually denotes a hypothalamic or stalk disorder, except when occurring following pituitary surgery.

GH deficiency

GH secretion is a continuous variable and a spectrum therefore exists from severe GH deficiency to mild GH insufficiency. Typically, the GH-deficient child has increased subcutaneous fat, especially around the trunk. The face is immature, with a prominent forehead and depressed mid-facial development; this is related to the lack of GH effect on endochondral growth at the base of the skull, occiput and the sphenoid bone. Dentition is delayed. In males, the phallus may be small, and the average age of pubertal onset is delayed in both boys and girls.

Over the last decade there has developed an increasing awareness of the role GH plays in adult life. The features of GH deficiency in adulthood are described in Table 2.4.

Gonadotrophin deficiency

Gonadotrophin deficiency may result from:

- deficient secretion of pituitary gonadotrophins
- faulty secretion of GnRH
- hyperprolactinaemia, which impairs the pulsatile release of GnRH and thus causes secondary hypogonadism.

Gonadotrophin secretion can also be reduced in some functional disorders, most commonly in women, i.e. excessive weight loss or exercise. The clinical features of secondary or hypogonadotrophic hypogonadism are similar to those of primary gonadal failure.

In *males*, the clinical features of gonadotrophin deficiency differ according to whether the deficiency was acquired before or after pubertal age. A eunuch is a male whose testes have been removed or have never developed.

Table 2.4   Severe GH deficiency in adults

Adverse changes in body composition	↑ per cent of body fat, predominant central distribution ↓ lean body mass ↓ extracellular fluid volume ↑ waist/hip ratio
Lipid profile	Modest ↑ in total plasma cholesterol ↑ LDL/HDL ratio ↑ fibrinogen levels ↑ plasminogen activator inhibitor levels
Insulin sensitivity	↑ fasting and postprandial plasma insulin levels ↑ insulin resistance
Bone mineral density	1–2 SD below the age-matched normal mean Evidence to suggest doubling of the fracture rate
Quality of life	More perceived health problems Lower perceived quality of life than controls Lack of energy – dominant complaint

LDL = low-density lipoprotein, HDL = high-density lipoprotein.

Patients with prepubertally acquired gonadotrophin deficiency demonstrate, in addition to those features found in patients who develop gonadotrophin deficiency postpubertally:

- underdeveloped penis and small testes
- eunuchoidal proportions (span exceeds height by greater than 5 cm).

Patients with postpubertally acquired hypogonadism demonstrate:

- reduction in testicular size
- loss of facial and body hair
- thinning of the skin, leading to the characteristic finely wrinkled facial skin of the 'ageing youth'
- ↓ muscle mass
- ↓ bone mass
- ↓ sexual function, libido and general well-being.

Azoospermia is an almost inevitable consequence of hypogonado-trophic hypogonadism; however, there are exceptions. In 'the fertile eunuch', partial LH deficiency may result in low circulating testosterone levels and gynaecomastia, but preserved fertility, as presumably intratesticular testosterone levels remain high enough to maintain spermatogenesis.

In the *female child*, hypogonadotrophic hypogonadism is associated with primary amenorrhoea and absent breast development. In the *adult woman* amenorrhoea/oligomenorrhoea, infertility, breast atrophy, vaginal dryness and dyspareunia are the result. Pubic and axillary hair remain unless ACTH deficiency is also present.

ACTH deficiency

- ACTH deficiency is the most life-threatening feature of hypopituitarism.

In addition to the other causes of pituitary failure discussed earlier, functional ACTH deficiency may occur following discontinuation of exogenous glucocorticoids or ACTH, even when these agents have only been administered for a few weeks. Isolated acquired ACTH deficiency has also been well documented, although its occurrence is rare. Although there are similarities, there are also important differences between the features of glucocorticoid deficiency due to ACTH deficiency and those of Addison's disease:

- *Weakness, tiredness, nausea and vomiting* are common, especially at the time of incidental disease. They may be less prominent in a chronic partial ACTH deficiency, but the patient is at risk with a minor illness which exposes failed ACTH rise with stress.
- *Weight loss* and *anorexia* may mimic anorexia nervosa or an underlying malignancy.
- Examination may reveal *pallor of the skin*, in contrast to the hyperpigmentation of Addison's disease and in females, particularly, there is *loss of secondary sexual hair*.
- In severe ACTH deficiency, particularly in childhood, *hypoglycaemia* can occur: cortisol deficiency results in increased insulin sensitivity and a decrease in hepatic glycogen reserves.
- *Hyponatraemia* occurs, particularly in the elderly, although it is less common in ACTH deficiency as there is preservation of aldosterone secretion compared with Addison's disease. Cortisol is needed for free water excretion; therefore the patient is water-expanded as well as salt-depleted.

Acute cortisol insufficiency should be considered in the differential diagnosis of a patient with a history of anorexia and weight loss, increasing fatigue, weakness, and nausea and vomiting. The

clinical features may include hypovolaemic shock, fever and an acute abdomen often precipitated by a separate problem. A history of an acute headache, pituitary surgery or irradiation may provide important pointers to the diagnosis.

TSH deficiency

TSH deficiency occurs late in most pituitary disorders. Symptoms, which include fatigue, weakness, inability to lose weight, constipation and cold intolerance, in keeping with those found in primary hypothyroidism, are, however, generally milder than those found in primary hypothyroidism. This is because the hypothyroidism is usually less severe, as on the whole there is some residual TSH secretion.

ADH deficiency

Polyuria and polydipsia with nocturia are the classical features of diabetes insipidus resulting from ADH deficiency. If the patient is unable to keep up with the fluid loss, hypotension and hypovolaemia ensue.

- The features of diabetes insipidus may be masked in the presence of ACTH deficiency, as the absence of cortisol is associated with reduced free water excretion. Only when cortisol replacement therapy is commenced may the polyuria and polydipsia of diabetes insipidus be revealed.

Diagnosis and Endocrine Assessment

- Clinical examination can provide important clues to the aetiology and duration of hypopituitarism and the adult physician in particular must not neglect an assessment of height, weight and pubertal status.
- Examination of the visual fields clinically is essential, and should be supported by either Goldmann or computer-assisted perimetry. The latter is more sensitive, detecting visual field defects that other techniques are unable to demonstrate.

Imaging of the pituitary fossa

Imaging of the pituitary fossa is indicated when there is clinical evidence of a visual field defect or biochemical evidence of hypopituitarism. CT and MRI scanning have superseded the plain X-ray. *MRI is the scanning technique of choice,* as it offers higher resolution than CT scanning and is able to demonstrate microadenomas as small as 3 mm in diameter. If a pituitary adenoma is demonstrated, careful note should be taken of any extension of the tumour outside the pituitary fossa. In diabetes insipidus, the normal high-intensity posterior pituitary signal may be absent, and other causes of hypopituitarism may show classical CT/MRI findings, e.g. craniopharyngioma.

- Incidental pituitary microadenomas (*'incidentalomas'*) are found in between 5 and 38% of normal individuals when CT or MRI scanning of the pituitary fossa is performed.

Empty sella

- An *empty sella* is a not uncommon finding. It refers to a cerebrospinal fluid-filled pituitary fossa, resulting from herniation of the arachnoid mata through an incomplete sellar diaphragm. The pituitary fossa may be enlarged or normal in size.
- An empty sella may be secondary to a congenital diaphragmatic defect (primary) or damage to the diaphragm by surgery, radiation or infarction of a pituitary tumour (secondary).
- The pituitary gland is usually flattened against the floor of the sella and the pituitary stalk may be laterally deviated.
- The majority of patients with primary empty sella have normal pituitary function; however, 15% have mild hyperprolactinaemia, and it has been described in association with headache, endocrine dysfunction (particularly GH deficiency in children) and visual disturbances.
- Patients with secondary empty sella more commonly have endocrine disturbances related to the underlying pathogenesis of the condition.

Endocrine testing

The endocrine assessment of a patient with suspected hypopituitarism usually involves the measurement of both baseline and stimulated hormone levels. Basal hormone levels yield much useful information; therefore, serum concentrations of prolactin, insulin-like growth factor-1 (IGF-I), TSH, thyroxine (T$_4$), cortisol, LH, FSH, testosterone in men, and oestradiol in women should be measured.

- Generally, suspected anterior pituitary hormone deficiency should be confirmed and corrected before possible ADH

deficiency is investigated, as ACTH deficiency can disguise the presence of ADH deficiency.
- Another important principle is that of retesting, which is important in two broad clinical contexts.

First, in young adults who received GH replacement in childhood. In studies in which these individuals are reassessed after completion of growth and puberty, GH status was considered normal in 20–87%. The original childhood diagnosis in the vast majority of the latter subjects was isolated idiopathic GH deficiency, whereas those young adults diagnosed as having organic GH deficiency in childhood as a consequence of either a mass lesion, pituitary surgery or irradiation to the hypothalamic–pituitary axis rarely reverted to normal GH secretory status. Hence, the aetiology of the childhood diagnosis of GH deficiency should logically affect the strategy of retesting. Patients with isolated GH deficiency should undergo two tests of GH secretory status, whereas those with additional anterior pituitary hormone deficits require only one test at reassessment.

The second cohort in whom retesting is indicated are those patients in whom progression of the hypopituitarism may be expected. This includes patients who were subject to irradiation of the hypothalamic–pituitary axis, following surgery, and in patients with an evolving pituitary or hypothalamic lesion.

Following irradiation, endocrine testing should be performed on a yearly basis until failure is apparent, for at least 10 years and then 5 yearly.

This is of particular importance because although the classical sequence of pituitary hormone deficits (GH, gonadotrophins, ACTH and TSH) occurs in the majority of patients, other patterns may occur, most notably ACTH deficiency before gonadotrophin deficiency.

GH deficiency

GH replacement therapy has been offered to GH-deficient children for more than 30 years, but it only became a licensed indication for GH-deficient adults in the UK in 1996.

The underlying pathophysiology differs in childhood-onset compared with adult-onset GH deficiency, with isolated idiopathic GH deficiency predominating in childhood, while in adulthood, GH deficiency is most frequently due to a pituitary adenoma and/or treatment with surgery or radiotherapy; isolated idiopathic GH deficiency acquired in adulthood has never been reported. In childhood, the differential diagnosis is dominated by alternative causes of poor growth, whereas difficulties in the diagnosis of adult-onset GH deficiency exist in the obese and elderly.

GH secretion is a spectrum between normality and abnormality and therefore, with rare exception, the diagnosis of GH deficiency must be made on arbitrary grounds. The more severe the GH deficiency, the less arbitrary the diagnosis, whereas the 'lesser degrees of GH deficiency' merge into normality. Today, in certain countries, children with all forms of GH insufficiency, from mild to severe, are considered for GH replacement, whereas in other countries only those with severe GH deficiency receive GH replacement.

In adulthood, however, it is only severe GH deficiency that has been proven to be associated with any benefit from GH replacement and thus in adulthood the purpose of investigation is to diagnose severe GH deficiency.

GH secretion is pulsatile and serum levels are low during many hours of the day. Therefore, a single basal GH estimation provides little useful information about GH secretory status. Twenty-four hour GH profiles with 20-min sampling are time consuming, expensive and there is controversy as to their scientific and practical value; thus, in reality, a 24-hour GH profile remains a research investigation. Provocative tests are the most popular method of determining GH secretory status.

At present the ITT (see Appendix 1) is the 'gold standard' for the biochemical diagnosis of severe GH deficiency.

The ITT provokes a pronounced GH response in normals, it allows the pituitary–adrenal axis to be tested at the same time and the morbidity associated with the performance of the test is low in experienced units.

A GH response of less than 9 mU/l to an ITT in which adequate hypoglycaemia has been achieved is diagnostic of severe GH deficiency.[7]

Nevertheless, each laboratory must establish its own diagnostic threshold values due to the lack of standardisation of GH assays rather than simply adopting the recommended cut-off level of 9 mU/l.

A number of other GH provocative tests are available, including the arginine stimulation test (see Appendix 1), glucagon stimulation test (see Appendix 1), etc. Each has advantages and disadvantages, either as an alternative to the ITT in patients in whom this test is contraindicated or as an adjunct in patients requiring a second provocative test. However, clonidine is unsuitable in adulthood and the GHRH–pyridostigmine test would be more attractive if the physician could be certain he was dealing with a pituitary rather than a hypothalamic defect.

It is crucial that the results of each provocative test must be interpreted in the context of normative values and local assays, as the 'cut-off' used for the ITT is not broadly applicable to all other provocative tests, which may be more or less potent stimulators of GH secretion.

Obesity and GH secretion

• *The pathophysiological state of obesity is difficult to distinguish from organic GH deficiency in an adult.*

Morbid obesity is accompanied by suppression of GH release, and substantial weight loss restores spontaneous and stimulated GH secretion. Even in clinically non-obese healthy adults, relative adiposity in the abdominal region, in particular, is a major negative determinant of stimulated GH secretion. In the obese individual with pituitary disease and no other pituitary deficit, a reduced GH response to any of the standard provocative tests may reflect organic GH deficiency or obesity itself and the distinction between the two is not easy at the present time.

Ageing and GH secretion. GH secretion in healthy elderly adults is reduced compared with that in young adults. GH secretion declines by approximately 14% per decade from young adult life. Normal ageing is associated with changes in body composition similar to those seen in patients with GH deficiency. In the clinical setting, this raises the question: Can the GH status of elderly patients with organic pituitary disease be distinguished from that of the normal elderly person? Toogood *et al.* (1996) have now established that GH secretion is significantly reduced in the elderly patient with pituitary disease compared with normal controls of similar age. This work suggested that the arginine stimulation test is a reasonable choice for assessing GH status in elderly patients with two or three additional pituitary hormone deficits, particularly in an age group in which an ITT carries an increased theoretical risk of morbidity or mortality. In an elderly patient with pituitary disease and with one or no additional pituitary hormone deficits, the distinction between GH deficiency and normality remains a challenge.

IGF-I in the diagnosis of GH deficiency. Serum IGF-I levels are stable throughout the day, mainly due to the complexing of IGF-I with a family of IGF-binding proteins. Thus, the potential for assessing GH status with a single estimation of the circulating IGF-I level, which is known to be GH-dependent, proved attractive and led to the hope that dynamic GH provocation tests would prove unnecessary.

- However, IGF-I levels are affected by number of other variables, including nutritional status, hepatic function, hypothyroidism, age and pubertal status, and thus matched control values must be used.
- Even then, there is considerable overlap between the values in GH-deficient and normal individuals, particularly in those patients who developed GH deficiency in adulthood or who were rendered GH deficient by irradiation.
- An IGF-I estimation is extremely useful for retesting young adults with a diagnosis of childhood-onset GH deficiency, moderately helpful (~30–50% positive predictive value) in middle-aged adults (25–55 years old) and rarely helpful in the elderly (over 60 years old).

How many tests? It is reasonable to perform only one provocative test of GH release in adult patients with two or three additional pituitary hormone deficiencies, as these patients are almost inevitably severely GH deficient. In the patient with pituitary disease and a possible diagnosis of adult-onset isolated GH deficiency or GH deficiency plus one additional pituitary hormone deficit, two provocative tests of GH release would be appropriate. The same strategy, which can be applied for reassessing the GH secretory status of young adults who received GH replacement for childhood GH deficiency, has been utilised for establishing a diagnosis of adult-onset GH deficiency. However, IGF-I estimation itself should be considered adequate in those in whom multiple pituitary hormone deficits exist, and should serve as one of the two tests of GH status in the much larger cohort of individuals with a putative diagnosis of isolated GH deficiency in whom retesting is required. For further discussion, see Shalet *et al.* (1998).

Gonadotrophin deficiency

In women, gonadotrophin deficiency is relatively easy to diagnose: in women of postmenopausal age, gonadotrophin levels are clearly low/undetectable, while in premenopausal women, amenorrhoea (or less commonly oligomenorrhoea), in addition to low oestradiol levels and low/normal gonadotrophin levels, provides sufficient evidence of the diagnosis.

In men, a similar picture of low testosterone levels and low/normal gonadotrophin levels is seen.

The most difficult distinction is between isolated gonadotrophin deficiency and constitutional delay of puberty in the male of peripubertal age.

Clinically delayed puberty is defined by failure to develop signs of puberty by the age of 14 years. Over 90% of 14+ year old boys with delayed puberty have no endocrine abnormality, and will go through puberty spontaneously at a later date. No biochemical tests reliably improve this epidemiological prediction. If during androgen therapy testicular volumes increase, the diagnosis of constitutional delay in growth and puberty rather than gonadotrophin deficiency is confirmed (see Chapter 9).

ACTH deficiency

In normal individuals, the highest plasma cortisol levels are found between 6 a.m. and 8 a.m. and the lowest before midnight. Plasma cortisol and ACTH concentrations are elevated in physical and emotional stress, including acute illness, trauma, surgery, infection and starvation.

• *If a 9 a.m. cortisol level is below 100 nmol/l, particularly in an unwell patient, cortisol deficiency is highly likely and many authors suggest that dynamic assessment of the hypothalamic–pituitary axis is unnecessary.*

A paired plasma ACTH level will help distinguish between primary and secondary glucocorticoid deficiency: in primary cortisol deficiency, i.e. Addison's disease, the ACTH level will be high; correspondingly, in secondary glucocorticoid deficiency, the ACTH level will be normal or low.

If cortisol deficiency is suspected in an unwell patient, baseline cortisol and ACTH samples should be taken; however, replacement therapy should be commenced immediately and provocative testing performed later if necessary.

The ITT is the gold standard for the assessment of the hypothalamic–pituitary–adrenal (HPA) axis and pituitary GH reserve. Neuroglycopenia occurs when the blood glucose is less than 2.2 mmol/l, resulting in the release of ACTH, cortisol and GH.

- *A serum cortisol response of greater than 550 nmol/l and a cortisol increment of greater than 170 nmol/l is considered to indicate a normal response in some laboratories.* It is important to take account of the local reference range.

The test is not without risk, and loss of consciousness and seizures are recognised complications. Thus, it is contraindicated in those with known ischaemic heart disease or a history of seizures; extreme age is a relative contraindication. However, when performed in an experienced endocrine unit the test is associated with a low risk of complications.

Other provocative tests useful for assessment of the HPA axis include the short Synacthen (tetracosactide) test and the (intramuscular) glucagon stimulation test (see Appendix 1). Each test has advantages and disadvantages, with some groups favouring the ITT and others the short Synacthen test. Of principal importance, however, is that the peak cortisol level (cut-off) achieved must be interpreted in the light of the provocative test used.

Even using these criteria, approximately 1 in 20 tests will produce misleading results.

When glucagon is used as the provocative agent, the peak cortisol response occurs later (the test should be continued for 180 min) and it is smaller in magnitude than that seen in response to an ITT, and in a number (up to 10%) of normal individuals a response is not seen.

As a consequence, while some patients can be classified as having *'barn door' ACTH deficiency* that requires glucocorticoid replacement therapy (i.e. cortisol response of < 400 nmol/l to an ITT), a proportion fall into *a grey zone* from which the results of testing must be interpreted in the light of clinical features; for example, patients with a cortisol response of between 400 and 550 nmol/l to an ITT may be advised only to take glucocorticoid replacement during an intercurrent illness or surgery.

- Tests of the HPA axis are not infallible, and consideration should be given to repeating a test if the results are at odds with the clinical picture.

TSH deficiency

In secondary hypothyroidism one might expect to find reduced concentrations of free and/or total thyroxine (T_4) in association with a serum TSH concentration below the normal range, analogous to the biochemical findings in secondary hypogonadism.

- However, this picture is only found in the minority of patients, the majority having normal or occasionally elevated TSH levels.

The mechanism behind this apparent contradiction is poorly understood, and a number of different explanations have been explored. One such, is that secondary hypothyroidism may be associated with TSH of reduced bioactivity.

The TSH response to thyrotrophin-releasing hormone (TRH) – TRH test – has been proposed as a tool to help differentiate between hypothalamic and pituitary hypothyroidism. Classically, in hypothyroidism secondary to a hypothalamic lesion and hence TRH deficiency, the TSH response is delayed (the 60-min response is greater than the 20-min response), while in hypothyroidism of pituitary origin, damage to the thyrotrophs results in an absent or impaired TSH response.

Studies have revealed no clear-cut differences between patients with hypothyroidism of pituitary and hypothalamic origin and, as such, the test cannot be used as the sole criterion to differentiate between these lesions. Furthermore, the information gained has no therapeutic implication.

ADH deficiency

- The diagnosis of ADH deficiency first requires confirmation of excess urine output.
- Polyuria is defined as the excretion of greater than 3 litres of urine in 24 hours (40 ml/kg in 24 hours).
- Any patient with normal serum sodium and plasma osmolality who has a fluid output of less than 2 litres in 24 hours is likely to be normal and does not warrant further investigation.

Once excess urine output is confirmed, the usual first-line investigation is an 8-hour fluid deprivation test (see Appendix 1). The basis for this test is the rise in plasma osmolality resulting from a lack of fluid intake for several hours, stimulating ADH secretion.

The test should be performed under strict observation as severe fluid and electrolyte depletion can occur.

Plasma osmolality, urine volume and osmolarity are measured hourly for 8 hours, following which a synthetic analogue of ADH (desmopressin) is given intramuscularly. The urine osmolality is then remeasured. In a patient without diabetes insipidus, ADH is secreted throughout the test, water is normally absorbed and there is a subsequent increase in urine osmolality. In diabetes insipidus the urine fails to concentrate (normal individuals achieve a urine osmolality at least twice the plasma osmolality) due to a lack of ADH; hence, plasma osmolality rises. Urine concentrates adequately only after administration of desmopressin. Sometimes in cases where there has been long-standing polyuria, failure of urine concentration in response to desmopressin occurs not because of nephrogenic diabetes insipidus, but because of a washout of interstitial solutes including urea. This may lead to diagnostic difficulties.

In cases where the results of a water deprivation test are inconclusive, the introduction of specific and sensitive radioimmunoassays for ADH has provided a further diagnostic avenue. Infusion of hypertonic saline (5%, 850 mmol) to increase plasma osmolality above 300 mOsm/kg appears to be a better osmotic stimulus for ADH release than water deprivation. A definitive diagnosis of ADH deficiency can therefore be established by infusing hypertonic saline for 2 hours, with regular 20–30 min blood sampling to estimate plasma osmolality and ADH.

The relationship between ADH level and urinary osmolality following a period of fluid restriction also provides useful information about the cause of diabetes insipidus.

In nephrogenic diabetes insipidus, ADH values are above the normal reference range, while in cranial diabetes insipidus, values are at the lower end or below the normal reference range.

Treatment of Hypopituitarism

The treatment of hypopituitarism can be separated into those therapies directed at the underlying disease process and endocrine replacement therapy (Table 2.5).

Therapies directed at the underlying cause of hypopituitarism will be discussed in the relevant chapters of this book.

- Endocrine replacement therapy should aim to mimic the normal hormonal milieu as far as possible, thus improving symptoms while avoiding over-treatment. It remains to be seen whether present regimes normalise the excess mortality in hypopituitary patients.

GH deficiency

Until 1989, the sole indication for GH therapy was in children with GH deficiency. With the availability of recombinant-DNA-derived

Table 2.5 Endocrine replacement therapy

Hormone deficiency	Replacement	Usual daily dose range
GH	Growth hormone	0.27–0.7 mg s.c. during evening
Gonadotrophins: Women	Oestradiol valerate *or* Conjugated equine oestrogens *plus* Progesterone	Oral: 1–2 mg daily Transdermally: 25–100 µg/24 hours Oral: 0.625–1.25 mg daily Progesterone dose depends on preparation
Men	*Intramuscular:* Testosterone ester, i.e. Sustanon (testosterone propionate, testosterone phenylpropionate and testosterone isocaproate)	250 mg i.m., every 2 to 3 weeks
	Transdermal: Testosterone	5–7.5 mg /24 hours
	Implant: Testosterone	600–800 mg every 4–6 months
TSH	Thyroxine	75–150 µg daily
ACTH	Hydrocortisone	10 mg morning, 5 mg noon, 5 mg evening to 10 mg t.d.s.
Prolactin	Nil	—
ADH	Desmopressin (DDAVP)	Intranasal 10–40 µg daily in two or three divided doses Oral 300–600 µg daily in two or three divided doses

ADH = antidiuretic hormone, ACTH = adrenocorticotrophic hormone, GH = growth hormone, TSH = thyroid-stimulating hormone.

GH, the situation has gradually changed, as the biological consequences of GH deficiency in adult life have been appreciated.

Effects of GH replacement therapy in adults

Body composition. GH replacement therapy in adulthood induces
favourable changes in body composition, with studies demonstrating
a 15.5% reduction in fat mass and a 6% increase in lean body mass
following 12 months therapy. Correspondingly, there is an improvement in indices of physical performance and maximal oxygen uptake.

Bone mineral density. In response to GH therapy the initial change
in bone mineral density (BMD) over the first 3–6 months is a
decrease, believed to be due to increased bone remodelling activity. Markers of bone formation and resorption are increased early,
and remain elevated at 1 year. The subsequent response of bone
differs in adults with childhood-onset and adult-onset GH
deficiency. By 6 months of treatment, the BMD is significantly
increased in childhood-onset GH deficiency and continues to rise
over 18 months of GH replacement. In adult-onset GH deficiency,
BMD is not increased at 12 months although there is a significant
increase at 24 months, which is more prominent in those with
lower baseline BMD scores.

Quality of life. There is evidence from placebo-controlled randomised studies that significant improvement in vitality, well-being
and overall quality of life occurs in GH-deficient adults in response
to GH replacement. The exact mechanism for the improved sense
of well-being remains controversial: possible explanations include
increased exercise capacity, improved hydration status with normalisation of extracellular volume or a direct central nervous
system effect.

Lipid profile. The effects of GH on the lipid profile are less clear. It
appears that GH therapy is associated with a decrease in serum
total cholesterol, triglyceride and low-density lipoprotein (LDL)
levels. A possible complicating factor is the apparent increase in
lipoprotein(a), an independent cardiovascular risk factor, although
the changes reported are assay-dependent.

Insulin resistance. GH-deficient adults are insulin-resistant. While
it is well established that earlier regimes using high-dose GH
replacement (> 2 IU daily) were associated with either a worsening
of the insulin-resistant state or no change, the data utilising more

physiological dose regimes are not available. In addition, it remains unclear whether the insulin-resistance described in hypo-pituitary patients is solely secondary to GH deficiency or whether supraphysiological glucocorticoid replacement therapy may play a role.

In clinical practice GH replacement remains the remit of the specialist physician. Current practice in our department is to con-sider GH replacement therapy only in severely GH-deficient patients who describe symptoms consistent with severe impairment of quality of life. Elsewhere, particularly in Scandinavia, GH replacement therapy is offered to all severely GH-deficient adults. The majority of modern regimes recommend a low starting dose, i.e. 0.27 mg/day (0.8 IU/day) as a single subcutaneous injection. This should then be increased every 4–6 weeks, based on clinical response and the IGF-I, until a steady replacement dose is reached.

Improvements in physiological well-being and quality of life do not occur in all GH-deficient patients on replacement therapy. It is therefore suggested that patients started on GH primarily for a quality of life indication should have an initial trial period of therapy; only those with definite improvement should continue treatment thereafter. Improvements in quality of life and body com-position often only occur after several months of maintenance therapy and therefore a trial of 6 months of GH at the correct main-tenance dose is necessary to determine if treatment is beneficial.

At the end of this trial, patients should be reassessed using a disease-specific questionnaire and measurements of body composi-tion and lipids. In patients with marked osteoporosis/osteopenia, GH therapy is reassessed following BMD estimation at 2 years. This therapeutic approach is rarely complicated by side effects, such as peripheral oedema, arthralgia and myalgia, reported when higher doses of GH replacement, particularly weight-based dosing regimes, were used. Monitoring of GH replacement should include regular measurement of weight, blood pressure, HbA1c, lipid profile, IGF-I, fat distribution (waist–hip ratio) and assessment of quality of life by disease-specific questionnaire and patient interview. In addition, a baseline MRI scan is mandatory for all patients previously treated for a pituitary or cranial tumour, or who received cranial irradiation.

Gonadotrophin deficiency

In both sexes, sex steroid status is important for the maintenance of normal body composition, BMD and sexual function. In patients not desirous of fertility, sex steroid replacement therapy is most appropriate. These topics are covered in Chapters 8 and 9.

Fertility

- In the hypogonadotrophic hypogonadal patient, fertility can be achieved with gonadotrophin therapy.

In males, excellent success rates can be achieved, provided primary testicular dysfunction does not coexist.

Testosterone replacement should be discontinued before initiating therapy. Female pituitary infertility is covered in Chapter 8.

ACTH deficiency

- *The decision to begin cortisol replacement therapy relies not only on the results of dynamic testing but also on clinical assessment.*

Which corticosteroid?

Hydrocortisone is the logical choice, as it directly replaces the missing hormone – cortisol. Alternatives include cortisone acetate which is metabolised to cortisol to achieve glucocorticoid activity and therefore cannot be monitored in the same way as hydrocortisone. Its onset of action is slower and biological activity is slightly longer, providing relative disadvantages and advantages over hydrocortisone, respectively. Other synthetic glucocorticoids, i.e. prednisolone and dexamethasone, have significant disadvantages: monitoring is difficult and, in the case of dexamethasone, the limited number of pharmaceutical preparations available makes dose titration impossible and overdosage more likely.

When?

Normal individuals have undetectable serum levels of cortisol and ACTH at midnight. There is a sharp rise at 6 a.m., a peak at 8–9 a.m. and, following this, a steady decline throughout the rest of the day. No existing oral glucocorticoid replacement regimen can mimic this pattern; therefore replacement is a compromise between theory, practicality and convenience.

Standard twice-daily regimens (Figure 2.3)

- Very low levels of cortisol from 4 p.m. to 6 p.m. and between midnight and 8 a.m.
- Low serum cortisol in the afternoon may be associated with nonspecific symptoms of tiredness.
- Low levels in the early morning may be responsible for overnight fuel deficiency, which may in turn be responsible for symptoms of lack of vigour, fatigue and early morning headache.

Thrice-daily regimens

- Associated with more 'normal' cortisol levels.
- Studies of small numbers of patients report higher quality of life scores on thrice-daily regimes.

How much?

- Estimations of daily cortisol production rates used to be in the region of 12–15 mg/m^2.
- More recent data suggest that actual daily production rates are much lower ~5 mg/m^2 (16 µmol/m^2). This equates to 10–12 mg/m^2/day of oral hydrocortisone (~17–20 mg/day).
- Thus, on traditional regimens of 30 mg hydrocortisone daily, many patients may be over-replaced.
- Further evidence exists to support this view.

Zelissen *et al.* (1994) demonstrated reduced BMD in men but not in women with Addison's disease, compared with age-matched controls. Those with low BMD scores were more likely to be taking higher doses of hydrocortisone.

Peacey *et al.* (1997) studied 32 patients, taking a mean hydrocortisone dose of 29.5 mg daily: 24 of 32 patients were judged to be over-replaced by day-curve criteria. The dosage of hydrocortisone was reduced to a mean of 21 mg daily. This 30% reduction in hydrocortisone dose led to a 19% increase in serum osteocalcin levels, suggesting increased bone formation. The authors concluded that even mildly excessive hydrocortisone replacement has adverse effects on bone formation.

Recommended starting cortisol replacement regimen:

Hydrocortisone 10 mg	**immediately on rising**
Hydrocortisone 5 mg	**lunch time**
Hydrocortisone 5 mg	**between 4 and 6 p.m.**

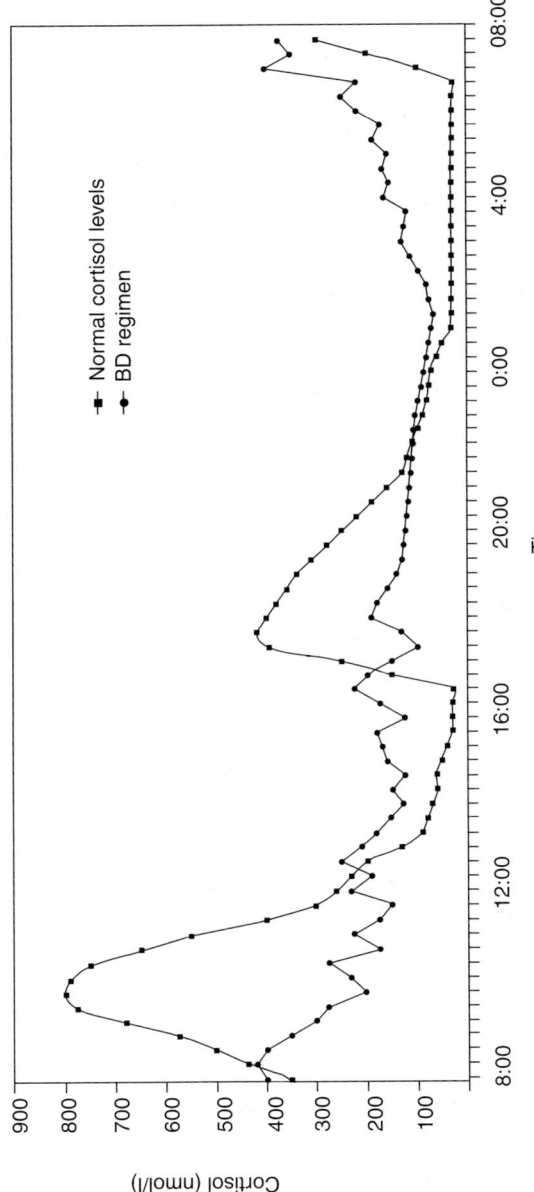

Figure 2.3 Twenty-four-hour cortisol levels in a normal individual and in a patient on a 'traditional' BD replacement regimen of hydrocortisone 20 mg morning and 10 mg in the afternoon.

Monitoring of therapy usually involves the use of an 8-hour hydrocortisone day curve or a modified three-point day curve, aiming to normalise cortisol levels.

- *Criteria:*
  9–12 a.m. peak < 650 nmol/l
  3–6 p.m > 50 nmol/l
  6–9 p.m. < 250 nmol/l
  mean 150–300 nmol/l

Such monitoring allows the detection of minor degrees of over- or under-replacement that are unlikely to be clinically obvious. Urinary free cortisol assessment cannot detect under-replacement with hydrocortisone and is probably best used as an initial screen to detect significantly over-treated individuals.

It is, however, crucial that the patient understands the need to increase his/her hydrocortisone dose if unwell due to an intercurrent illness or because he/she has to undergo a minor procedure; under the circumstances, the dose of hydrocortisone will need to be increased two- to three-fold. The possibility of a vomiting component to the illness means that all such patients should be advised to carry an emergency hydrocortisone pack containing hydrocortisone for intramuscular administration.

TSH deficiency

Secondary hypothyroidism is treated in the same way as primary hypothyroidism with T_4 replacement therapy. The normal starting dose in a young patient without evidence of cardiac disease is 100 µg daily; however, in the elderly or in a patient with evidence of ischaemic heart disease, therapy should be started at lower doses, i.e. 25–50 µg daily.

A complicating factor in this situation, however, is that measurement of serum TSH is obviously unhelpful in the monitoring of T_4 replacement therapy. Thus, the objective biochemically should be to restore the serum free T_4 concentration to the normal range. TSH-deficient female patients will commonly also be on oestrogen replacement therapy, with a consequent increase in thyroxine-binding globulin level, and thus the total T_4 level may be misleading. Over-replacement with T_4 over long periods may be associated with reduced BMD, an increased risk of osteoporotic fracture and an increase in the rate of development of atrial fibrillation; thus, excessive doses of T_4 should be avoided.

- *In a patient with suspected hypopituitarism, T_4 therapy should be delayed until ACTH deficiency has been excluded or treated, as there is a risk of worsening the features of cortisol deficiency.*

ADH deficiency

Desmopressin is the drug of choice for the treatment of ADH deficiency. It is a synthetic analogue of arginine vasopressin with two minor alterations in its molecular structure: a switch of arginine from the L to the D form in position 8, and deamination of cysteine in position 1. This results in a two- to four-fold increase in the antidiuretic activity, prolongation of the biological half-life to 6–8 hours and elimination of pressor activity. This latter effect results in an absence of the side effects noted with arginine vasopressin, including hypertension, renal colic, coronary artery spasm and abdominal colic.

Desmopressin is available in a number of preparations, including oral, intranasal and parenteral. Dosages vary widely, up to 10-fold between individuals, with no apparent relationship to age, sex, weight or degree of polyuria. The drug should be started at a low dose and increased gradually until the urine output is controlled. Overdosage carries a risk of hyponatraemia, and sodium levels should be checked after commencing therapy or dosage changes.

Strategies to Prevent Hypopituitarism

Hypopituitarism increases morbidity and mortality in affected patients, requires therapy with complex drug regimes and incurs significant cost to the health care provider. The development of GH replacement therapy has, in particular, exacerbated the problem, with a yearly cost of £3000 to £4000 per patient. Thus, attention has turned to strategies that might reduce the incidence of hypopituitarism.

Pituitary tumours are treated by surgery, radiotherapy and medically. Given that two modalities of therapy may achieve the same cure rate of the primary disorder, it is possible that the modality of therapy associated with the least risk of inducing hypopituitarism may be chosen for cost–benefit reasons.

One area worthy of consideration is the routine use of radiotherapy following surgery for non-secreting pituitary adenomas. There is now little remaining doubt that postoperative radiotherapy reduces the risk of tumour recurrence very significantly. A study was made of 126 patients with non-functioning pituitary adenomas who received radiotherapy as an adjuvant treatment postoperatively. Within this cohort, the progression free survival rate was 93% at both 10 and 15 years. In contrast, a long-term follow-up was made of a subgroup of patients with non-functioning adenomas who did not receive radiotherapy. These were patients with complete tumour removal as judged by the surgeon, without radiological and surgical evidence of spread into the parapituitary structures or evidence of rapid tumour growth. Among these individuals, there was an 82% recurrence-free survival at 5 years. Recurrence rates increased with time, however, and by 10 years, the percentage of patients who were recurrence-free had dropped to 56%.

It should also be pointed out that surgical results are highly operator-dependent, in terms of tumour recurrence, and that regular clinical and radiological surveillance is mandatory. Nonetheless, by avoiding radiotherapy as a routine procedure, the incidence of long-term hypopituitarism will be significantly reduced. Thus, particularly in the young adult with normal pituitary function postoperatively and desirous of fertility in the future, the possibility of avoiding radiation-induced hypopituitarism is very attractive and justifies the approximately 50% risk of tumour recurrence over the next 10 years. After all, if a recurrence does occur, it remains treatable by radiotherapy at this later point in time.

Medical therapy offers an alternative to radiotherapy or surgery in patients with prolactinomas and now in patients with acromegaly. Dopamine agonist drug therapy can shrink prolactinomas in size and restore normoprolactinaemia in many patients: 70% of macroadenomas shrinking by 25% or more, and restoration of normoprolactinaemia and normal gonadal function occurring in a least 75% of patients with prolactin-secreting microadenomas or macroadenomas.

Whether these agents are also associated with a restoration of other aspects of pituitary function is less clear; variable recovery from both ACTH and TSH deficiency has been described, but the data regarding GH status, particularly in adults, are scanty.

Somatostatin analogues as an adjunct therapy following surgery for acromegaly have potential advantages over radiotherapy, as they are unlikely to be associated with a further deterioration in pituitary function. Few data are available as yet to confirm the effects of this modality of treatment on recurrence rates and, furthermore, it is unknown whether acromegalic patients 'cured by' somatostatin analogues are rendered functionally GH deficient. In addition, long-term side effects of somatostatin analogues have not been fully determined.

Increasingly in the years to come, the therapeutic ratio of benefit to side effects will contribute to the choice of treatment for patients with pituitary disease.

Further Reading

Arafah BM. Reversible hypopituitarism in patients with large non-functioning pituitary adenomas. *J Clin Endocrinol Metab* 1986;**62**(6):1173–9.

Bates AS, Van't Hoff W, Jones PJ *et al*. The effect of hypopituitarism on life expectancy. *J Clin Endocrinol Metab* 1996;**81**(3):1169–72.

Bengtsson B, Johannsson G, Shalet SM, Simpson H, Sonken PH. Treatment of growth hormone deficiency in adults, *J Clin Endocrinol Metab* 2000;**85**:933–7.

Bulow B, Hagmar L, Mikoczy Z *et al*. Increased cerebrovascular mortality in patients with hypopituitarism. *Clin Endocrinol (Oxf)* 1997;**46**(1):75–81.

Carroll PV, Christ ER, Bengtsson BA *et al*. Growth hormone deficiency in adulthood and the effects of growth hormone replacement: a review. Growth Hormone Research Society Scientific Committee. *J Clin Endocrinol Metab* 1998;**83**(2):382–95.

Gittoes NJ, Bates AS, Tse W *et al*. Radiotherapy for non-function pituitary tumours. *Clin Endocrinol (Oxf)* 1998;**48**(3):331–7.

Growth Hormone Research Society. Consensus guidelines for the diagnosis and treatment of adults with growth hormone deficiency: summary statement of the Growth Hormone Research Society Workshop on Adult Growth Hormone Deficiency. *J Clin Endocrinol Metab* 1998;**83**(2):379–81.

Littley MD, Shalet SM, Beardwell CG *et al*. Hypopituitarism following external radiotherapy for pituitary tumours in adults. *Q J Med* 1989;**70**(262):145–60.

Peacey SR, Guo CY, Robinson AM *et al*. Glucocorticoid replacement therapy: are patients over treated and does it matter? [see comments]. *Clin Endocrinol (Oxf)* 1997;**46**(3):255–61.

Rosen T, Bengtsson BA. Premature mortality due to cardiovascular disease in hypopituitarism. *Lancet* 1990;**336**(8710):285–8.

Shalet SM, Beardwell CG, Pearson D *et al*. The effect of varying doses of cerebral irradiation on growth hormone production in childhood. *Clin Endocrinol (Oxf)* 1976;**5**(3):287–90.

Shalet SM, Toogood AA, Rahim A *et al.* The diagnosis of growth hormone deficiency in children and adults. *Endocrine Rev* 1998;**19**(2):203–23.

Toogood AA, O'Neill PA, Shalet SM. Beyond the somatopause: growth hormone deficiency in adults over the age of 60 years. *J Clin Endocrinol Metab* 1996;**81**(2):460–5.

.Turner HE, Stratton IM, Bryne JV, Adams CB, Wass JA. Audit of selected patients with nonfunctioning pituitary adenomas treated without irradiation – a follow-up study. *Clin Endocrinol (Oxf)* 1999;**51**(3):281–4.

Zelissen PM, Croughs RJ, van Rijk PP *et al.* Effect of glucocorticoid replacement therapy on bone mineral density in patients with Addison disease [see comments]. *Ann Intern Med* 1994;**120**(3):207–10.

3

Prolactin and Prolactinomas

Ayesha Siddiqi and Diana F Wood

Introduction

Prolactin is a peptide hormone secreted by the lactotroph cells of the anterior pituitary gland. It belongs to a multigene family that includes growth hormone (GH) and the chorionic somatomammotrophin genes. Prolactin binds with two molecules of its membrane-bound receptor to initiate biological activity.

Hyperprolactinaemia is one of the most common pituitary abnormalities. Although it is detected in less than 1% of the general population, it has been found in up to 25% of patients with secondary amenorrhoea.

Physiology

Prolactin release is under negative control by the hypothalamic 'prolactin-inhibiting' hormone dopamine. Dopamine inhibits prolactin release by activating D2 dopamine receptors, which are negatively coupled with adenyl cyclase activity in lactotroph cells. Prolactin is secreted in a pulsatile manner with a frequency of 95 min, with a major nocturnal peak soon after the onset of sleep.

In chronic hyperprolactinaemia, oestradiol levels in women and testosterone levels in men are reduced. High prolactin levels stimulate dopamine release in the hypothalamus, which in turn stimulates β-endorphin secretion. This opioid inhibits hypothalamic gonadotrophin-releasing hormone (GnRH) release, resulting in reduced luteinising hormone (LH) pulses. In women, positive feedback of oestrogens on LH secretion fails and there is no ovulatory

LH rise. Together with the abnormality at the hypothalamic level, hyperprolactinaemia may also induce direct inhibition of oestradiol and progesterone synthesis in the ovary and inhibit peripheral conversion of testosterone to 5-dihydrotestosterone.

Role of Prolactin

Prolactin is primarily involved in the initiation and maintenance of lactation. It may also be important in regulating reproductive function; homozygous prolactin receptor 'knockout' female mice are infertile, while males have reduced fertility. In the male, prolactin increases sensitivity of the testes to LH, potentiating the effect of androgens on male accessory glands, influencing sperm motility and fertilising capacity. In females, prolactin may be needed for optimal corpus luteal function in addition to regulation of lactation. Recently, roles in osmoregulation, especially in the fetus, and in immune modulation have been postulated.

Disorders of prolactin secretion mainly relate to hyperprolactinaemia, since the syndrome of prolactin deficiency has not been described. Hyperprolactinaemia can be caused by numerous physiological and pathological factors (Table 3.1).

Hyperprolactinaemia

Prolactinomas

Prolactinomas are the most common form of functioning pituitary adenomas, accounting for 25–30% of such tumours. They may be classified as either macroadenomas (>10 mm in diameter) or microadenomas (<10 mm). They mostly occur sporadically, but rarely can be associated with parathyroid and pancreatic tumours as part of the syndrome of multiple endocrine neoplasia (MEN 1). The prevalence of prolactinomas in unselected post-mortem studies is around 10%, with an equal sex distribution. Clinically, microprolactinomas are much more common in women, while a higher proportion of adenomas in men are macroadenomas. This difference is probably related to delayed diagnosis in men due to lack of easily identifiable symptoms and a higher tumour growth velocity, but the precise reason remains unknown. The age of diagnosis in women is usually between 15 and 44 years, whereas in the majority of men it ranges from 45 to 75 years. Hyperprolactinaemia may also be secondary to other tumours or granulomatous disease in the region of the hypothalamus as a result of functional disinhi-

Table 3.1 Causes of hyperprolactinaemia

Physiological
Pregnancy
Nipple stimulation, suckling
Neonatal
Sleep
Coitus
Stress (hypoglycaemia, surgery)

Pituitary disease
Prolactinoma
Other intrasellar tumours causing stalk compression/'pseudoprolactinoma'
(pituitary adenoma, meningioma, germinoma)
Empty sella
Lymphocytic hypophysitis

Drugs
Dopamine antagonists (neuroleptics, e.g. haloperidol and chlorpromazine;
metoclopramide, sulpiride)
Antidepressants (imipramine, amitriptyline)
Antihypertensives (α-methyldopa, verapamil)
Oestrogens (high-dose oral contraceptives)
Opiates
Cimetidine (parenteral)

Hypothalamic disease
Tumour (craniopharyngioma, glioma, germinoma, metastasis)
Granulomatous disease (sarcoidosis, histiocytosis X, tuberculous meningitis)
Cranial irradiation
Pseudotumour cerebri

Miscellaneous
Primary hypothyroidism
Polycystic ovarian syndrome
Chronic renal failure
Macroprolactinaemia
Cirrhosis
Chest wall lesion (injury, herpes zoster)
Ectopic prolactin secretion (bronchogenic carcinoma, hypernephroma)
Grand mal fit
Idiopathic

bition. In these cases, dopaminergic input to the anterior pituitary is thought to be disrupted, resulting in excessive prolactin secretion from normal pituitary lactotrophs.

Aetiology

The pathogenesis of all pituitary tumours is unclear. A primary pituitary origin for prolactinomas is suggested by the presence of lactotroph hyperplasia in the para-adenomatous pituitary tissue. In addition, X-chromosomal deletion studies have found many of these tumours to be monoclonal, suggesting a genetic mutation in a progenitor cell with subsequent clonal expansion. Alternatively, other studies have documented abnormal dopaminergic neuro-transmission, suggesting that hypothalamic function may also play a role in the aetiology.

Malignant prolactinomas are very rare. As it is often difficult to distinguish benign from malignant prolactinomas, histologically for a pituitary neoplasm to be designated as malignant, there must be proven metastases either within the central nervous system or to other sites.

Non-pituitary hyperprolactinaemia

As shown in Table 3.1, there is a wide range of non-pituitary causes of hyperprolactinaemia.

Drugs

Drugs are an important cause of hyperprolactinaemia because of the large numbers of patients treated with dopamine antagonist therapy. Since dopamine is the physiological prolactin inhibitory factor, the most common pharmacological causes of hyperprolactinaemia are centrally acting compounds that interact with dopamine release. Thus, all drugs that block dopamine receptors (phenothiazines), deplete central catecholamine stores (reserpine) or interfere with dopamine synthesis (methyldopa) cause hyperprolactinaemia. H_2 antagonists (cimetidine) may reduce dopamine tone in the hypo-thalamus, whereas opiates probably reduce dopamine release in the median eminance. Newer antipsychotic agents, e.g. sulpiride, commonly raise prolactin levels. Tricyclic antidepressants and mono-amine oxidase inhibitors have only rarely been reported to cause hyperprolactinaemia and galactorrhoea.

However, the new subgroup of antidepressants, the selective serotonin reuptake inhibitors (SSRIs), have recently been introduced and have gained increasing popularity among psychiatric as well as general physicians. The SSRIs, such as fluoxetine and paroxetine, activate serotoninergic pathways and stimulate prolactin release, mainly via the hypothalamus. In the last 5 years these drugs have been frequently reported to cause hyperprolactinaemia, probably via the action of type 2A serotonin receptors. They are associated with an approximately eight times risk of non-puerperal lactation when compared with other antidepressants such as tricyclic antidepressants and monoamine oxidase inhibitors.

Other identifiable non-pituitary causes of hyperprolactinaemia are shown in Table 3.1.

Idiopathic hyperprolactinaemia

Idiopathic hyperprolactinaemia describes the presence of raised serum prolactin concentrations in patients who have no demonstrable pituitary/hypothalamic disease and in whom no other recognised cause of hyperprolactinaemia is present. It is a heterogenous condition that includes different entities.

A relatively recently described condition is macroprolactinaemia in which elevated levels of macro- or large molecular weight prolactin give rise to overall hyperprolactinaemia. Prolactin exists in the circulation in multiple molecular forms: monomeric prolactin (MW 23 kDa), big prolactin (MW 50–60 kDa) and big–big prolactin or macroprolactin (MW 150–170 kDa). Macroprolactin forms a complex with an immunoglobulin G (IgG) autoantibody which has a prolonged half-life, leading to apparent hyperprolactinaemia. In hyperprolactinaemic patients, 16–26% of prolactin has been shown to be macroprolactin. The clinical impact of macroprolactinaemia remains controversial. Although some reports document associated galactorrhoea and menstrual disturbance, others suggest that patients remain asymptomatic. However, in general, macroprolactin has reduced bioavailability, and patients with macroprolactinaemia do not require treatment.

Clinical signs and symptoms of hyperprolactinaemia

Table 3.2 summarises the clinical signs and symptoms (%) in patients with prolactinoma.

Gonadal dysfunction

In women, chronic hyperprolactinaemia may induce primary or secondary amenorrhoea, oligomenorrhoea, a short luteal phase or infertility. Dyspareunia and loss of libido are also associated with

Table 3.2   Clinical manifestations of hyperprolactinaemia

Symptoms and signs	Per cent in patients with prolactinoma
Gonadal dysfunction	
Oligospermia and other sperm abnormalities	100
Impotence	91
Oligomenorrhoea	54
Secondary amenorrhoea	40
Primary amenorrhoea	2
Galactorrhoea	
Females	70
Males	20
Neurological features	
Headache	56
Hirsutism and acne	25
Visual field defects in macroadenomas	18
Other endocrine abnormalities	
Hypopituitarism	2
Hirsuitism	25
Acne (females)	5

long-term oestrogen deficiency. Hyperprolactinaemia may also be secondary to polycystic ovary syndrome and hence may be associated with hirsutism and acne.

In men, loss of libido, impotence, infertility and a decrease in seminal fluid are described. Gynaecomastia is rare, and galactorrhoea is less frequent than in the female patients, probably because of lower levels of oestrogens in the circulation.

Complications of long-standing hyperprolactinaemia and the ensuing hypogonadism include a reduction in bone mineral density. Up to 50% of such patients have decreased bone density compared to age-matched normal subjects.

Galactorrhoea

Galactorrhoea is found in 30–80% of female patients, depending partly on the intensity with which it is sought. However, only 50% of women with galactorrhoea also have hyperprolactinaemia: thus, galactorrhoea is a poor marker for the presence of hyperprolactinaemia in females. Both oestrogen and prolactin are necessary for the development of galactorrhoea, so galactorrhoea is less common than amenorrhoea alone, as chronic hyperprolactinaemia is associated with hypo-oestrogenism.

Galactorrhoea may be present in 5–10% of normal menstruating women, but in the majority serum prolactin levels are normal. The cause of such *normoprolactinaemic galactorrhoea* in normally menstruating women is not known. Several explanations have been proposed such as increased prolactin release in response to stress or sleep, which may cause high prolactin levels at certain times of the day. Other possible explanations include increased sensitivity of prolactin receptors in the breasts and hyper-responsive serotonin receptors in the hypothalamus, causing elevated intermittent prolactin release. Increased GH secretion, especially of a low molecular weight isoform, has been found in some patients with galactorrhoea and normal prolactin levels. Patients with normoprolactinaemic galactorrhoea may have a positive family history of this condition. When no cause can be found, treatment with dopamine agonists is often effective.

Neurological features

When hyperprolactinaemia is due to a macroadenoma, tumour-mass-dependent symptoms can occur. Headaches occur commonly in patients with pituitary adenomas, particularly those with macroadenomas. However, for reasons which are unclear, headaches also appear to occur frequently in women with hyperprolactinaemia due to microadenoma with minimally abnormal radiological findings. Cranial nerve lesions depend on tumour extension: compression of the optic chiasm can lead to visual field defects (typically bilateral hemianopia) and optic nerve atrophy, and lateral extension of the tumour with infiltration of the cavernous sinuses can lead to cranial nerve paralysis (III, IV and VI).

Endocrine abnormalities

Secretion of other anterior pituitary hormones may be affected due to tumour compression by macroprolactinomas, leading to hypopituitarism. Diabetes insipidus is not a feature, being more characteristic of hypothalamic lesions. Other endocrine abnormalities include hirsutism and acne, which are thought to be due to effects of prolactin on adrenal androgen production.

Diagnosis

Clinical evaluation of the patient with hyperprolactinaemia

Clinical evaluation should involve a careful history designed to exclude non-pituitary causes including details of the drug history, menstrual cycle, libido, infertility and impotence. Clinical examination, including breast examination for galactorrhoea (Table 3.3) and visual field testing (with confrontation and/or Goldmann perimetry), should be performed; in certain cases, recordings of visual evoked potentials can be helpful.

Biochemical evaluation

Confirmation of hyperprolactinaemia

Prolactin is secreted in a pulsatile fashion, so three samples taken on consecutive occasions or 30 min apart may occasionally be needed to make the diagnosis of pathological hyperprolactinaemia. Unless a prolactin-secreting adenoma is cystic or necrotic, the levels of prolactin in serum accurately reflect tumour size. Macroprolactinomas are often associated with prolactin levels above 8000 mU/l, while levels can rise to 1,000,000 mU/l or more in larger tumours. Levels between 1000 and 8000 mU/l may be associated with either a pro-

Table 3.3 Cause of hyperprolactinaemia in relation to serum prolactin level

Prolactin level (mU/l)	Cause
< 1000	Non-tumorous aetiology
	Pseudoprolactinoma
	Macroprolactinaemia
1000–4000	Microprolactinoma
	Pseudoprolactinoma
	Non-tumorous aetiology
	Macroprolactinaemia
4000–8000	Microprolactinoma
	Macroprolactinoma
	Pseudoprolactinoma
8000	Macroprolactinoma

lactinoma or pituitary stalk compression from another tumour. Macroadenomas with prolactin levels < 1000 mU/l are probably not prolactinomas (Table 3.3). The availability of the α-subunit assay in specialised centres may be of help in detecting non-functioning tumours. Polycystic ovary syndrome is associated with prolactin levels up to 2000 mU/l in possibly 7% of cases.

Exclusion of secondary causes

Attention should be paid to testing for renal impairment, polycystic ovary syndrome and hypothyroidism.

Assessment of anterior pituitary function

Co-secretion of other hormones or hypopituitarism should be excluded. Initial measurements should include 9 a.m. cortisol and GH, insulin-like growth factor-1 (IGF-1), luteinising hormone/follicle-stimulating hormone (LH/FSH), thyroxine (T_4) and thyroid-stimulating hormone (TSH).

Radiological evaluation

If a non-pituitary cause for the hyperprolactinaemia is not apparent, pituitary imaging is indicated. This has been revolutionised by high-resolution computed tomography (CT) scanning and magnetic resonance imaging (MRI). MRI combined with the administration of gadolinium is superior to CT, because it allows visualisation of the optic chiasm and cavernous sinus regions, thus defining the superior and lateral borders of a mass. Microadenomas usually appear as hypodense lesions on T1-weighted images; macroadenomas tend to have signal characteristics similar to the normal gland and may contain cystic or haemorrhagic areas. High-resolution CT images with contrast administration and coronal and sagittal reconstruction pictures are also very valuable in the diagnosis of pituitary adenomas, particularly for visualisation of possible bone erosion caused by the tumour. It should be borne in mind when interpreting pituitary radiology that microadenomas are present in a significant proportion of the normal population, and focal abnormalities have been demonstrated in 30% and 40% of healthy females on high-resolution CT and MRI, respectively. Conversely, a normal scan does not exclude the presence of a small prolactinoma. The radiological findings should always be interpreted with caution and correlated with the clinical and biochemical findings.

Treatment

Non-pituitary hyperprolactinaemia

The main thrust of management is to correct and treat the underlying cause. For example, hypothyroidism will require thyroxine replacement and polycystic ovary syndrome weight reduction or oestrogen/antiandrogen therapy to regulate menstrual disturbances and modify androgen action, respectively. However, if correction of the underlying cause is not possible or the patient has symptoms attributable to hyperprolactinaemia, medical therapy is indicated.

Prolactinomas

The treatment of prolactinomas includes medical, surgical and radiation therapy alone or in combination. In selected and carefully monitored cases, observation is also a viable option.

Medical Therapy

Effects of drug therapy

The introduction of dopamine agonist therapy (Box 3.1) has been a major advance in the treatment of patients with hyperprolactinaemia and prolactinoma. Dopamine agonists reduce prolactin secretion and the volume of prolactinomas by interference with transcriptional regulation of the prolactin gene and hence messenger RNA synthesis.

The evidence is now unequivocal that dopamine agonist drugs not only reduce prolactin release but also may actually shrink prolactinomas. This effect can occur within hours, and visual field defects may reverse within days of primary medical therapy. Thus, the clinical presentation of a patient with visual impairment is no longer an absolute indication for surgery.

Box 3.1   Dopamine agonist drugs currently available

Bromocriptine
Cabergoline
Quinagolide
Pergolide (listed indication Parkinson's disease)

Prolactin levels are lowered in over 90% of prolactinomas and valuable shrinkage achieved in well over 90% of microadenomas and 60–65% of macroprolactinomas, especially in the first 6–12 weeks of therapy. Even very large macroadenomas extending well outside the pituitary fossa may dramatically shrink into the pituitary fossa, with relief of local complications such as visual field defects or oculomotor nerve palsies. If hypopituitarism is present before treatment, it resolves in about 50% of patients as the tumour shrinks.

In pituitary tumours other than prolactinomas, the excessive prolactin comes from normal pituitary cells which always express dopamine receptors. This prolactin is extremely sensitive to dopamine agonist therapy but, while a rapid fall in elevated prolactin levels may occur with restoration of gonadal function, the size of the tumour rarely ever changes on dopamine agonist therapy.

Management of patient after commencing medical therapy

Following commencement of dopamine agonist therapy as primary treatment for a large pituitary tumour, the patient should be carefully assessed in the following weeks for the incidence of headache and its resolution, and for improvement in any visual field defects. Serum prolactin levels should be checked twice a week initially. In the absence of clinical improvement, imaging should be repeated after 2–4 weeks. If there is no sign of tumour shrinkage, surgical treatment should be advised.

If clinical improvement occurs, imaging should be repeated after 6–12 weeks to check shrinkage of the tumour. If the tumour shrinks back to the pituitary fossa, then long-term medical therapy is advised, bearing in mind that cessation of therapy will usually cause re-expansion of the tumour. For this reason, patients on medical therapy require indefinite treatment. If after 3–6 months of dopamine agonist therapy an extrasellar extension persists, then surgery is indicated. Pituitary irradiation may be necessary in cases of aggressively growing tumours or in patients who are resistant to or intolerant of medical therapy.

A rare but important complication of dopamine agonist therapy can occur with shrinkage of tumours invading the sphenoid sinus: as the tumour shrinks in response to dopamine agonist therapy the 'plug' is pulled and a cerebrospinal fluid (CSF) leak appears as clear white fluid dribbling from the nose. This phenomenon may also occur after radiotherapy. To prove that this discharge is CSF, a sample collected in a tube with fluoride and a corresponding peripheral blood sample should be sent to the laboratory for glucose measurement. CSF has about 50% glucose concentration of blood, while true nasal mucosal discharge is practically devoid of glucose. MRI after injection of intrathecal contrast may reveal a CSF leak.

Resistance and intolerance to dopaminergic therapy

True prolactinomas occasionally show relative or absolute resistance to dopamine agonist treatment in terms of a decrease in serum prolactin levels and shrinkage of tumour size. Resistance does not correlate with the level of hyperprolactinaemia or the size of the tumour. The percentage of patients with resistance to bromocriptine therapy varies from 5 to 18% in different series. Variable drug absorption and abnormal drug pharmacokinetics might explain the resistance in some patients, but this has not been consistently demonstrated and intramuscular bromocriptine is no more effective than oral preparations. In other patients, the prolactin-secreting adenomas may be relatively or absolutely deficient in type 2 dopamine receptors, as shown in studies on pituitary tissue removed from the resistant patients during transsphenoidal surgery.

Intolerance has been found in about 10% of patients treated with bromocriptine, and 3% of patients taking cabergoline. Box 3.2 lists some of the more common side effects of dopamine agonists. Careful prescription of the drug prevents or reduces side effects in many patients. A suggested regimen, with cautious dose increments, is shown in Box 3.3. Occasionally, a patient who is intolerant of one drug may be more tolerant of another. Recently, it has been shown that cabergoline may be able to restore normal prolactin levels in 70% of patients refractory to bromocriptine *and* quinagolide therapy. Cabergoline possesses a greater affinity for dopamine-binding sites and occupies D2 receptors for a longer time than bromocriptine. Cabergoline may also be more effective because of its greater tolerability compared with bromocriptine or quinagolide which allows dose increments in patients with relatively hyporesponsive tumours. It also has a longer duration of action (7–21 days) and the weekly regime helps improve compliance.

Box 3.2   Side effects of dopamine agonists

- Postural hypotension
- Dizziness
- Nausea and vomiting
- Constipation
- Weakness
- Nasal stuffiness
- Somnolence
- Psychological symptoms: hallucinations, delusions and mood changes
- Alcohol intolerance

Box 3.3   Administration of commonly used dopamine agonists

Bromocriptine
Starting dose: 0.625–1.25 mg taken in the middle of evening meal
Dose increments of 0.625–1.25 mg every 2–3 days
Average dose: 10 mg daily
Range: 1.25–30 mg daily

Cabergoline
Starting dose: 250 µg once weekly
Dose increments of 250 µg every 2–3 weeks
Average dose: 250 µg twice weekly
Range: 250 µg once weekly – 500 µg daily

Surgery

Pituitary surgery is discussed in Chapter 1. Indications for surgery in prolactinomas are listed in Box 3.4.

Box 3.4   Indications for surgery in prolactinomas

Failure of medical therapy due to resistance or intolerance
Non-compliance with long-term medication
Continuing symptoms despite medical therapy
Persisting suprasellar extension despite medical therapy
Macroadenomas in women desiring fertility to avoid pregnancy-induced tumour enlargement

The surgical cure rate for microprolactinomas is 80% immediately postoperatively but the recurrence rate rises to 10–50% within 5 years and is progressively higher afterwards. Preoperative prolactin levels provide an excellent prediction of outcome, but postoperative prolactin measurements are even better predictors; an unmeasurable serum prolactin 1 or 2 days after surgery predicts a cure of 90%, and higher values within the normal range are inversely related to the probability of cure. Postoperative values even slightly above the normal range indicate incomplete removal of the adenoma.

The surgical recurrence rate for macroprolactinomas at 10 years is nearly 100% even when the immediate postoperative levels are normal. This is because of microscopic tumour infiltration into the surrounding tissues. For this reason, surgery for macroprolactinomas is usually combined with medical treatment or radiotherapy. If surgical cure is not possible because of extrasellar spread, surgery has the focused objective of reducing the mass of the adenoma. This may allow prolactin production to be reduced into a desirable range by a tolerated dose of dopamine agonist and also relieve symptoms of compression and reduce the bulk of the adenoma before irradiation.

Complications of surgery are covered in Chapter 1.

Radiotherapy

Radiotherapy is an important tool in the management of pituitary adenomas. It is seldom needed for prolactinomas and is covered in Chapter 1.

Observation

In carefully selected cases of pituitary prolactinomas with no mass effect or other clinical disturbance, observation is a possible choice of management. These patients should be regularly reviewed clinically and for serum prolactin levels and occasional imaging. However, every woman should be offered a trial of dopamine agonist therapy, as other subtle disturbances of mood or libido may be greatly improved. Premenopausal women with amenorrhoea and no interest in fertility need oestrogen replacement with careful monitoring of prolactin levels. Postmenopausal women may or may not choose oestrogen replacement therapy.

Special Situations

Prolactinomas and pregnancy

Once a woman has received effective treatment for hyperprolactinaemia, fertility is usually restored often before the complete normalisation of prolactin levels. This may occur extremely rapidly, such that the patient may become pregnant even before the onset of menses. Patients with suppressed prolactin levels and regular cycles have theoretically and practically the same chance of achieving pregnancy as normal women. In contrast, patients with untreated pituitary adenomas appear to have an increased risk of miscarriage, with an incidence of 27–32%. When pregnancy is confirmed, treatment with dopaminergic drugs is usually discontinued.

The volume of the normal pituitary increases by approximately 30–70% during pregnancy. In the presence of a prolactinoma, tumour growth needs to be excluded. Microprolactinomas have a 1% or less risk for the development of complications related to tumour growth but still need careful clinical evaluation throughout the pregnancy. In untreated macroprolactinomas the risk of expansion with pregnancy is 15–35%. In patients with unresponsive adenomas or who are intolerant to dopamine agonist therapy, irradiation or surgery is indicated before conception; however, spontaneous ovulation is unusual in such patients. In patients who responded to dopamine agonists prior to the pregnancy, the risk of tumour expansion during pregnancy is reduced to less than 10%. These women require regular clinical assessment, with visual field examination and assessment of headache: dopamine agonist therapy can be reintroduced if indicated.

Alternatively, dopamine agonists may need to be administered throughout the pregnancy. No increase has been found in the risk of spontaneous abortion or congenital abnormalities of the baby in women taking bromocriptine. This is currently the only drug licensed in the UK for treatment of women with hyperprolactinaemia who wish to get pregnant. However, increasing evidence suggests that cabergoline and quinagolide can also be used safely in this patient group.

Patients with prolactinoma usually find it easy to breast-feed their babies and there is no contraindication if the patient is monitored regularly. Indeed there may be difficulties in cessation of lactation.

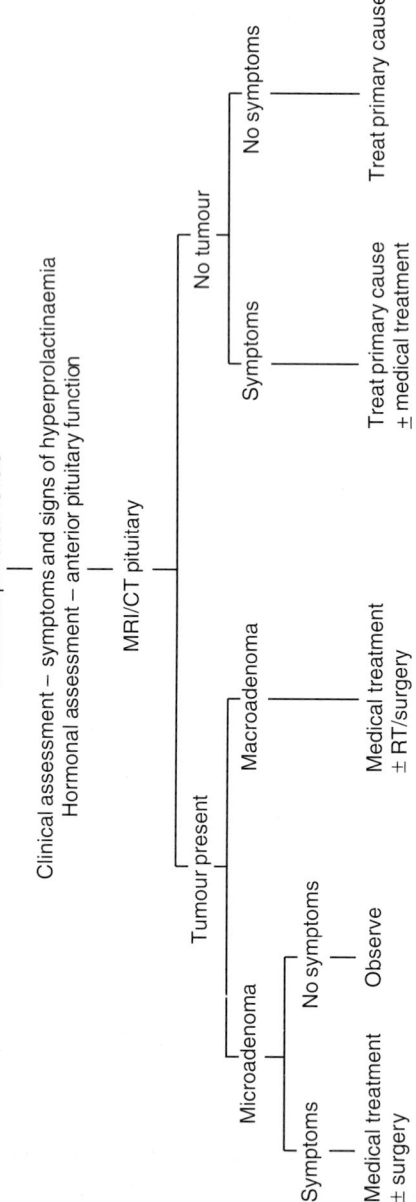

Figure 3.1 Suggested plan for the management of hyperprolactinaemia.

Hyperprolactinaemia and oestrogens

Oestrogens induce prolactin-secreting tumours in animals, and oestrogen administered to young women and postmenopausal subjects leads to an increase in prolactin levels. Oestrogen may decrease the ability of dopamine agonist drugs to inhibit prolactin secretion or may induce increased prolactin release from the pituitary. In women with hyperprolactinaemic amenorrhoea when fertility is not an issue, oestrogens are attractive options for their beneficial effects on the skeletal and cardiovascular system. However, it must be remembered that the safety of chronic oestrogen therapy in patients with prolactinoma is yet to be established.

Summary

In a patient with hyperprolactinaemia the cause of the elevated prolactin levels should be first established with the help of physical examination, biochemical tests and imaging techniques (Figure 3.1). True prolactinomas have to be carefully distinguished from other tumours in the pituitary/hypothalamic region. Medical treatment with dopamine agonists is indicated as first-line therapy in any type of true prolactinoma. In patients with microprolactinomas, this remains the only form of treatment required unless intolerance or resistance occur, when surgery is the preferred option. Patients with macroprolactinomas should be carefully reviewed to check the resolution of hyperprolactinaemia and the shrinkage of the tumour. Macroprolactinomas successfully treated with medical therapy showing shrinkage back to the pituitary fossa should be treated either with radiotherapy or with long-term dopamine agonist therapy to prevent recurrence of the tumour. Transsphenoidal surgery is reserved for patients with intolerance or resistance to dopamine agonist therapy or for patients with tumours other than true prolactinomas.

Further Reading

Besser M. Criteria for medical as opposed to surgical treatment of prolactinomas [Review] [11 refs]. *Acta Endocrinol (Copenh)* 1993;**129**(Suppl 1): 27–30.

Camanni F, Ciccarelli E. Prolactinomas. In: Grossman AB (ed), *Clinical Endocrinology*. Oxford: Blackwell Scientific Publications, 1992:132–47.

Ciccarelli E, Camanni F. Diagnosis and drug therapy of prolactinoma [Review] [63 refs]. *Drugs* 1996;**51**:954–65.

Colao A, Di Sarno A, Sarnacchiaro F *et al.* Prolactinomas resistant to standard dopamine agonists respond to chronic cabergoline treatment. *J Clin Endocrinol Metab* 1997;**82**:876–83.

Molitch ME, Thorner MO, Wilson C. Management of prolactinomas. *J Clin Endocrinol Metab* 1997;**82**:996–1000.

Plowman PN, Grossman AB. Non-surgical management of pituitary tumours. In: Lynn J, Bloom SR (eds), *Surgical Endocrinology*. Oxford: Butterworth Heinemann, 1993:146–9.

Reber PM. Prolactin and immunomodulation [Review]. *Am J Med* 1993;**95**:637–44.

Vance ML, Thorner MO. Prolactin: hyperprolactinaemic syndromes and management. In: DeGroot LJ (ed.), *Endocrinology*, 3rd edn. Philadelphia: WB Saunders, 1995:394–405.

Webster J, Scanlon MF. Prolactinomas. In: Sheaves R, Jenkins PJ, Wass JAH (eds), *Clinical Endocrine Oncology*. London: Blackwell Science, 1997:189–94.

4

Acromegaly

Paul J Jenkins

Introduction

The term acromegaly, first described by Pierre Marie in 1886, is derived from the Greek words *akron* (extremities) and *megas* (large), which sums up some of its essential clinical features. It is a disease characterised by excessive secretion of growth hormone which, in more than 99% of cases, is due to a benign pituitary growth hormone secreting adenoma. Extremely rarely it may be due to ectopic secretion of growth hormone releasing hormone (GHRH) from a metastatic neuroendocrine tumour, or from excessive hypothalamic GHRH secretion. Approximately 5% of cases are associated with the multiple endocrine neoplasia type 1 (MEN1) syndrome. Acromegaly is a rare disease, with approximately 2500 cases in the UK and an annual incidence of 3–4 per million. It affects both sexes equally, with the majority of cases becoming clinically apparent between the ages of 40 and 60. Younger patients tend to have more aggressive disease with larger invasive tumours.

Growth Hormone Physiology

Growth hormone is a 191 amino acid single-chain protein containing two disulphide bonds. It has considerable structural homology with prolactin. Approximately 70% circulates as a 22 kDa protein, 10% as a 20 kDa isoform and the remainder as dimers or sulphated and glycosylated isoforms. An important point is that pituitary growth hormone is secreted in pulsatile bursts, approximately 4 and 11 pulses in 24 hours, especially at night, with extremely low or undetectable levels occurring in the nadir between pulses. Thus, a random single serum measurement is invalid as a means of assessing the overall level of secretion, which requires either frequent sampling over a 24-hour period, or more pragmatically, the mean level of five serum measurements taken over 10–12 hours – a growth hormone day curve. Pituitary growth hormone release is controlled by both secretory and inhibitory hypothalamic factors. Growth hormone releasing hormone and the recently identified and cloned ghrelin act by distinct receptors to stimulate release, while the 14 amino acid somatostatin exerts marked inhibitory effects on its release. Both of these stimulatory and inhibitory factors are subject not only to higher influences within the brain but also to peripheral signals such that the overall secretion of growth hormone can vary widely with different stimuli (Table 4.1).

Growth hormone circulates in blood bound to its binding protein, which comprises the extracellular portion of its receptor. The growth hormone receptor is very widely distributed and is present in most tissues, where its activation can lead to the production of insulin-like growth factor-I (IGF-I) (Figure 4.1). Although classical endocrinology states that it is hepatic-synthesised IGF-I acting in an endocrine manner that is responsible for most, if not all, of the effects of growth hormone, it is becoming increasing clear that local production of IGF-I acting either in a paracrine (nearby cells) or autocrine (on the same cell) manner also plays an important role.

Elegant gene 'knock-out' experiments have demonstrated that animals with selective hepatic IGF-I loss have a normal phenotype and growth, despite serum IGF-I levels being extremely low. Thus, rather than being the sole effector of growth hormone, serum IGF-I should more accurately be regarded as a marker of serum growth hormone concentrations. Both the local and systemic IGF-I bioactivity are influenced by insulin-like growth factor binding proteins (IGFBPs), of which six have currently been identified, although

Table 4.1   Physiological factors increasing GH secretion

Sleep (slow waves)
Malnutrition and fasting (IGF-I is low)
Stress
Exercise
Fall in blood glucose
Type 1 diabetes mellitus, if uncontrolled (IGF-I is low)
Cirrhosis of the liver

IGF-I = insulin-like growth factor-I.

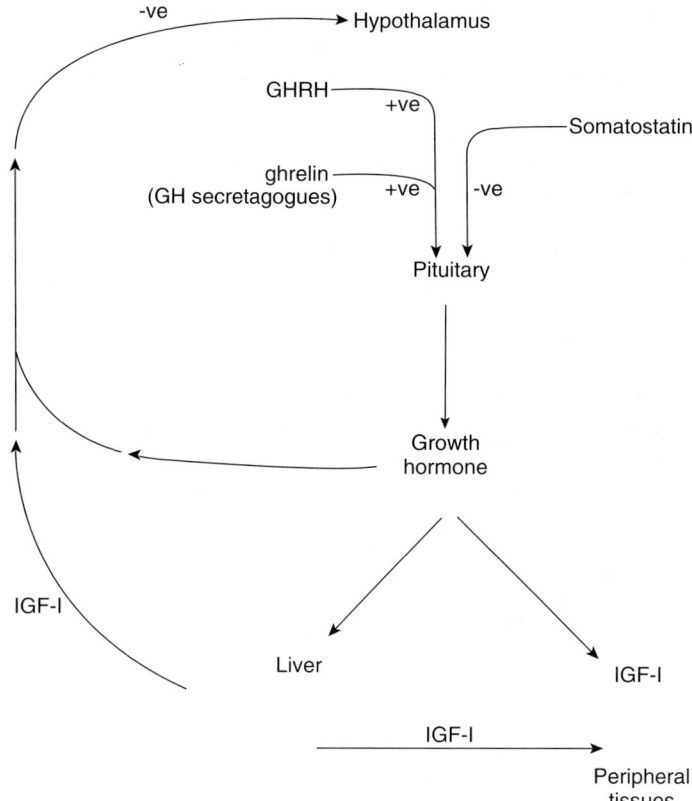

Figure 4.1   The growth hormone/insulin-like growth factor-1 (GH/IGF-I) axis. GHRH = growth hormone releasing hormone.

IGFBP-3 preferentially binds the vast majority of IGF-I (> 95%). IGF-II is independent of growth hormone, acting via a separate receptor.

IGF-I exerts negative feedback effects at both the hypothalamus and pituitary level; the former is also subject to negative feedback by growth hormone.

Clinical Symptoms and Signs

In common with other pituitary tumours, a growth hormone secreting pituitary adenoma may be associated with local mass effects such as headache (often severe and out of proportion to the size of the pituitary tumour), hydrocephalus, visual field defects or ophthalmoplegia. Deficiencies of other anterior pituitary hormones can also occur. Hypogonadism, presenting as decreased libido, infertility or oligo/amenorrhoea is a common finding at presentation; it may be due to both gonadotrophin deficiency as well as hyperprolactinaemia, either from coexistent excessive secretion of prolactin or from stalk compression. The occurrence of diabetes insipidus in relation to a pituitary adenoma is extremely rare and almost always suggests an alternative pathology. The systemic effects of acromegaly relate to the elevated levels of circulating growth hormone, either from its direct actions or from the systemic and local production of IGF-I (Table 4.2). However, their insidious nature of onset means that there is usually a considerable delay of about 6–8 years before the condition is diagnosed.

Overall, patients complain of generalised weakness and lethargy. The most characteristic feature and one that usually precipitates the diagnosis is a change in appearance, comprising coarsening of the facial features and broadening of the nose. This is accompanied by thickening of the lips and prominence of the supraorbital ridges. There is elongation of the jaw, with progna-

Table 4.2   Clinical symptoms and signs of acromegaly

Symptoms and signs at presentation	Overall prevalence (%)
Facial change, acral enlargement and soft-tissue swelling	100
Excessive sweating	83
Acroparaesthesia / carpal tunnel syndrome	68
Tiredness and lethargy	53
Headaches	53
Oligo- or amenorrhoea, infertility	55[a]
Erectile dysfunction and/or decreased libido	42[b]
Arthropathy	37
Impaired glucose tolerance/ diabetes	37
Goitre	35
Ear, nose, throat and dental problems	32
Congestive cardiac failure/ arrhythmia	25
Hypertension	23
Visual field defects	17

[a]   Percentage of female patients.
[b]   Percentage of male patients.

thism, which may result in malocclusion of the teeth, accompanied by interdental separation, and temporomandibular joint pain. Greasiness of the skin is a frequent finding, with excessive sweating, perhaps one of the most sensitive signs of growth hormone excess. Musculoskeletal changes are a common cause of morbidity; excessive growth hormone secretion before fusion of the bony epiphyses results in gigantism, although nowadays this is a rare event due to earlier diagnosis and treatment. Accelerated degenerative changes, particularly of the weight-bearing joints – hips and knees – are a common occurrence, leading to osteoarthritis.

Symptomatic carpal tunnel syndrome is present in approximately 60% of patients at diagnosis but about 80% will have electrophysiological evidence of median nerve neuropathy. Interestingly, it appears that the pathophysiology is due to swelling of the median nerve itself within the carpal tunnel rather than extrinsic compression from the increased volume of the carpal tunnel contents. Growth of the vertebral cartilage may result in kyphoscoliosis. There is increased total lean body mass and muscle hypertrophy, although the muscles themselves are weaker. Increase in soft tissues results in the other classical clinical manifestations. There is enlargement of the hands, resulting in their characteristic 'spade-like' appearance and soft dough-like consistency of the palms. Ring size increases – a sensitive objective assessment of disease activity and response to treatment. Similar changes occur in the feet, which become wider with increase in shoe size. Hypertrophy of the soft tissues of the upper airway results in deepening of the voice and often obstructive sleep apnoea, although a third of patients with sleep apnoea have a central cause. Skin tags are a frequent finding, perhaps related to epithelial cell hyperproliferation in response to IGF-I. While generalised organomegaly is commonly stated to occur in acromegaly, careful analysis of the data leaves it questionable. However, there is no doubt that goitres are common; these tend to become nodular with time. Cardiomegaly has also been documented, as has enlargement of the colon.

Complications

The complications of acromegaly are usually an extenuation of the clinical symptoms and signs. Overall, acromegaly is associated with considerable increased morbidity and mortality, with the latter being at least two-fold that of the general population. In early epidemiological reviews, more than 50% of patients had died by the age of 60 years, usually as a result of diabetes, cardiovascular or cerebrovascular disease. With improved treatment of both the underlying disease and these complications, patients are now surviving longer, although they may then be susceptible to other complications such as malignancy (Table 4.3).

Growth hormone results in insulin resistance and many patients will exhibit either impaired glucose tolerance or frank diabetes mellitus. Cardiovascular complications are common and are the principal cause of death; cardiomegaly and cardiomyopathy frequently occur, due to both a direct effect of growth hormone itself or the accompanying hypertension. The precise pathogenesis of the latter remains uncertain although it is related to increased total body sodium and an expanded plasma volume as it does not always

Table 4.3 Complications of acromegaly

Local
Headache
Visual field loss
Cranial nerve lesions
Hydrocephalus
Temporal lobe epilepsy

Systemic
Cardiovascular
Ischaemic heart disease
Cardiomyopathy
Congestive cardiac failure
Arrhythymias
Hypertension

Respiratory
Kyphosis
Obstructive sleep apnoea

CNS
Stroke

Metabolic
Diabetes mellitus
Impaired glucose tolerance (insulin resistance)
Hyperlipidaemia (triglycerides)

Neoplastic
Colorectal
Breast and prostate – uncertain

respond to reduction in growth hormone levels. Patients are at increased risk of ischaemic heart disease and cerebrovascular disease, due to the hypertension, diabetes and abnormal lipid profile.

In addition to these established complications, in recent years it has become increasingly apparent that patients with acromegaly are also at increased risk of developing neoplasia, particularly colorectal tubular adenomas and carcinoma. Although some of these studies are hampered by a lack of matched control groups, the increased risk for colorectal cancer appears to be at least three-fold and may be as high as 14-fold. It is related to disease activity, with patients with elevated serum growth hormone and IGF-I levels being particularly prone to developing colonic adenomas. Although the exact pathogenesis of these tumours remains uncertain, it is likely to involve altered homeostasis of cell numbers within the colonic epithelial crypts; increased proliferation and decreased apoptosis within the crypts of patients with acromegaly have both been documented.

Given these findings, patients with acromegaly should be regarded as a high-risk group for colorectal cancer, and regular colonoscopic screening should be offered to all patients. Current evidence suggests that this should begin at the age of 40 years, with the subsequent interval depending both on disease activity and the findings at the original colonoscopic screening. In the presence of a tubular adenoma or elevated serum IGF-I levels, screening should be repeated after 3 years, while a normal colonoscopic screening, presence of a hyperplastic/metaplastic polyp or serum IGF-I level within the normal range suggests screening every 5 years may be appropriate. As approximately 30% of lesions occur at the caecum or in the ascending colon, total full-length colonoscopy is required. This should be performed by an experienced colonoscopist, as the caecum is reached in only about 70% of patients in inexperienced hands. Due to their slow bowel transit time and elongated colon, patients with acromegaly require rigorous bowel preparation; a total of 6 litres of Klean-Prep (Norgine Ltd, Middlesex, UK), with 2 litres drunk at 6, 4 and 2 hours prior to the procedure together with a liquid-only diet for 24 hours beforehand, is usually sufficient. Failure to visualise the caecum necessitates a repeat colonoscopy or, failing this, a barium enema or virtual CT colonoscopy.

Whether patients with acromegaly are also prone to other malignancies remains controversial. Certainly there is epidemiological evidence in the non-acromegalic population that serum IGF-I levels in the upper part of the normal range are associated with an increased risk of breast and prostate cancer and some reviews have shown the former to be increased in acromegaly. However, to date, these findings have not generally been confirmed in other large series, although it may be that, as with colorectal cancer, the demonstration of an increased prevalence of these tumours will only now become apparent as patients are surviving longer from other causes of morbidity.

Investigations

Confirmation of diagnosis

Failure of suppression of serum growth hormone to a glucose load remains the gold standard for the diagnosis of acromegaly: 75 g of oral glucose (e.g. 250 ml of Lucozade) is given at 9 a.m. and serum glucose and growth hormone levels are measured at baseline, 30, 60, 90, 120 and 150 min thereafter. In normal subjects, growth hormone should suppress to undetectable levels, while in acromegaly serum growth hormone remains detectable or in approximately 30% of cases there is a paradoxical increase. The use of this test also detects those patients with impaired glucose tolerance or frank diabetes mellitus. Due to the pulsatile nature of its secretion, a single growth hormone measurement is of no use in either monitoring or confirming the diagnosis of acromegaly. The assessment of growth hormone hypersecretion requires the mean value of serial samples taken throughout the day (e.g. five samples over a 12-hour period). In normal subjects, the majority of values throughout the day are undetectable, but in acromegaly all are usually elevated.

A single serum IGF-I level has been advocated as being an alternative test for the diagnosis of acromegaly, as it is elevated in the majority of subjects. However, as previously indicated, it is an indirect assessment of growth hormone secretion, with approximately 25% of patients having a discrepancy between the mean value of a growth hormone day curve and an IGF-I level. IGF-I secretion is subject to several influences, including liver and renal dysfunction, nutrition and diabetes mellitus, and the presence of a statistical correlation between its levels and those of growth hormone should not be used as proof that they are interchangeable. However, despite these limitations, from a practical point of view, an elevated serum IGF-I measurement may be useful as confirmatory evidence, assuming that age- and sex-matched normal ranges are used, and for monitoring treatment.

In cases of remaining doubt about the diagnosis of acromegaly, a TRH test can be used (200 µg of thyrotrophin-releasing hormone given intravenously with serum measurement at 0, 20 and 60 min). In normal subjects, TRH inhibits growth hormone secretion with a fall in serum concentration, while approximately 60% of acromegalics will show a paradoxical rise in growth hormone levels.

In the rare patient in whom a non-pituitary aetiology is suspected, measurement of serum GHRH may be performed, although it can be normal if originating from a hypothalamic source.

Radiological assessment

A skull X-ray remains a quick and easy preliminary assessment that can offer useful information, providing it is taken correctly with alignment of the posterior clinoid processes. Enlargement or ballooning of the pituitary fossa is seen, in addition to increased size of the frontal air sinuses and increased bony thickness of the skull vault.

More detailed information regarding the presence and size of a pituitary mass requires either a computed tomography (CT) or a magnetic resonance imaging (MRI) scan, with the latter generally being preferable. The advantages of MRI are the absence of ionising radiation, the ability to image in any desired plane and demonstration of the inherent contrast between tissues. Not only is it able to accurately determine the shape and dimensions of the anterior and posterior pituitary lobes – the latter has a high signal on T1-weighted images in over 90% of normal subjects – but it also delineates the hypothalamic region and optic chiasm. MRI allows accurate assessment of the size of the pituitary adenoma, detecting lesions as small as 2 mm. It also determines the extent of any invasion superiorly, inferiorly or laterally into the cavernous sinuses. On T1-weighted images the pituitary adenoma tends to be of lower signal intensity than the surrounding normal gland and enhances less briskly than the normal gland after injection with intravenous gadolinium contrast.

Neuro-ophthalmological assessment

Neuro-ophthalmological assessment is mandatory in all cases of acromegaly. At the initial consultation visual acuity should be assessed with the use of Snellen charts and fundoscopy performed to exclude optic atrophy, retinal vein engorgement or papilloedema from pressure on the visual pathways. Visual fields may be assessed by confrontation using a red pin. Patients with any clinical symptoms or evidence of optic chiasmal compression from imaging studies require formal assessment of visual fields with Goldmann perimetry or visual evoked responses, stimulating each half-field in turn.

Although permanent loss of vision and/or visual field defects usually result from long-standing optic chiasmal compression, the shorter the time of compression the easier and more complete is the reversal of any visual field deficit. Surgical decompression may result in rapid improvement in visual fields within hours or days, although the presence of optic atrophy reduces the likelihood of this occurring. Because onset is often insidious, patients may be unaware of any alteration in their vision, although once documented its presence requires them to inform the vehicle licensing authority as driving ability may be impaired. An exception to this usual gradual deterioration is pituitary haemorrhage when visual loss may be sudden with a loss of central vision and development of bitemporal field defects and possible ophthalmoplegia often accompanied by changes in mental function.

Pituitary function tests

Assessment of the other pituitary axes needs to be performed by a combination of the appropriate basal and dynamic tests (see Chapters 1 and 2).

Management

Given its chronic nature and associated significant increased morbidity and mortality, treatment is required for almost all patients. Three modalities of treatment are available: surgery, pituitary irradiation and medical therapy. All of these have advantages and disadvantages and more than one modality is frequently needed, often all three. The decision as to whether to treat and the modality employed must be based on a number of factors, including patient age and general health, severity of disease and any associated complications, and the risk/benefit ratio of the proposed treatment modality. The aims of treatment are several-fold (Table 4.4).

While the general principles of these aims are accepted by all endocrinologists, there remains considerable controversy as to the degree of growth hormone reduction that should be the target and what level should be regarded as normal. The use of sensitive growth hormone assays has demonstrated that abnormal patterns of growth hormone secretion remain despite reduction in mean circulating concentrations to extremely low levels, and thus complete

Table 4.4   Aims of treatment

Removal of the pituitary tumour and resolution of mass effects
Relief of the symptoms and signs of acromegaly
Restoration of growth hormone secretion and IGF-I levels to normal
Maintenance of anterior pituitary function
Prevention of recurrence
Assessment and treatment of chronic complications

IGF-I = insulin-like growth factor-I.

restoration to normality is unlikely to be achieved. Early epidemiological reviews, particularly those documenting the results of
surgery, tended to regard a mean level of less than 10 mU/l as being
satisfactory. It has become clear in recent years that the excess mortality associated with acromegaly can be significantly reduced and
indeed restored to that of the normal population by aggressive
treatment and reduction of serum growth hormone concentrations
to a mean level of less than 5 mU/l and/or a normal serum IGF-I.
Thus, rather than using the word 'cure', it is more appropriate to
consider a concentration of less than 5 mU/l (2.5 ng/ml) as representing that of a 'safe' level. Alternatively, a nadir level of less than
2 mU/l after a glucose tolerance test is also regarded by some
clinicians as representing a 'safe' level (Figure 4.2).

Transsphenoidal surgery

Transsphenoidal surgery is the initial treatment of choice for most
patients with acromegaly (Chapter 1). Although different series
have often used different criteria to determine success rates, in
experienced hands postoperative mean growth hormone levels of
less than 5 mU/l should be achieved in 70–90% of microadenomas
and 30–50% of macroadenomas. In a series of 100 patients with
acromegaly operated on at St Bartholomew's Hospital, new
hypopituitarism occurred in 21% of patients following surgery, but
with 35% having hypopituitarism preoperatively.

Pituitary irradiation

Pituitary irradiation is usually used as an adjunct to pituitary
surgery when growth hormone levels remain elevated. Numerous
studies have confirmed the efficacy of such megavoltage irradiation with a 50% fall in growth hormone values occurring in the
first 2 years, regardless of basal levels, followed by a continuing

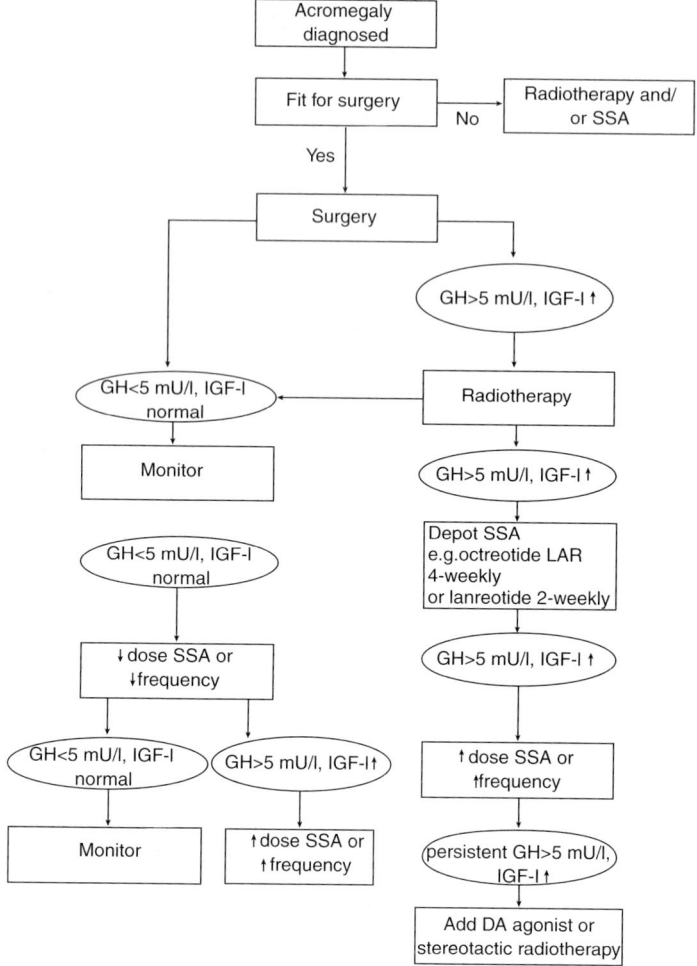

Figure 4.2 Algorithm for the management of acromegaly. DA = dopamine agonist, GH = growth hormone, IGF-I = insulin-like growth factor-1. SSA = somatostatin analogue. Assessment of prevailing growth hormone status requires a minimum of 3 months off depot SSAs.

exponential decline thereafter. The majority of patients therefore do eventually achieve a level of less than 5 mU/l, although the interval to reach this depends on the baseline levels. A similar response is seen with IGF-I, with more than 50% of patients eventually achieving a normal serum level after 10 years. At St Bartholomew's Hospital, it is currently reserved as a second-line therapy for patients who have persisting active disease despite surgery and conventional irradiation.

Medical therapy

Three different types of medical therapy are currently used in the treatment of acromegaly – dopamine agonists, somatostatin analogues and, more recently, growth hormone antagonists.

Dopamine agonists

From their discovery and synthesis in 1971 until the introduction of somatostatin analogues in the mid-1980s, dopamine agonists, such as bromocriptine, were the sole medical therapy for acromegaly. However, they are relatively ineffective and, while approximately 60% of patients will show a reduction in growth hormone levels, only about 10–15% achieve a mean level of less than 5 mU/l. Furthermore, the doses required, often 20–30 mg of bromocriptine/day, are much higher than those needed for prolactinomas. Consequently, the side effects of nausea, headache, dizziness, postural hypotension and nasal stuffiness tend to be worse, although they can be minimised by taking the drug in the middle of a main meal to slow absorption and most patients will demonstrate tachyphylaxis. Unlike prolactinomas, there may be a slight reduction in tumour size, but this is usually insignificant. Cessation of treatment results in rebound growth hormone hypersecretion. Other dopamine agonists have a similar effect, but with the long-acting cabergoline tending to be the most preferred due to its reduced side effects, although again high doses of up to 1 mg/day may be needed. There are no accurate predictive tests as to which patients will respond to dopamine agonists, but mixed growth hormone and prolactin secreting tumours with elevated serum prolactin levels tend to respond the most favourably.

Somatostatin analogues

The development of octreotide (Sandostatin, Novartis, Basel, Switzerland), a synthetic somatostatin analogue, represented a major advance in the treatment of acromegaly. In contrast to the short half-life of native somatostatin (approximately 90 s), the 8 amino acid octreotide has a half-life of about 2 hours. Following a single 100 µg dose, there is prolonged suppression of growth hormone, which lasts for several hours, and indeed this response to a single dose can be used to predict the long-term efficacy of octreotide. It is administered by subcutaneous injection and thus a thrice-daily regime results in stable drug concentrations and maximal effect. More than 90% of patients show a reduction in growth hormone levels, with approximately 50–60% achieving levels of less than 5 mU/l and a normal serum IGF-I level. The usual doses are between 100 and 200 µg three times daily although occasional patients may require higher doses. This biochemical improvement is matched by rapid clinical improvement.

Octreotide also has additional and independent, but poorly understood, analgesic properties on the headache associated with acromegaly. Such an effect is unrelated to the slight reduction in tumour size that is observed in approximately 50% of patients. It has also been claimed that tumours become softer in consistency, perhaps facilitating surgical removal.

In the last couple of years, depot formulations of somatostatin analogues have become available. These consist of the active drug incorporated with microspheres of biodegradable polylactide and polyglycolide polymers which allow the slow release of analogue after intramuscular injection. There are currently two such preparations available – octreotide LAR (Sandostatin LAR, Novartis), which is given at a variable dose of 10 mg , 20 mg or 30 mg at recommended 4-weekly intervals, and lanreotide (Somatuline LA, Ipsen Biotech, Paris, France), which is given as a single dose of 30 mg at 7–14 day intervals. However, there is great variation in individual patient's sensitivity to these analogues and more than 90% of patients who achieve adequate control with 4-weekly octreotide LAR injections will also do so with 6-weekly injections. Consequently, careful dose titration needs to be performed on each patient. This is particularly important given the cost of these depot formulations: in the UK, the approximate annual cost of octreotide LAR given 4-weekly is £8000 for 10 mg injections, £11,000 for 20 mg and £14,000 for 30 mg, while the cost for lanreotide given every 14 days is £8600 per annum, which increases to £17,000 if given every 7 days.

While these novel formulations represent an advance in terms of patient convenience, their efficacy is similar to that of subcutaneous octreotide. However, more potent and selective analogues for the type 2 and 5 somatostatin receptors present on growth hormone secreting pituitary tumours are under development, as are novel delivery systems which may allow for even more intermittent administration. The side effects of somatostatin analogues relate mainly to the gastrointestinal system, comprising colicky abdominal pain, diarrhoea, flatulence and nausea, although these tend to resolve with time. In the long term, gastritis occurs in a significant proportion of patients and perhaps, most significantly, gallstones form in approximately 50% of patients after 2 years of use. This is due to both an inhibition of gall bladder contraction and alterations in the composition of bile with cholesterol supersaturation. However, perhaps due to the gall bladder paresis, the majority of these remain asymptomatic. There is no effect in the long term on glucose homeostasis.

With their improved patient convenience, there have been suggestions that these depot formulations should be used as a first-line treatment for acromegaly. However, their increased cost and the need for continuing treatment should be borne in mind. At present, there remains a general consensus that while these analogues may have a role prior to surgery in trying to decrease tumour size, their major place is as an adjunct to irradiation while waiting for growth hormone levels to fall. Patients who remain uncontrolled despite the use of these somatostatin analogues may gain occasional extra benefit with the addition of a dopamine agonist, but this is the exception rather than the rule.

Pegvisamont

One of the most exciting developments in the medical therapy of acromegaly is the recent development of the growth hormone antagonist, pegvisamont. This is a recombinant modified growth hormone molecule which has increased affinity to the first growth hormone receptor binding site but with decreased affinity to the binding site on the second receptor. Thus, receptor dimerisation and subsequent signal transduction is prevented. Its conjugation with polyethylene glycol (PEG) increases its molecular size and prolongs its half-life. Although growth hormone levels cannot be measured, as the drug itself interferes with growth hormone assays, serum IGF-I levels are normalised in approximately 90% of patients. It is currently administered as a daily subcutaneous injection of approximately 1 ml in volume. There remain some theoretical concerns about the increase in circulating growth hormone levels due to the loss of any negative feedback effects on the tumour, a situation analogous to Nelson's syndrome, although to date there have been no cases of any tumour growth. Pegvisamont is generally well tolerated, although abnormalities of liver function have been reported in some patients. It is due to become marketed in the near future, although its cost remains uncertain, and while there is no doubt that it will represent a major advance, its role as first-line therapy remains to be determined.

Further Reading

Bates AS, Van't Hoff W, Jones JM, Clayton RN. An audit of outcome of treatment in acromegaly. *Q J Med* 1993;**86**(5):293–9.

Duncan E, Wass JA. Investigation protocol: acromegaly and its investigation. *Clin Endocrinol* 1999;**50**(3):285–93.

Ezzat S, Forster MJ, Berchtold P, Redelmeier DA, Boerlin V, Harris, AG. Acromegaly. Clinical and biochemical features in 500 patients. *Medicine (Baltimore)* 1994;**73**(5):233–40.

Jenkins PJ, Fairclough PD, Richards T *et al.* Acromegaly, colonic polyps and carcinoma. *Clin Endocrinol* 1997;**47**(1):17–22.

Jenkins PJ, Besser GM, Fairclough PD. Colorectal neoplasia in acromegaly. *Gut* 1999;**44**:585–7.

Lancranjan I, Atkinson AB, and Sandostatin LAR Group. Results of a European multicentre study with Sandostatin LAR in acromegalic patients. *Pituitary* 1999;1105–14.

Melmed S, Ho K, Klibanski A, Reichlin S, Thorner M. Clinical review 75: Recent advances in pathogenesis, diagnosis, and management of acromegaly. *J Clin Endocrinol Metab* 1995;**80**(12):3395–402.

Melmed S, Jackson I, Kleinberg D, Klibanski A. Current treatment guidelines for acromegaly. *J Clin Endocrinol Metab* 1998;**83**(8):2646–52.

Orme SM, McNally RJ, Cartwright RA, Belchetz PE. Mortality and cancer incidence in acromegaly: a retrospective cohort study. *J Clin Endocrinol Metab* 1998;**83**:2730–4.

Plowman PN. Radiotherapy for pituitary tumours. *Baillière's Clin Endocrinol Metab* 1995;**9**(2):407–20.

Robbins RJ. Depot somatostatin analogs – a new first line therapy for acromegaly. *J Clin Endocrinol Metab* 1997;**82**(1):15–17.

Sheaves R, Jenkins P, Blackburn P *et al.* Outcome of transsphenoidal surgery for acromegaly using strict criteria for surgical cure. *Clin Endocrinol* 1996;**45**(4):407–13.

Swearingen B, Barker FG, Katznelson L *et al.* Long-term mortality after transsphenoidal surgery and adjunctive therapy for acromegaly. *J Clin Endocrinol Metab* 1998;**83**(10):3419–26.

5

Cushing's Syndrome

John DC Newell-Price and Ashley Grossman

Introduction

Since Harvey Cushing's original description of his eponymous syndrome, this condition has continued to fascinate endocrinologists. The diagnosis and differential diagnosis of Cushing's syndrome remains a challenge in clinical endocrinology. In some circumstances diagnosis and differential diagnosis is straightforward: for example, the classically 'cushingoid' man with a cortisol-secreting adrenal adenoma. On the other hand, however, endocrinologists are increasingly called upon to consider the diagnosis at an early stage in the natural history of the disease, when there may be a much more subtle phenotype.

This may test our clinical skills and diagnostic tools to the limit. Moreover, the differential diagnosis of adrenocorticophic hormone (ACTH)-dependent Cushing's syndrome is frequently complex, requiring all the skill of endocrinologists, chemical pathologists and radiologists. Treatment can only be commenced once an accurate diagnosis has been made. Whereas surgery for adrenal and ectopic ACTH causes of Cushing's syndrome is often highly successful, the overall cure rate following transsphenoidal surgery for Cushing's disease is disappointing. We discuss the diagnosis, differential diagnosis and treatment options available to provide an overall framework for management.

Definitions

Cushing's syndrome is a term applied to the clinical state that results from prolonged, and inappropriate, exposure to excessive circulating free glucocorticoid. Pseudo-Cushing's syndrome refers to conditions that may manifest a similar clinical phenotype, such as primary depression or alcohol dependence. However, in contrast to Cushing's syndrome, treatment of the depression or withdrawal of alcohol will lead to improvement of the cushingoid state.

Aetiology

A cushingoid phenotype is most commonly caused by the use of supraphysiological amounts of exogenous glucocorticoids. Endogenous Cushing's syndrome (Table 5.1) is more common in women than men, with ACTH-dependent causes accounting for approximately 80% of cases. Of the ACTH-dependent cases, 80% are due to pituitary adenomas (Cushing's disease), with the remainder being due to ectopic ACTH secretion (Table 5.2). When the source of ACTH is apparent on simple imaging, this is referred to as the overt ectopic ACTH syndrome and is almost uniformly due to rapidly progressing small cell lung cancer. In contrast, a clinical phenotype almost indistinguishable from Cushing's disease may result from ectopic ACTH secretion from carcinoid tumours, most commonly bronchial in origin.

Non-ACTH-dependent Cushing's syndrome is due to benign adrenal adenomas in 60% and carcinomas in 40% of cases. Very rare causes of adrenal-dependent Cushing's syndrome are bilateral primary pigmented nodular hyperplasia, macronodular adrenal

Table 5.1 Aetiology of Cushing's syndrome in 320 patients seen at St Bartholomew's Hospital, 1969–1999

Cause of Cushing's syndrome	Female	Male
ACTH-dependent:		
Cushing's disease	170	50
Ectopic ACTH syndrome	16	16
Unknown source of ACTH	14	3
ACTH-independent:		
Adrenal adenoma	20	6
Adrenal carcinoma	12	8
Nodular adrenal hyperplasia	1	4
Total	233	87

ACTH = adrenocorticotrophic hormone.

Table 5.2   Aetiology of the ectopic ACTH syndrome causing clinical Cushing's syndrome in patients seen at St Bartholomew's Hospital, 1969–1999

Site of secretion	Female	Male
Bronchial carcinoid tumor	11	2
Small cell lung cancer	1	5
Medullary thyroid carcinoma		3
Pancreatic carcinoid tumor	1	2
Thymic carcinoid tumor		1
Disseminated carcinoid tumor		1
Mesothelioma	1	
Pancreatic carcinoma		1
Colonic carcinoma	1	
Phaeochromocytoma		1
Gall bladder carcinoma	1	
Total	16	16

ACTH = adrenocorticotrophic hormone.

hyperplasia, the ectopic actions of G-protein coupled receptors (such as gastric-inhibitory peptide receptor or the adrenergic receptor), the McCune–Albright syndrome and Carney's complex.

Clinical Features (Table 5.3)

Commonly quoted clinical features such as truncal obesity, lethargy, menstrual irregularity, weakness, loss of libido, hirsutism, acne, depression and psychosis, although frequently present, are of low specificity for diagnosis. The signs that most reliably distinguish Cushing's syndrome from pseudo-Cushing's syndrome are the presence of thin skin, easy bruising or proximal myopathy. Proximal myopathy is best demonstrated by requesting the patient to rise from a squat with their arms crossed. In children, weight gain and growth retardation are particularly common. Osteopenia and osteoporosis, particularly in the absence of other predisposing factors to these conditions, may provide useful corroborative evidence of glucocorticoid excess. Over 70% of patients with Cushing's syndrome may present with psychiatric symptoms, ranging from anxiety to frank psychosis, and if depressed this is often agitated in nature. Some degree of depression often persists following cure of Cushing's syndrome. In the overt ectopic ACTH syndrome, the high circulating levels of ACTH cause pigmentation.

Table 5.3 The frequency of clinical signs and symptoms of Cushing's syndrome in five series of adults (1952–1982) and two of children (1994, 1995)

Sign/symptom (%)	Plotz 1952 n = 33	Sprague 1956 n = 100	Soffer 1961 n = 50	Urbanic 1981 n = 31	Ross 1982 n = 70	Magiakou 1994 n = 67	Weber 1995 n = 12
Obesity or weight gain	97	84	86	79	97	90	93
Decreased linear growth						83	80
Hypertension	84	90	88	77	74	51	
Plethora	89	81	78		94		
Rounded face	89	92	92		88		
Hirsutism	73	74	84	64	81	81	58
Thin skin				84			
Abnormal glucose tolerance	94		84	39	50		
Easy bruising	60	62	68	77	62	27	16
Weakness	83		58	90	56	45	58
Osteopenia or fracture	83		56	48	50		
ECG changes or atherosclerosis (men/women)	66/89		34		55		
Menstrual changes	86	35	72	69	84	81	8
Decreased libido (men/women)	86		100/33	55	100		
Depression or emotional lability	67		40	48	62		
Headache	58				47		25
Striae	60	64	50	51	56	63	58
Edema	60		66	48	50		
Acne	82	64		35	21	52	58
'Buffalo hump'			34		54		
Female balding		67	51		13		8
Lipid abnormalities	39						
Decreased wound healing	42						
Delayed bone age						14	
Pigmentation							16

Adapted from Yanovski JA, Cutler GB Jr. Glucocorticoid action and clinical features of Cushing's syndrome. In Aron DC, Tyrrell JB (eds), Endocrinology and Metabolism Clinics of North America, Cushing's Syndrome. Philidelphia: WB Saunders, 1994.

Diagnosis of Cushing's Syndrome

It is essential that the diagnosis of Cushing's syndrome be established before any attempt at differential diagnosis: failure to do so results in misdiagnosis and inappropriate management. Three principal diagnostic tools are commonly employed to establish a diagnosis of Cushing's syndrome:

- the low-dose dexamethasone-suppression test (LDDST)
- the midnight plasma cortisol
- 24-hour urinary free cortisol (UFC).

Low-dose dexamethasone-suppression test

In Cushing's syndrome, there is a loss of the normal feedback of the hypothalamo–pituitary–adrenal axis. Dexamethasone tests are designed to demonstrate this; in normal individuals, dexamethasone (which is not measured in cortisol RIAs) causes suppression of ACTH and thence cortisol.

The overnight dexamethasone-suppression test is frequently used as a screening test, and is easily performed as an outpatient. It involves the administration of 1 mg of dexamethasone at 23.00 h, with measurement of plasma cortisol at 08.00 h. Lack of suppression is consistent with Cushing's syndrome. Some patients, particularly with Cushing's disease, show unusual suppressibility of plasma cortisol following dexamethasone. Therefore, to avoid false negatives, it is recommended that a post-dexamethasone cut-off value of 50 nmol/l is used, above which is *consistent* with a diagnosis of Cushing's syndrome: this cut-off point will help to avoid missing mild cases. However, using this criterion the specificity of the test is only 87%.

Because of this, it is our routine clinical practice to use the 48-hour 2 mg/day LDDST for all patients considered for the diagnosis of Cushing's syndrome.

With adequate written instructions, the test is performed reliably even as an outpatient, and in normal subjects the cortisol value at 48 hours is below 50 mmol/l.

This test has a sensitivity and specificity approaching 100%, and is superior to the overnight test. Particular caution needs to be exercised if patients are on drugs that increase hepatic clearance of dexamethasone; these include carbamazepine, phenytoin, phenobarbital or rifampicin; ideally, these drugs should be stopped prior to investigation. Other common interfering drugs are oral oestrogens, which increase the corticosteroid-binding globulin (CBG) and therefore give a falsely elevated level of cortisol on most routine radioimmunoassays (which measure total rather than free cortisol). Therefore, if possible, oestrogens should be stopped for a period of 6 weeks prior to investigation, in order that the CBG may return to basal values.

Midnight plasma cortisol

Normally, levels of plasma ACTH begin to rise between 03.00 h and 04.00 h, reaching a peak between 06.00 h and 08.00 h: levels then fall away during the rest of the day. The plasma cortisol values mirror this, with levels being highest at 08.00–09.00 h, falling to less than 50 nmol/l at midnight while asleep in the unstressed state. This circadian rhythm is disturbed in patients with Cushing's syndrome.

A single sleeping midnight plasma cortisol of greater the 50 nmol/l is the most sensitive indicator of Cushing's syndrome, and in our experience is present in every case, but does not allow ready discrimination between aetiologies (Figure 5.1). For the test to be performed adequately, admission for a period of 48 hours is required to allow restoration of the normal circadian rhythm in unaffected individuals, and thus avoid false positives. It is one of the harder tests to perform correctly, and requires that the patients be instructed to retire no later than 22.30 h.

To avoid an elevated cortisol as a result of anticipation of the test, it is recommended that patients under investigation are not warned that the sample is going to be taken. It is crucial that documentation is made as to whether the patient is awake or asleep when sampling was made, since, if the patient is awake, the test is not readily interpretable. The sample should be drawn within 15 min of waking the patient. Unfortunately, the specificity of this test is liable to be rather low, as individuals with acute illness, such as sepsis or heart failure, will exhibit a blunted circadian rhythm with elevated levels of midnight cortisol. This is seen in its most extreme on the intensive care unit, where the circulating levels of cortisol commonly remain persistently elevated, with an entirely absent circadian rhythm.

Urinary free cortisol

Excess circulating cortisol saturates circulating binding proteins and is excreted in the urine as free cortisol; therefore, UFC provides an integrated estimation of the prevailing level of circulating corti-

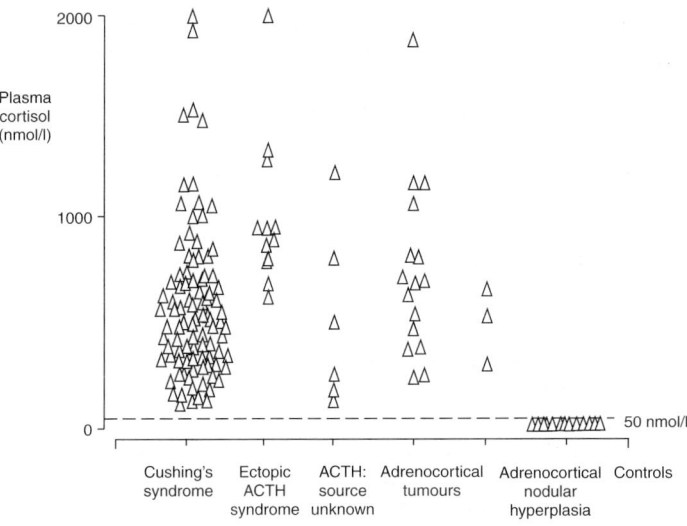

Figure 5.1 Sleeping midnight plasma cortisol values in patients with Cushing's syndrome and normal volunteers. (Reproduced with permission from Newell-Price *et al.*, *Clin Endocrinol (Oxf)* 1995;**43**(5):545–50.)

sol. Although this test is in widespread use, it has a low sensitivity and requires at least three or four collections to be performed to miss mild disease. The specificity is also poor, illustrated by complete overlap in the levels seen with those patients with pseudo-Cushing's syndrome, and frequently overlap in the levels seen in individuals with depression and the polycystic ovarian syndrome. Further limitations include the adequacy of the 24-hour urine collection, although expressing a UFC/creatinine ratio can improve the test. If three or four 24-hour UFC collections are within the normal range, Cushing's syndrome is very unlikely. If factitious Cushing's syndrome is suspected, high-performance liquid chromatography (HPLC) of urine samples may detect synthetic glucocorticoid. Conversely, if the level is more than four times the upper limit of normal, then Cushing's syndrome is highly probable.

Pseudo-Cushing's syndrome

Two well-characterised conditions that result in pseudo-Cushing's syndrome are alcohol dependence and depression. Admission of patients with suspected alcohol dependence may be extremely useful as alcohol may be detected in the blood, and the sleeping midnight plasma cortisol value has been demonstrated to become undetectable within 5 days of observed abstinence. The more common presentation that needs to be differentiated from true Cushing's syndrome is depression, and this is frequently a more challenging problem. A trial of antidepressants may, on occasion, be the only means to establish the diagnosis.

Tests that may help in the differentiation between pseudo-Cushing's syndrome and Cushing's syndrome are the insulin tolerance test (ITT) and the dexamethasone-suppressed cortico-trophin-releasing hormone (CRH) test. Depressed patients usually have an intact cortisol response to an insulin-induced hypogly-caemia, whereas such a response is seen in only 18% of patients with Cushing's syndrome. If performing this test, 0.3 U/kg of soluble insulin, rather than 0.15 U/kg, should be administered to overcome the insulin-resistant effects of high levels of circulating cortisol. The dexamethasone-suppressed CRH test involves per-forming a standard 48-hour 2 mg/day LDDST, which is immedi-ately followed by a CRH test (see below). A plasma cortisol 15 min after administration of CRH of greater than 38 mmol/l has been reported as being consistent with Cushing's syndrome. It should be noted, however, that many cortisol RIAs demonstrate poor preci-sion at this level, and caution is needed in the widespread appli-cation of this test.

Cyclical Cushing's syndrome

For unknown reasons, certain patients with Cushing's syndrome exhibit cyclical secretion of cortisol that may fluctuate and remit spontaneously, sometimes over many years. The signs and symp-toms of Cushing's syndrome such as myopathy, hypertension and diabetes may fluctuate with the circulating level of cortisol. Such dynamics can cause considerable diagnostic difficulty, and rein-vestigation at intervals, and on several occasions, may be required. It is crucial that any assessment of the differential diagnosis is made only when there is an established prevailing hypercortisolaemia. Repeated admissions to an endocrine unit may be necessary. One potential strategy is the use of salivary cortisol estimates: timed sali-vary samples may be sent in capped tubes to the endocrine unit through the post. If the salivary cortisol levels are high, the patient can be rapidly admitted for formal investigation.

Summary

We routinely use the 48-hour LDDST and sleeping midnight plasma cortisol in the investigation of Cushing's syndrome. Because of low sensitivity and specificity, we rarely use UFC as a diagnostic tool.

Differential Diagnosis of Cushing's Syndrome

Following confirmation of Cushing's syndrome and prevailing hypercortisolaemia, the next step is to measure plasma ACTH. The handling of samples is crucial. ACTH is rapidly degraded and, to avoid falsely low values, samples need to be handled carefully, cold-centrifuged immediately after sampling and 'flash-frozen' prior to storage for later assay.

Plasma ACTH

Patients with primary adrenal causes of Cushing's syndrome will have plasma ACTH suppressed to levels below 5 pg/ml, and attention can be turned to imaging the adrenal with computed tomography (CT) or magnetic resonance imaging (MRI). Levels of ACTH persistently above 15 pg/ml can confidently be ascribed to ACTH-dependent pathologies and require investigation as detailed below. ACTH values between 5 and 15 pg/ml require cautious interpretation as, on occasion, a patient with Cushing's disease may have a plasma ACTH below 10 pg/ml. It is recommended that at least two–three plasma ACTH estimations are made to avoid inappropriate classification of certain patients with Cushing's disease.

ACTH-dependent Cushing's syndrome

Differentiating between pituitary and non-pituitary sites of ACTH remains one of the most difficult challenges in clinical endocrinology. Carcinoid tumours may mimic many of the clinical features of Cushing's disease, and to a certain extent this reflects similar tumour biology. These features are compounded by the fact that these ectopic tumours are frequently less than 1 cm in diameter and, consequently, may be difficult to visualise, even with modern axial imaging. Moreover, during investigation, radiological abnormalities may be disclosed that do not necessarily have functional significance. These 'incidentalomas' can complicate interpretation, and it is for this reason that reliance should be placed on biochemical evaluation, rather than imaging, for the differentiation between pituitary and non-pituitary sources of ACTH.

In ACTH-dependent Cushing's syndrome, 9 out of 10 cases will be due to Cushing's disease. It is against this pre-test likelihood that the diagnostic performance of the tests has to be judged. No single test has 100% diagnostic accuracy and, indeed, such a property would presuppose an invariant difference between the biology of the tumours causing pituitary and non-pituitary ACTH secretion, and this does not appear to be the case. Therefore, several tests need to be used to gather evidence to favour the site of ACTH secretion. Since pituitary surgery is routinely used for Cushing's disease, the response criteria of the tests are set such that inappropriate transsphenoidal surgery is avoided in those with evidence of ectopic secretion.

Basal testing

Plasma ACTH

The circulating levels of plasma ACTH are usually lower in patients with Cushing's disease compared with those with ectopic secretion. There is, however, considerable overlap, and this trend is not useful for discrimination between groups.

Plasma potassium

The ectopic ACTH syndrome is usually associated with higher circulating levels of cortisol than Cushing's disease. These high levels saturate the 11β-hydroxysteroid dehydrogenase type II enzyme, allowing cortisol to act as a mineralocorticoid in the kidney. Consequently, hypokalaemia with alkalosis is more frequently seen in the ectopic ACTH syndrome. However, it is important to remember that this simply represents severity of disease rather than any specific aetiology, and approximately 10% of patients with Cushing's disease present with hypokalaemia.

Dynamic testing

The high-dose dexamethasone-suppression test (HDDST)

Corticotroph adenomas typically retain some responsiveness to the suppressive effects of glucocorticoids, whereas tumours causing the ectopic ACTH syndrome usually do not. This forms the rationale for the HDDST. The commonest form of this test is for dexamethasone 2 mg to be administered strictly 6 hourly, with estimation of plasma cortisol basally and at 48 hours. Since this is a high dose of dexamethasone, the test should be conducted as an inpatient with careful observation, since a proportion of patients with active Cushing's syndrome experience either a deterioration in their psychological state, or in some circumstances frank psychosis, during the test. Approximately 80% of patients with Cushing's disease will demonstrate suppression of the cortisol to less that 50% of the basal level. It is important to realise the 50% cut-off criterion has no intrinsic validity, and simply represents the threshold that has been established in large series of patients to most reliably distinguish pituitary from non-pituitary disease. By itself, the diagnostic accuracy of this test falls short of the pre-test likelihood, but when the results are considered in the light of the response to CRH (see below) it remains a useful test. The alternative 8 mg overnight HDDST is inferior.

Corticotrophin-releasing hormone (CRH) test

CRH stimulates the release of ACTH from the corticotrophs of the anterior pituitary. The CRH test is well tolerated, with side effects consisting of a metallic taste in the mouth and mild short-lived facial flushing and transient sinus tachycardia. The test is performed with the patient in the recumbent position. Following basal samples drawn from an indwelling forearm venous catheter at −15 and 0 min, CRH (100 μg) is administered as a single intravenous bolus dose. Plasma cortisol and ACTH are then sampled at 15-min intervals thereafter, for 1 hour. Patients with Cushing's disease typically show an excessive rise in plasma cortisol, whereas those with ectopic ACTH secretion usually do not. Analysis of large series reveals that a plasma cortisol rise of 20% or more above baseline is seen in over 85% of cases of Cushing's disease. It is apparent, therefore, that in isolation this test also falls short of the pre-test diagnostic likelihood of Cushing's disease. If, however, the results of the HDDST and CRH test are analysed for the same individual, it is our experience that virtually every patient can be correctly classified.

Bilateral inferior petrosal sinus sampling (BIPSS)

BIPSS is the most reliable test for differentiating between pituitary and non-pituitary sources of ACTH. The pituitary effluent drains into the petrosal sinuses via the cavernous sinuses, and therefore a gradient of the value of plasma ACTH from this sampling position compared with a simultaneous peripheral plasma sample indicates a central source of ACTH. Clearly, this would be the case in normal individuals, whereas in those with ectopic disease, the normal pituitary corticotrophs should be adequately suppressed by the circulating plasma cortisol and therefore there should be no gradient. Therefore, it is essential that the patient has active and ongoing hypercortisolaemia for the test to be properly interpreted. If there is evidence that the patient has 'cycled out', then the test should be deferred and performed on a later occasion.

This highly skilled, invasive, technique involves the placement of fine catheters in both inferior petrosal sinuses via a femoral approach by an experienced radiologist. Confirmation of position by fluorography in two dimensions is mandatory to ensure that successful catheterisation has been achieved. The diagnostic accuracy of the test is increased by the use of CRH stimulation. In most series a basal central-to-peripheral gradient of ACTH of more than 2 to 1 or a stimulated gradient of more than 3 to 1 is indicative of Cushing's disease. Analysis of all published series indicates that the sensitivity of this test is of the order of 96% at a specificity of 100%. Sampling directly from the cavernous sinuses is a technically more demanding procedure, requiring access to more expensive catheters, and obviates the need for CRH stimulation. Furthermore, it is debatable whether cavernous sinus sampling is an improvement over more widely applied BIPSS.

Complications of BIPSS include transient discomfort in both ears during catheter placement. The very rare complication of brainstem stroke has been reported, and this appears to relate to catheter design. It is recommended that heparinisation of patients is performed once the catheters are *in situ*. In centres of excellence, the complication is very low.

Whereas this technique is extremely good at distinguishing between a central or peripheral source of ACTH, it is not of as great utility in the lateralisation of ACTH secretion from within the pituitary fossa in patients with Cushing's disease. If a pituitary adenoma is not evident on imaging, and no tumour is apparent at surgery, hemihypophysectomy may be recommended in an attempt to remove micoadenomas. However, if based on the lateralisation results from BIPSS, these recommendations should be cautiously applied, since in approximately 30% of cases the source of ACTH secretion within the fossa is incorrectly localised by this technique.

Radiology

Pituitary

MRI is superior to CT for imaging of the pituitary gland. The majority of corticotroph adenomas have a hypo-intense signal on MRI, which fails to enhance with gadolinium. However, since approximately 5% of pituitary microadenomas enhance following gadolinium, pre- and post-contrast images are essential. More recently, dynamic MRI, in which very rapid signal acquisition is achieved following gadolinium administration, may disclose a higher number of corticotroph adenomas. With standard MRI protocols, corticotroph microadenomas are not visualised in up to 50% of cases.

Adrenal

CT scanning remains the imaging modality that gives the greatest special resolution for adrenal anatomy. It is not possible to distinguish between cortisol-secreting adenomas and carcinomas, although lesions of more than 6 cm in diameter should certainly be considered to be malignant. This is particularly true if there is evidence of vascular invasion associated with an adrenal tumour of any size. A functioning cortisol-secreting tumour will cause suppression of plasma ACTH. Therefore, the contralateral gland will undergo atrophy. In ACTH-dependent Cushing's syndrome adrenal glands undergo bilateral hyperplasia, with the size reflecting the prevailing level of cortisolaemia, driven by ACTH. Nodular hyperplasia may result from ACTH-dependent disease, and distinguishing this from primary adrenal tumours is aided by establishing whether or not there is hypertrophy, as opposed to atrophy, of the remaining limbs. This is an important management point, as therapy directed towards the pituitary may be more appropriate in some circumstances.

Imaging in ectopic ACTH secretion

The commonest site of ectopic ACTH secretion is from small cell lung cancer and bronchial carcinoid tumours. With the advent of rapid diagnosis, and chemotherapeutic intervention, the overt ectopic ACTH syndrome associated with small cell lung cancer is less commonly seen by endocrinologists. It is likely, however, that these patients represent a large cohort that is not referred for consideration of the diagnosis of Cushing's syndrome. In contrast, currently, most presentations to endocrinologists of the ectopic ACTH syndrome are due to ACTH-secreting bronchial carcinoid tumours. These are usually very small (< 1 cm) and difficult to visualise. High-definition spiral CT scans of the chest are required and, typically, carcinoid tumours enhance following intravenous radiographic contrast media. Differentiation between vascular markings within normal lung may be problematic. One means of differentiating between tumour and vascular marking is to scan the patient in both supine and prone positions: vascular markings will tend to disappear in the prone position. Thymic carcinoid tumours associated with Cushing's syndrome have been shown to be greater than 2 cm in diameter at presentation, and are usually easily disclosed on CT scanning. If no lesion is disclosed by imaging the lung, extensive imaging of the abdomen may also be required. Selective body catheter sampling for plasma ACTH has not been shown to be a useful technique other than in occasional cases.

Carcinoid tumours frequently express somatostatin receptors and may be visualised on radiolabelled octreotide or lanreotide scintigraphy. Careful analysis of published literature reveals that the lesions thus disclosed are usually apparent with conventional axial imaging. Thus, it is likely that this technique will not disclose 'occult' ACTH-secreting tumours that have not been disclosed on careful axial imaging. The value of positron emission tomography (PET) scanning remains to be established.

Summary

In ACTH-dependent Cushing's syndrome the best means of differentiating between pituitary and ectopic sources of ACTH is BIPSS, and it is our routine practice to rely most heavily on this test. Some centres prefer to routinely use noninvasive testing with HDDST and CRH testing together with imaging, reserving BIPSS for cases of doubt. Figure 5.2 illustrates an algorithm for diagnosis and differential diagnosis.

Treatment

Associated medical conditions such as hypertension and diabetes mellitus will require treatment on their own merits. To allow tissue recovery from the effects of high levels of circulating glucocorticoid, it is recommended that any patient with severe Cushing's syndrome be treated medically to lower the level of cortisol for a period of at

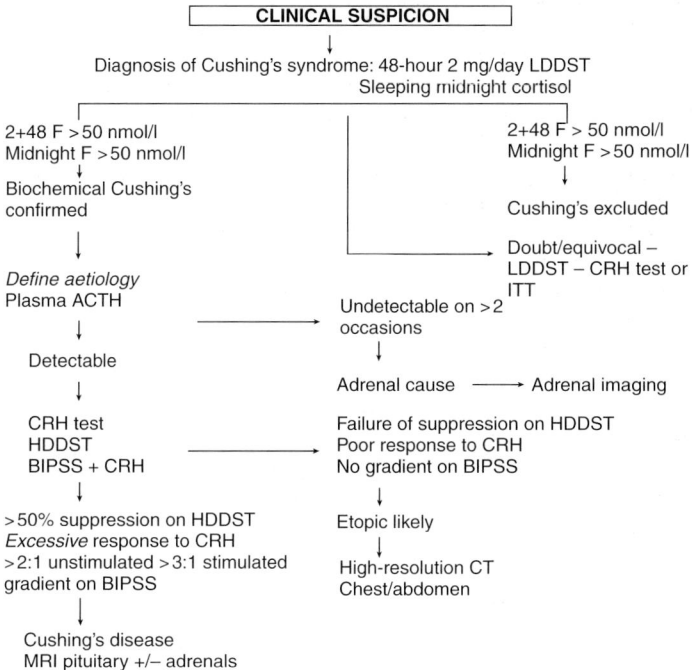

Figure 5.2   Diagnostic algorithm for the investigation of Cushing's syndrome. F = plasma cortisol. For other abbreviations, see text.

least 6 weeks before any operative intervention, although with mild disease and transsphenoidal surgery this may not be necessary. Two specific problems merit discussion.

Hypokalaemia

In some circumstances, life-threatening hypokalaemia will require urgent therapy with potassium supplementation and the use of potassium-sparing drugs such as trimaterene (50 mg two to three times daily).

Psychosis

Whereas this usually responds rapidly to the cortisol-lowering, it may be necessary to use anti-psychotic medication during investigation.

Medical Therapy to Lower Cortisol

Metyrapone

Metyrapone inhibits the secretion of cortisol by blocking the final step in the cortisol synthetic pathway. This is effective in controlling hypercortisolaemia in 80% of patients with Cushing's disease and adrenal tumours and in up to 70% of cases of the ectopic ACTH syndrome. Cortisol levels fall within 2 hours of starting treatment, but since metyrapone has a short duration of action it requires to be administered three times daily. Treatment is usually commenced at a dose of 500 mg three times daily. Response is monitored by sampling plasma cortisol at five points during the day between 09.00 h and 21.00 h. Dose titration is performed at 72-hour intervals until a mean plasma cortisol level of 150–300 mmol/l is achieved. This equates to the normal cortisol production rate. The average daily dose of patients with Cushing's disease and the ectopic ACTH syndrome is 2 g and 4 g, in divided doses, respectively. Since metyrapone causes an increase in steroid androgenic precursors, hirsutism is a major adverse effect in women. Moreover, there is a rapid and large increase in the level of circulating 11-deoxycortisol, which may crossreact in some cortisol RIAs, and care is required in the interpretation of the values of cortisol.

Ketoconazole

Ketoconazole is an imidazole antifungal agent that also blocks the adrenal steroid synthesis at several points. In contrast to metyrapone, treatment with ketoconazole does not cause a build up of androgenic precursors and hirsutism is not a side effect. However, in some instances, ketoconazole may induce hepatocellular dysfunction, and monitoring of liver biochemistry is mandatory. Treatment is instigated at a dose of 200 mg three times daily, with the mean dose required in Cushing's disease being 1.2 g/day in divided doses. The onset of action of ketoconazole is slower than that of metyrapone, and dose increments should be made at 2–3 weekly intervals. In some circumstances it may be necessary to use both drugs in combination, and frequently the dose of each may be lower than that required when used as monotherapy. On occasion it may be useful to start ketoconazole and metyrapone together, and subsequently withdraw metyrapone at a later date: metyrapone will allow rapid control, but in some circumstances it can be withdrawn after a few weeks, leaving a maintenance dose of ketoconazole, and thus avoiding hirsutism.

Hypoadrenalism is an important side effect following treatment with both metyrapone and ketoconazole, but is more common following treatment with the former. Occasionally, and particularly with cyclical disease, it may be necessary to instigate a 'block and replace' regime with high doses of metyrapone and/or ketoconazole and replacement doses of dexamethasone.

o,p'-DDD (Mitotane)

o,p'-DDD appears to have a direct adrenolytic action on adrenocortical cells and also blocks cortisol synthesis. It has a slow onset of action, taking up to 6 weeks to be fully effective. A major side effect is that of hypercholesterolaemia, which may be treated with the statin class of cholesterol-lowering drugs. At high doses, such as those formerly used for adrenocortical carcinoma (9 g/day), there are often associated significant side effects such as anorexia and ataxia.

Etomidate

Etomidate is a short-acting intravenous anaesthetic agent and is the only parenteral drug that can be used for hypercortisolaemia. At nonsedative doses, it has been used in the acute control of severe hypercortisolaemia, especially while on ITU. Doses of between 1.2 and 2.5 mg/h will usually lower serum cortisol levels to undetectable levels, and the patients may be treated with a 'block and replace' regime with an intravenous infusion of hydrocortisone of 1–2 mg/h.

Surgery for Cushing's Syndrome – Definition of Cure

High levels of circulating glucocorticoid will suppress the synthesis and secretion of ACTH from normal corticotroph tissue. Therefore, selective removal of any cause of Cushing's syndrome should result in a circulating plasma cortisol that is undetectable, i.e. less that 50 nmol/l in most routine RIAs (Figure 5.3). Merely lowering the plasma cortisol to 'normal levels' postoperatively is suboptimal, and, without adjuvant therapy, is likely to result in recurrence of disease.

Transsphenoidal surgery

Transsphenoidal selective microadenomectomy by an experienced surgeon is the treatment of choice for the vast majority of patients

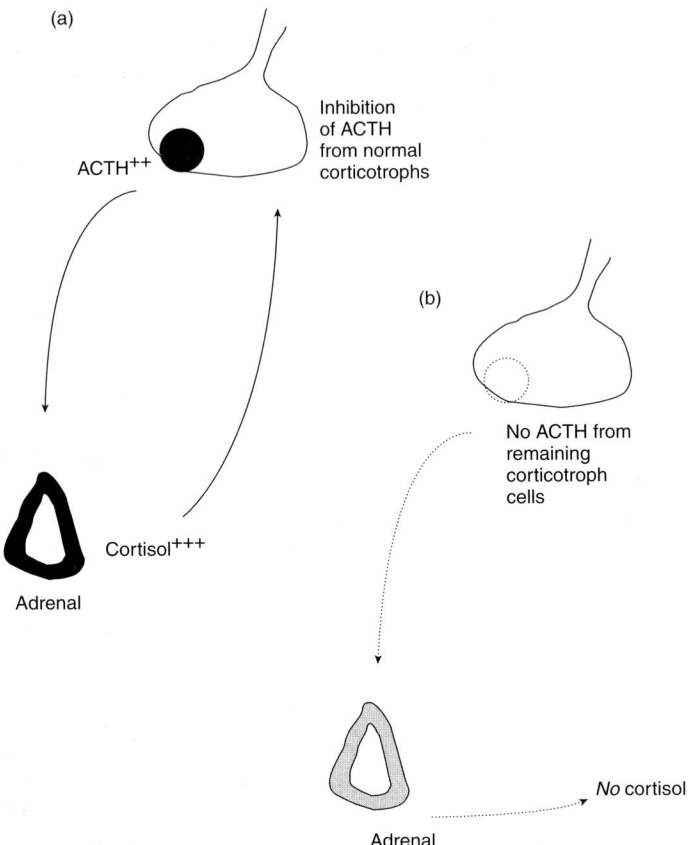

Figure 5.3 Outcome of curative transsphenoidal hypophysectomy for Cushing's disease. (a) ACTH-secreting pituitary adenoma; (b) surgical cure.

with Cushing's disease. When successfully performed, this surgery results in a long-lasting cure without other pituitary hormonal deficiency. However, even in the best centres, only 50% of patients are cured, with approximately a further 30–40% achieving clinical remission; this statistic emphasises the need for surgery to be performed in specialised centres. Complications of cerebrospinal fluid (CSF) leakage (less that 5%) or meningitis (less than 2%) are unusual in experienced hands.

Prompt postoperative assessment of the pituitary–adrenal axis is essential. If there is persisting hypercortisolaemia, reoperation within 7–10 days may cure a further 50% of those undergoing re-operation. Preservation of remaining pituitary function is a priority in the younger patient, whereas in the more elderly, particularly if there are coexistent medical problems, the emphasis should shift more towards cure at the first operation: this may involve recommendation of total hypophysectomy rather than an attempt at selective microadenomectomy.

In those patients who have been cured by surgery, glucocorticoid therapy may be required for several years, since the remaining normal corticotrophs often remain suppressed for this period of time. Repeated re-evaluation is required to establish when the pituitary–adrenal axis has 'woken up'; this may be achieved by admitting the patient, stopping his glucocorticoid therapy, and assessing his 09.00 h cortisol. Once this value is above 100 mmol/l, these individuals may undergo an ITT to assess if they have achieved an adequate restoration of their axis.

Adrenal Surgery

Unilateral adrenalectomy is the treatment of choice for patients with an isolated adrenal adenoma. Laparoscopic adrenalectomy is associated with a shorter hospital stay and less morbidity than open adrenalectomy. Since the contralateral adrenal gland may remain suppressed for many years, glucocorticoid cover is necessary for the procedure and should be given at replacement doses following recovery from surgery, whereas mineralocorticoid replacement will not be required. The prognosis following removal of adrenocortical cortisol-secreting adenomas is good. In contrast, the prognosis is almost uniformly very poor in patients with adrenocortical carcinomas, which frequently present with metastases, and patients often die within months of diagnosis. Regrettably, these tumours are poorly radiosensitive or chemosensitive.

In any case of ACTH-dependent Cushing's syndrome, bilateral adrenalectomy may be required to achieve adequate control of the circulating levels of cortisol. This should result in a dramatic improvement in the clinical state. With adequate preparation using cortisol-lowering drugs, modern anaesthesia and laparoscopic approaches, the morbidity can be extremely low. Following surgery, patients will require lifelong glucocorticoid and mineralocorticoid treatment. A major concern following bilateral adrenalectomy in patients with refractory Cushing's disease is the development of Nelson's syndrome. In this syndrome there develops a locally aggressive pituitary tumour that secretes high levels of ACTH, resulting in pigmentation. The tumour itself may be treated with further surgery and radiotherapy, but these rarely cure the disease. Radiotherapy to the pituitary at the time of bilateral adrenalectomy has been demonstrated to be the most effective means of preventing the onset of this syndrome.

Pituitary Radiotherapy

Following transsphenoidal surgery, persisting hypercortisolaemia may be treated with pituitary radiotherapy. This should be considered in all patients with mean postoperative cortisol levels above 150 nmol/l. The long-established means of delivering radiotherapy to the pituitary, which has a high safety record, is by giving 25 fractions of 180 cGy in three fields – a total dose of 4500 cGy – over a period of 35 days. Over several years the circulating levels of cortisol fall and the dose of cortisol-lowering medical therapy can be reduced. Progressive anterior pituitary failure is the major side effect and, in particular, growth hormone deficiency is virtually uniform 10 years after treatment whereas gonadotrophin deficiency is present in about 15% of patients. Approximately 4 years after treatment, 80% of patients are in remission with respect to their circulating plasma cortisol levels.

Stereotactic radiosurgery is an alternative form of radiotherapy in which a highly focused radiotherapy is administered as a single dose. However, there are no large cohort long-term follow-up data on the outcomes of patients with Cushing's disease treated with this mode of therapy, although it probably has a more rapid mode of cortisol-lowering action.

Conclusions

Patients presenting with Cushing's syndrome require specialist assessment and treatment, and warrant a referral to major centres. Accurate diagnosis is a prerequisite for effective management. Cyclical disease may be particularly challenging. In the differentiation between pituitary and non-pituitary sources of ACTH, reliance should be placed on biochemical evaluation prior to imaging. Medical therapy is often used preoperatively to lower levels of plasma cortisol, and postoperatively to control levels in those patients not cured, and until the mean level of plasma cortisol falls to 150–300 nmol/l following radiotherapy after non-curative transsphenoidal surgery. Transsphenoidal surgery with microadenomectomy is the treatment of choice for Cushing's disease, whereas laparoscopic bilateral adrenalectomy is being used increasingly in refractory cases. More data are needed on the most effective means of delivering radiotherapy to the pituitary.

Further Reading

McCance DR, Besser M, Brew-Atkinson A. Assessment of cure after transsphenoidal surgery for Cushing's disease. *Clin Endocrinol* 1996;**44**,1–6.

Newell-Price J, Grossman A. Diagnosis and management of Cushing's syndrome. *Lancet* 1999;**353**(9170):2087–8.

Newell-Price J, Trainer P, Perry L, Wass J, Grossman, A, Besser M. A single sleeping midnight cortisol has 100% sensitivity for the diagnosis of Cushing's syndrome. *Clin Endocrinol (Oxf)* 1995;**43**(5):545–50.

Newell-Price JDC, Trainer PJ, Besser GM, Grossman AB. The diagnosis and differential diagnosis of Cushing's syndrome and pseudo-Cushing's states. *Endoc Rev* 1998;**19**(5):647–72.

Rees LH, Besser GM, Jeffcoate WJ, Goldie DJ, Marks V. Alcohol-induced pseudo-Cushing's syndrome. *Lancet* 1977;**1**(8014):726–8.

Trainer PJ, Besser GM. Cushing's syndrome. Therapy directed at the adrenal glands. *Endocrinol Metab Clin North Am* 1994;**23**(3):571–84.

Trainer PJ, Besser GM. *The Barts Endocrine Protocols.* London: Churchill Livingstone, 1995.

Trainer PJ, Lawrie HS, Verhelst J *et al.* Transsphenoidal resection in Cushing's disease: undetectable serum cortisol as the definition of successful treatment. *Clin Endocrinol (Oxf)* 1993; **38**(1):73–8.

Wajchenberg BL, Mendonca BB, Liberman B *et al.* Ectopic adrenocorticotropic hormone syndrome. *Endocr Rev* 1994;**15**(6):752–87.

Wood PJ, Barth JH, Freedman DB, Perry L, Sheridan B. Evidence for the low dose dexamethasone suppression test to screen for Cushing's syndrome – recommendations for a protocol for biochemistry laboratories. *Ann Clin Biochem* 1997;**34**(Part 3):222–9.

Yanovski JA, Cutler GB Jr, Chrousos GP, Nieman LK. Corticotropin-releasing hormone stimulation following low-dose dexamethasone administration. A new test to distinguish Cushing's syndrome from pseudo-Cushing's states *JAMA* 1993;**269**(17):2232–8.

Yanovski JA, Cutler GB Jr, Doppman JL *et al.* The limited ability of inferior petrosal sinus sampling with corticotropin-releasing hormone to distinguish Cushing's disease from pseudo-Cushing states or normal physiology. *J Clin Endocrinol Metab* 1993;**77**(2):503–9.

6

Addison's Disease

Jean O'Connell and Donal O'Shea

Introduction

Addison's disease is a condition of primary adrenal insufficiency, resulting from destruction or removal of the adrenal cortex. Secondary causes of hypoadrenalism include deficient pituitary adrenocorticotrophic hormone (ACTH) secretion or deficient hypothalamic secretion of corticotrophin-releasing hormone (CRH).

Thomas Addison first described the condition in 1855 when he published 'Diseases of the suprarenal capsules', a paper detailing the clinical features and postmortem findings of 11 cases of primary adrenocortical failure. At that time tuberculosis was responsible for the majority of cases, but since then in the developed world there has been a shift towards autoimmune disease as the main aetiological factor, and with this an overall female preponderance of 2:1.

Although a rare condition, with an estimated incidence of 40–110 cases per million adults, once considered, Addison's disease is reliably diagnosed and easily treated. The introduction of therapeutic synthetic cortisone in 1949 represented a breakthrough in the successful long-term management of Addison's disease.

The main pitfall is the initial diagnosis of the illness, as clinical symptoms and signs are vague and common to many conditions. Misdiagnosis is potentially fatal, so it is important to include Addison's disease in a differential if there is any uncertainty.

Hormone Physiology

ACTH is a 39-amino acid peptide synthesised primarily in the anterior pituitary gland from a larger precursor glycoprotein known as

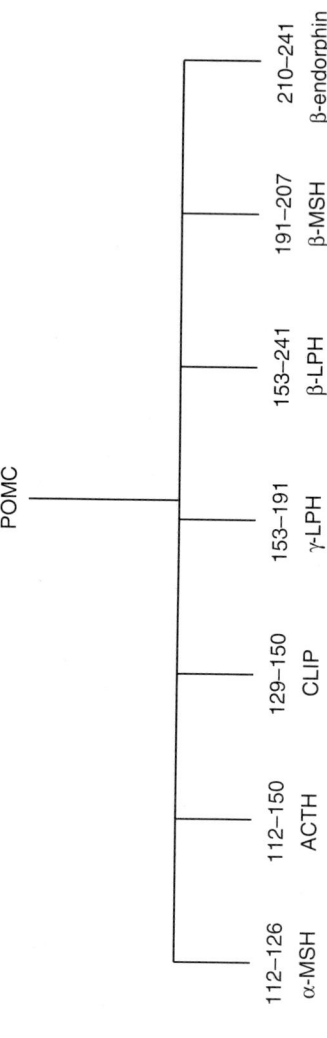

Figure 6.1 Differential cleavage of pro-opiomelanocortin (POMC) into active hormones. Letters represent hormones produced: MSH – melanocyte-stimulating hormone (the α-subunit has the most melanocyte-stimulating activity); ACTH – adrenocorticotrophic hormone; LPH – lipotrophic hormone; CLIP – corticotrophin-like intermediate peptide.

pro-opiomelanocortin (POMC). POMC undergoes differential cleavage into active hormones in various tissues, as seen in Figure 6.1.

Control of ACTH secretion is under the influence of hypothalamic CRH, which in turn is stimulated by emotion, stress or trauma, and both are then affected by negative feedback from glucocorticoids. In the absence of this negative feedback, as occurs in Addison's disease, the resulting high levels of ACTH – and the co-produced melanocyte-stimulating hormone (MSH) – lead to a characteristic darkening of the skin.

Hormones secreted in the hypothalamic–pituitary–adrenal (HPA) axis follow a circadian rhythm (i.e. they exhibit a pattern based on the 24-hour cycle; circadian is from the latin *circa* = about; *dies* = day). This synchronisation with the solar day is in response to external cues from the light–dark cycle. Understanding this pattern of hormone secretion is important when interpreting results of blood samples taken at different times of the day or night.

The concentration of ACTH (and therefore cortisol) is lowest around midnight, increases until a morning 6–8 a.m. peak, and thereafter slowly declines. Under stressful conditions such as pain, fear, fever or hypoglycaemia, secretion of CRH, ACTH and cortisol increases and the circadian variation is blunted.

Any glucocorticoid can suppress ACTH secretion, but the degree of suppression depends on the dose, potency and duration of action of the steroid as well as the duration and time of its administration. The shorter the interval before the normal early morning peak of ACTH secretion, the greater the suppressive effect on the HPA axis. After withdrawal of chronic pharmacological doses of glucocorticoids, the axis may remain suppressed for weeks to months.

Aetiology (see Table 6.1)

Autoimmune

Autoimmune or 'idiopathic' Addison's disease accounts for approximately 75–80% of cases of adrenal destruction. As with other autoimmune conditions, the majority of patients are female, particularly when the condition occurs as part of the polyglandular autoimmune syndrome (PGA). However, in the setting of isolated adrenal insufficiency this is only the case from the fourth decade onward, with a definite male preponderance in the first two decades of life. The reason for this is unclear but could be partly explained by early presentations of adrenomyeloneuropathy.

Table 6.1   Aetiology of Addison's disease

Autoimmune adrenalitis:

- Sporadic
- Polyglandular autoimmune syndrome type I
  (*primary manifestations*: Addison's disease, primary
  hypoparathyroidism, mucocutaneous candidiasis)
- Polyglandular autoimmune syndrome type II
  (*primary manifestations*: Addison's disease, thyroid disease,
  primary hypogonadism, diabetes mellitus type 1, vitiligo)

Infectious adrenalitis:

- Tuberculosis
- Disseminated fungal infection: histoplasmosis,
  paracoccidioidomyosis
- Acquired immune deficiency syndrome (AIDS): cytomegalovirus,
  cryptococcus, tuberculosis, *Mycobacterium avium-intracellulare*,
  Kaposi's sarcoma, lymphoma
- Syphilis

Bilateral adrenal haemorrhage:

- Septicaemia (meningococcal, *Pseudomonas*)
- Anticoagulant therapy/coagulopathy
- Trauma
- Thrombosis, embolism, vasculitis

Bilateral adrenalectomy

Infiltration:

- Carcinoma/lymphoma
- Sarcoid
- Amyloid

Medication:

- Enzyme inhibition (ketoconazole)
- Enzyme induction (rifampicin)

Inherited disorders:

- Adrenoleukodystrophy/adrenomyeloneuropathy
- Congenital adrenal hypoplasia
- Familial glucocorticoid deficiency

The classic pathological feature of autoimmune destruction is
early lymphocytic infiltration of the adrenal cortex. This progresses
to total loss of the normal architecture of all three cortical zones,
with sparing of the adrenal medulla.

Autoantibodies

The importance of circulating adrenocortical antibodies has been long suspected but until recently their exact pathogenetic significance had not been established. Recent studies have investigated the involvement of various antibodies in both isolated Addison's disease (IAD) and adrenal insufficiency as part of the polyglandular autoimmune syndromes (PGA I and PGA II):

- Adrenal cortex autoantibodies (ACA): these antibodies are detected by a standard immunofluorescence test and are found in the serum of 60–70% of patients with primary adrenal insufficiency. Patients with positive ACA serology may not have Addison's disease but have been shown to develop the condition at a rate of up to 19% per year.
- Adrenal P450 enzyme antibodies: adrenal enzymes 21-hydroxylase (21OH), 17α-hydroxylase (17OH) and side chain cleavage enzyme (SCC) represent major target antigens, and antibodies directed against them are detected by immunoprecipitation assay. A high prevalence of 21OH antibodies (21OH-A) is seen in patients suffering from IAD or PGA II: this was 76% and 85%, respectively, in one study.
- Autoantibodies against aromatic L-amino acid decarboxylase (AADC): these antibodies are found in about 50% of patients with PGA I but are absent in sera from patients with other organ-specific autoimmune diseases such as diabetes mellitus type 1, Hashimoto's thyroiditis and Graves' disease.
- There is disagreement in the literature over the significance of the level of antibody titres and the degree of adrenal dysfunction. However, it is possible that production of high levels of 21OH-A signal the destructive phase of the disease process and it appears that levels progressively decrease with disease duration.
- In children with organ-specific autoimmune diseases without adrenal insufficiency, the presence of ACA/21OH autoantibodies are important predictive markers for the development of Addison's disease.

Isolated Addison's disease

In this patient group the prevalence of adrenal autoantibodies is lower than in patients with other associated endocrine diseases. There is no clinical evidence of gland dysfunction elsewhere, but serology may still be positive for parathyroid, thyroid or islet-cell antibodies. Development of an associated endocrinopathy is therefore a possibility in later years.

Associated endocrine disorders

The incidence of other endocrine autoimmune diseases in patients with autoimmune adrenal insufficiency is increased as follows:

1. Thyroid disease:
   * thyroid microsomal antibodies occur in ~ 50% of patients but only half of these have overt hypothyroidism
   * thyrotoxicosis occurs in about 8%.
2. Gonadal failure:
   * primary ovarian failure is very common in female patients (~20%)
   * testicular failure is rare in males (< 2%).
3. Diabetes mellitus type 1 (~10%).
4. Hypoparathyroidism (~5%).

The incidence of other autoimmune disorders such as vitiligo (melanin-producing cell antibodies), pernicious anaemia (intrinsic factor antibodies) and atrophic gastritis (parietal cell antibodies) is also increased.

Polyglandular autoimmmune syndromes

The polyglandular autoimmune syndromes describe well-recognised clinical conditions of two or more dysfunctional endocrine glands as well as associated nonendocrine manifestations.

PGA I is a paediatric disorder, inherited in an autosomal recessive pattern, with all manifestations present by the age of 15 years. The clinical manifestations of PGA I are summarised in Table 6.2.

PGA II (Schmidt's syndrome) occurs in adulthood; adrenal insufficiency is the primary manifestation. Thyroid disease and diabetes mellitus are the other main features. About half the cases are familial and there is a 2:1 female preponderance. It appears to be associated with the human leucocyte antigen HLA-DR3. The clinical manifestations of PGA II are summarised in Table 6.3.

Genetics

Autoimmune adrenal insufficiency is more likely to be familial if it occurs as part of a polyglandular syndrome (~50%) than when it is an isolated condition (~30%).

Table 6.2 Clinical manifestations of PGA I

Disorder	Prevalence (%)
Hypoparathyroidism	93
Chronic mucocutaneous candidiasis	83
Adrenal insufficiency	73
Gonadal failure	43
Malabsorption syndromes	15
Alopecia	37
Pernicious anaemia	15
Thyroid disease	10
Chronic active hepatitis	20
Vitiligo	15
Diabetes mellitus type 1	2

Table 6.3 Clinical manifestations of PGA II

Disorder	Prevalence (%)
Adrenal insufficiency	100
Autoimmune thyroid disease	70
Diabetes mellitus type 1	50
Gonadal failure	5–50
Vitiligo	4

The defect in immune regulation leading to sensitisation to autoantigens is thought to arise from a gene in the histocompatibility antigen (HLA) region. Autoimmune endocrine disease has been mainly linked to the class II HLA genes (DR3 & DR4, DQ8 & DQ2) but also to HLA B8. These associations are similar to those of type 1 diabetes mellitus, but are not found in other organ-specific diseases such as pernicious anaemia or primary gonadal failure. This would suggest other, non-HLA-associated genes are responsible and this could also be true for PGA I, in which no HLA association has been found.

Infection

Tuberculosis (TB) was the leading cause of adrenal deficiency in the 1920s and 1930s. At that time it accounted for approximately 80% of cases but, since the introduction of effective prevention and treatment of tuberculosis, this figure has decreased to only 20% (prevalence is higher in countries where TB is still endemic). A high proportion of patients with extrapulmonary TB will have adrenal involvement, but only a minority will develop clinical adrenal insufficiency. Destruction of the gland is gradual and may be incomplete or affect mainly the medulla. Nodules of caseous necrosis replace the normal architecture of the glands and eventually they become atrophied and calcified.

Fungal infections can also invade the adrenal gland, and antifungal therapy is usually ineffective in preventing progression to Addison's disease. Histoplasmosis and paracoccidioidomycosis are common causes in endemic areas as they have a predilection for the adrenals. Cryptococcosis and blastomycosis are much less common.

Syphilis can also cause adrenal insufficiency as part of a multisystem spirochaete invasion.

Patients with human immunodeficiency virus (HIV) very commonly have adrenal gland involvement, particularly secondary to cytomegalovirus (CMV) infection, but this may also be due to HIV directly. Infection with toxoplasmosis, atypical tuberculosis and cryptococcosis can also be responsible as well as lymphoma and Kaposi's sarcoma.

As with tuberculosis, in HIV patients, despite a high incidence of adrenal infection, overt Addison's disease is unusual: in fact, cortisol levels are often elevated, possibly a stress response to chronic illness.

Partial adrenal insufficiency can be unmasked during treatment for opportunistic infections. Drugs such as ketoconazole (sometimes used in the treatment of Cushing's disease) and rifampicin interfere with hepatic cortisol metabolism and can precipitate an adrenal crisis.

Metastatic infiltration

Metastasis of cancer to the adrenals is very common, but overt adrenal disease is not, as this requires bilateral and complete cortical destruction. Lung, breast, stomach and colon cancer as well as melanoma, Hodgkin's and non-Hodgkin's lymphoma have all been documented as sources of the primary neoplasm.

Symptoms of adrenal insufficiency may be mistakenly attributed to the cancer and this may contribute to the low incidence of diagnosis in this setting.

Adrenal haemorrhage

Bilateral adrenal haemorrhage is a potential cause of acute, rapid loss of glucocorticoid and mineralocorticoid production. Recent advances in imaging techniques have improved diagnostic pick-up and hence prognosis in this condition.

In children, meningococcal or *Pseudomonas* septicaemia are the commonest causes and in adults over 50 years anticoagulant therapy or spontaneous coagulopathy are the main precipitants.

There is an extensive list of more unusual causes, including adrenal vein thrombosis, malignancy, lymphoma, renal failure, trauma and severe burns.

Adrenoleukodystrophy and adrenomyeloneuropathy

These diseases are inherited in an X-linked recessive pattern and therefore primarily affect males. Because of an abnormality in their metabolism, long-chain fatty acids accumulate in the spinal cord, brain, adrenals and other organs. Adrenoleukodystrophy develops in adolescence with rapid progression of neurological dysfunction. Adrenomyeloneuropathy presents later, usually after age 21, and has a milder and slower course. It is not uncommon for adrenal insufficiency to present before neurological symptoms manifest and therefore these disorders should be considered in young males with hypoadrenalism.

Adrenal hypoplasia

This is a rare inherited condition where there is failure of development of the adrenal cortex. The condition presents shortly after birth with one of several variants that have been described: e.g. sporadic form associated with pituitary hypoplasia, an X-linked form associated with hypogonadotrophic hypogonadism.

Familial glucocorticoid deficiency

A rare autosomal recessive disorder characterised by adrenocortical unresponsiveness to ACTH. Mineralocorticoid function is usually preserved.

Drugs

A number of drugs inhibit cortisol synthesis, usually by means of enzymatic inhibition. Examples include ketoconazole (antifungal), suramin (antiparasitic), aminoglutethimide, etomidate (induction anaesthethic agent) and metyrapone. This is normally balanced by increased ACTH production so that clinical adrenal insufficiency is uncommon except in the setting of pre-existing reduced adrenal reserve.

Other drugs act by induction of hepatic oxygenases, leading to increased metabolism of cortisol and other steroids. Rifampicin, phenytoin and other barbiturates have this effect. Similarly, symptomatic adrenal disease only occurs if adrenal function is already compromised.

Glucocorticoids

Exposure to long-term glucocorticoids may cause HPA axis suppression. There is both CRH with ACTH deficiency and resultant adrenal atrophy.

Clinical Features (see Table 6.4)

The spectrum of symptoms in Addison's disease is broad, ranging from the hyperpigmented, asymptomatic individual to the critically ill patient suffering an addisonian crisis. At either end of this spectrum complaints are often nonspecific and common to many other conditions. Anorexia, weight loss, malaise and generalised weakness may be a background to more specific features.

Gastrointestinal symptoms such as nausea, vomiting, abdominal pain and diarrhoea are common and may herald the onset of an addisonian crisis. It is essential this is not misdiagnosed as an acute abdomen, as surgical intervention could be fatal.

Postural hypotension, with associated dizziness and syncope, may predate low blood pressure and in the setting of adrenal crisis profound hypotension (shock) is an almost universal finding. Salt or liquorice craving is a significant feature in some cases and occasionally persists even after diagnosis and treatment.

Hyperpigmentation is a characteristic feature of most but not all patients with primary adrenal deficiency. Increased levels of POMC peptides stimulate melanocytes, resulting in a generalised darkening of the skin. Although characteristically diffuse, pigmentation is prominent in sun-exposed areas and areas subject to chronic friction or pressure, such as the elbows, knees, waist (belt) and shoulders (bra straps). It also occurs in the palmar creases, mucous membranes, axillae, areolae and perineum. Existing freckles become darker, new

Table 6.4   Clinical features in chronic adrenal insufficiency

Pathophysiology	Symptom/sign	Per cent frequency
Glucocorticoid deficiency	Weight loss	100
	Malaise/fatigue	100
	Weakness	100
	Nausea	86
	Vomiting	75
	Anorexia	100
	Abdominal pain	31
	Diarrhoea	16
	Postural syncope	12
	Hypoglycaemia	18
Mineralocorticoid deficiency	Hypotension/shock	88
	Salt craving	19
Increased ACTH levels (or related peptides)	Hyperpigmentation	92
Adrenal androgen deficiency	Loss of body hair in women	~50
	Reduced libido	
Others	Vitiligo	10–20
	Auricular cartilage calcification	5

freckles may appear and recently acquired scars become permanently pigmented. A rare but notable exception known as 'white Addison's disease' describes the absence of hyperpigmentation even with raised levels of circulating MSH. A skin biopsy from one such case showed a high degree of melanosome degradation in secondary lysosomes ('compound melanosomes') which overwhelmed the increased stimulation of the skin pigmentation.

Psychiatric symptomatology is present in many adult-onset cases and can be one of the earliest features of the disease. Symptoms can range from memory and cognitive impairment to depression, delirium, mania or psychosis. Most symptoms disappear within days of initiating treatment but psychosis may persist for longer.

Although the clinical picture is similar in both sexes, features of androgen deficiency are more prominent in women because the adrenal gland is the main source of androgens. This leads to complaints of decreased axillary and pubic hair as well as reduced libido. Amenorrhoea may occur, possibly secondary to weight loss or chronic illness. Autoimmune-related primary gonadal failure should be excluded, however, as there is an increased incidence of this condition.

Adrenal insufficiency may present in association with other conditions:

- Vitiligo occurs in 10–20% of cases of autoimmune adrenalitis. The presence of these patchy areas of depigmentation may assist in diagnosis in an otherwise nonspecific clinical picture.
- Diabetes mellitus type 1 is more common in Addison's disease and may present as recurrent severe hypoglycaemia, unexplained reduction in insulin requirements and new onset of hypoglycaemia unawareness. These problems are reversed with adequate glucocorticoid replacement.
- Coeliac disease should be considered if gastrointestinal symptoms persist, particularly chronic diarrhoea, which is a well-recognised initial symptom of Addison's disease but should resolve with treatment.

Investigations

Blood tests

There are many biochemical abnormalities commonly attributed to Addison's disease (Table 6.5), but the diagnosis is suggested by an inappropriately low basal (8 a.m.) plasma cortisol (< 50 nmol/), and confirmed by demonstrating a failure to rise after administration of synthetic tetrocosactrin/ACTH (Synacthen). It is clear that a biochemical diagnosis should be made before prescribing long-term steroid replacement. The patient may need emergency treatment on clinical suspicion before the results are available.

Plasma ACTH

In primary adrenal insufficiency, basal plasma ACTH levels are always elevated and therefore clearly differentiate Addison's from pituitary or hypothalamic disease. The blood sample must be obtained and handled correctly and the assay must be reliable – all of which is frequently not the case. The sample should be collected in a tube containing 7.5% ethylenediaminetetraacetic acid (EDTA) and transferred on ice to the laboratory, where it is spun and frozen within 1 hour.

Table 6.5   Biochemical abnormalities in Addison's disease

Test	Finding
FBC	Normocytic anaemia (macrocytosis if associated pernicious anaemia), eosinophilia
U&E	Hyponatraemia, hyperkalaemia High urea (dehydration)
Glucose	Hypoglycaemia (particularly if acute illness, also commoner in children)
Calcium	Occasionally high (can mask hypocalcaemia if associated hypoparathyroidism)
LFTs	Rarely hypertransaminasaemia
Cortisol	Undetectable, low or normal
ACTH	Always high (> 80 ng/l)
Renin	Usually high (mineralocorticoid function can be preserved in autoimmune adrenalitis)
Aldosterone	Low or normal
Thyroid	Moderate elevation of TSH (usually <3 × ULN) – possibly secondary to loss of steroid suppression, sick euthyroid or autoimmune diease
Autoantibodies	Adrenal, thyroid, insulin, intrinsic factor

ACTH = adrenocorticotrophic hormone; FBC = full blood count;
LFTs = liver function tests; TSH = thyroid-stimulating hormone;
U&E = urea and electrolytes; ULN = upper limit of normal.

Accurate assessment of ACTH levels has led to a reduction in the need for further tests to confirm the diagnosis.

Short Synacthen test

This is the most widely used test for assessing the HPA axis even though it is a test only of adrenal responsiveness, not of the entire axis. The procedure involves administration of 250 µg of Synacthen intravenously/intramuscularly with blood samples taken at 0, 30 and 60 min.

The discussion on HPA axis testing is covered in Chapter 2 (hypopituitarism). A suggested protocol for management of the patient who is attempting discontinuation of therapeutic glucocorticoids is given in Box 6.1. The plasma cortisol should rise by at least 170 nmol/l to a peak of 580 nmol/l; the actual values will depend on the local laboratory. An impaired response confirms adrenal insufficiency but does not discriminate the level of the lesion in the axis.

Box 6.1   Protocol for management of the patient who is attempting discontinuation of therapeutic glucocorticoids

Most patients are able to discontinue steroids under supervision without endocrine tests. Occasionally, you will be asked by rheumatologists, neurologists or chest physicians about patients who have taken steroids for several years:

- Patient must be taking 5 mg prednisolone (or equivalent) or less a day
- Attempt alternate day steroids and test 48 hours after last dose
- Short Synacthen test. If failed response, give blue steroid card and repeat test in 4 months (the axis is likely to recover)
- Ensure patient is not taking 'topical', inhaled or intranasal steroids

---

Long Synacthen test

This test is now rarely used. It is indicated to confirm a diagnosis of primary adrenal insufficiency. Depot ACTH 1 mg is administered and serum cortisol is checked at 0, 30, 60 and 120 min and at 4, 8, 12 and 24 hours. In the setting of secondary adrenal deficiency, plasma cortisol levels fail to rise normally in the first hour but slowly rise to a peak at 24 hours as the atrophied adrenal glands recover secretory function. Table 6.6 demonstrates a normal response.

If glucocorticoid replacement is required in the lead up to metabolic testing, dexamethasone is the recommended supplement as it does not interfere with the cortisol assay. It should be discontinued 24 hours prior to the metabolic tests being performed.

Radiological tests

Radiological investigation is essential when dealing with secondary or tertiary adrenal insufficiency. It is of less importance in the management of Addison's disease with the following exceptions.

Table 6.6   Serum cortisol levels

Time	Serum cortisol, nmol/l (95% confidence limits)
60 min	605–1265
120 min	750–1520
4 hours	960–1650
8 hours	1025–1600
24 hours	609–1496

X-ray

Chest X-ray films are useful in the setting of TB or histoplasmosis and also frequently reveal a small heart.

CT abdomen

The computed tomography (CT) findings in TB or other granulomatous diseases are typically those of bilateral adrenal involvement: usually enlarged glands if TB is active and classically atrophic and calcified when non-active. Areas of non-enhancing necrosis and preserved contours of the glands are other common features. Enlarged adrenal glands or the presence of calcium excludes an autoimmune cause; however, absence of these features does not exclude TB.

Bilateral metastatic disease or adrenal haemorrhage is also demonstrated with a CT scan.

Echocardiogram

Reversible cardiomyopathy associated with Addison's disease has been reported in the literature and echocardiographic findings studied before and after replacement therapy. Left ventricular end-systolic and end-diastolic dimensions were significantly reduced in comparison to controls and there was an increase in the incidence of mitral valve disease. Echocardiographic and clinical findings resolved after steroid substitution.

It is postulated that a valvular–ventricular disproportion secondary to the hypovolaemic state may be responsible.

Pituitary imaging

Early reports of sella turcica enlargement on plain X-ray have been superseded by CT scan/magnetic resonance imaging (MRI), confirming increased pituitary size in patients with Addison's disease.

Microbiological tests

Tuberculosis. If this diagnosis is suspected because of clinical or radiological findings, confirmation of the diagnosis can be achieved with urine culture, tuberculin skin testing and polymerase chain reaction.

Fungal infections. Complement fixation titres for histoplasmosis should be obtained, as well as for more unusual fungal infections such as paracoccidioidomycosis, coccidioidomycosis, cryptomycosis and blastomycosis.

HIV. HIV and cryptococcal antibodies, CMV titres and culture for *Mycobacterium tuberculosis* and *M. avium-intracellulare.*

Electrocardiogram

Abnormalities reported on electrocardiogram (ECG) include those secondary to hyperkalaemia and also flattened or inverted T waves, prolonged QT interval and low QRS voltage, all of which resolve with steroid replacement.

Differential Diagnosis

The symptomatology of Addison's disease is many and varied, leading to an exhaustive list of differential diagnoses. Some features of adrenal failure are similar to those of chronic fatigue syndrome. The diagnosis should be confirmed biochemically in order to avoid the unindicated use of glucocorticoid therapy. It is important to clinically distinguish primary from secondary adrenal failure and to consider the diagnosis of anorexia nervosa.

Primary adrenal vs. secondary adrenal insufficiency

Hyperpigmentation is not seen in secondary or tertiary adrenal insufficiency because ACTH secretion is inadequate.

The other main difference is the presence of an intact adrenal zona glomerulosa that produces aldosterone in response to the renin–angiotensin system. Volume depletion, dehydration and shock are rarely encountered and therefore acute adrenal crisis is not a feature.

Hyperkalaemia does not occur in the presence of normal aldosterone levels; however, hyponatraemia is commonly seen, as cortisol has an important role in free water clearance.

Anorexia nervosa

Addisonian and anorexic patients exhibit clinical similarities, including nausea, vomiting, weight loss, abdominal pain, cold intolerance, hypothermia and orthostasis. They also display prolonged PR and QT intervals on ECG and generalised slowing on electroencephalogram (EEG). Clinical differences include a brown hyperpigmentation in Addison's disease in contrast to a yellowish colour in anorexia. Biochemical features that differ include hypocortisolism, hypoglycaemia and hyperkalaemia in a case of hypoadrenalism, as opposed to hypercortisolism, hyperglycaemia and hypokalaemia seen in anorexia.

Causes of generalised hyperpigmentation

1. Sun exposure
2. Liver disease (haemochromatosis, primary biliary cirrhosis)
3. Endocrine diseases (Cushing's syndrome, acromegaly, hyperthyroidism)
4. Pregnancy/oral contraceptive pill (OCP)
5. Carcinomatosis
6. Renal failure
7. Systemic sclerosis
8. Drugs (chloroquine, chlorpromazine, tetracycline, heavy metals)
9. Primary adrenal failure

Management

Acute addisonian crisis

Adrenal crisis is a medical emergency. The classical presentation is of a shocked, hypovolaemic, hypoglycaemic patient who requires immediate treatment that should not be delayed by laboratory investigations.

A blood sample should be taken for serum electrolytes, glucose and cortisol, followed by administration of high-dose intravenous glucocorticoids. Additional essential therapy includes volume replacement, correction of glucose and electrolyte abnormalities and treatment of coexisting or precipitating disorders.

The glucocorticoid of choice is hydrocortisone (100 mg, 6 hourly), with a tapering of this dose to maintenance levels after 1–3 days if progress is satisfactory. Some authors advocate the administration of a single dose of dexamethasone (4 mg) during the initial resuscitation. Dexamethasone has a long duration of action and does not interfere with subsequent cortisol assays.

Mineralocorticoids are not useful in the acute situation because they take several days to influence sodium retention, and adequate sodium replacement is achieved with intravenous saline. High doses of glucocorticoids used initially have sufficient mineralocorticoid effect. Mineralocorticoid therapy should be commenced when the hydrocortisone dose is below 50–60 mg/day.

After the initial resuscitation, precipitating conditions should be investigated and treated appropriately. This is commonly a bacterial infection or viral gastroenteritis, either in a previously undiagnosed patient or a patient with established adrenal insufficiency who does not or cannot increase his medication dose during a period of physiological stress. When stable, investigations such as the ACTH stimulation test or autoimmune assays can be performed as necessary.

The above guidelines can be summarised using the five S's of management: salt, sugar, steroids, support and search for a cause.

Chronic adrenal insufficiency

A combination of medical therapy and comprehensive education of the patient and his family allows for a full and active life with a normal life span (Box 6.2).

Box 6.2   Treatment of Addison's disease

1. Make diagnosis. A cortisol and ACTH will be useful, even if a short Synacthen test cannot be performed
2. Saline, may be 5–8 litres deficient, but treatment should not be too rapid as there may be a plasma : CSF (cerebrospinal fluid) osmolality difference
3. Glucocorticoid: hydrocortisone, 100 mg three times a day to start
4. Mineralocorticoid: not required at beginning, as glucocorticoid will suffice until replacement levels
5. Treat cause of Addison's disease (e.g. tuberculosis)
6. Treat precipitant of addisonian crisis (e.g. pneumonia)
7. Educate

Education

Patients should at all times wear a medical alert bracelet and carry a steroid information card with details of diagnosis and dose of steroid. The patient should understand the nature of the illness and replacement medications, with particular advice about the following situations.

Times of stress. Double or triple the glucocorticoid dose is necessary for mild to moderate infections. In the case of severe infection or major surgical procedures intravenous hydrocortisone is usually required (the dose is adjusted to the degree of surgical stress).

Gastroenteritis/vomiting. May require hospital admission for parenteral steroids.

Maintenance therapy

Glucocorticoid replacement therapy was traditionally given in the form of cortisone acetate (25–37.5 mg/day) or hydrocortisone (15–25 mg/day) in two or three divided doses. This regimen attempts to simulate the normal circadian rhythm with morning and post-lunch peaks and a trough between 6 p.m. and 3 a.m. Unfortunately, oral ingestion of hydrocortisone leads to a surge in serum cortisol levels that exceeds the capacity of cortisol-binding globulin (CBG) and therefore results in a rapid clearance within approximately 80 min. This may be responsible for complaints of symptoms of fatigue and nausea between doses as well as persistent hyperpigmentation secondary to inadequately suppressed ACTH.

For these reasons, long-acting glucocorticoids, such as dexamethasone (0.25–0.75 mg/day) or prednisone (2.5–7.5 mg/day), are often preferred. A smoother hormone profile is achieved and if taken at bedtime this regimen provides adequate cortisol activity on awakening and effective suppression of morning plasma ACTH levels.

Several studies have shown that a high proportion of patients on steroid replacement therapy are overtreated. There is not much hard evidence in the literature that excessive glucocorticoid replacement in this setting leads to adverse effects such as osteoporosis but it may exacerbate a tendency in those already predisposed to it. Individual assessment of replacement therapy is therefore not routinely advised. The goal of therapy is to ensure the patient receives the minimum dose necessary and has good symptom control. This may be evaluated using serial measurements of urinary cortisol excretion or a cortisol day curve, but there is no evidence to suggest this is better than clinical assessment of response to dose adjustments.

Mineralocorticoid replacement is usually required in cases of primary adrenal insufficiency. The natural hormones are aldosterone and 11-deoxycorticosterone (DOC) but these are not used as they are rapidly degraded by hepatic metabolism. The drug of choice is a synthetic mineralocorticoid, fludrocortisone given as a daily dose of 0.05–0.2 mg. If hydrocortisone is the glucocorticoid used, the dose required is lower, as this has some mineralocorticoid activity. During the summer, or exposure to high temperatures, the dose may need to be increased.

Routine monitoring includes standing/lying blood pressures and serum electrolytes, and some centres suggest plasma renin activity (PRA).

Oral dehydroepiandrosterone (DHEA) has recently been proposed as a potentially routine treatment for women with Addison's disease.

Traditionally, the lack of androgen production in adrenocortical failure has not been treated. One large study has shown a positive correlation between levels of DHEA and functional status and expressed sense of well-being in the elderly.

Another recent study demonstrated that DHEA levels were restored to normal in patients receiving 50 mg daily without any serious side effects. This was associated with a marked increase in psychological well-being in about half of the women studied. There was no significant change in insulin sensitivity, LDL/HDL (low-density lipoprotein/high-density lipoprotein) ratio or body mass composition. Within the next 10 years it is possible that females with Addison's disease will receive routine androgen replacement.

Exposure to long-term glucocorticoids

Patients with difficult-to-control asthma may have prolonged courses of oral prednisolone or other steroids. Recent advances in the management of chronic asthma (with methotrexate and inhaled corticosteroids with low systemic bioavailability) mean that patients may be slowly weaned. These patients may have adrenal atrophy, although this is secondary to exogenous steroid suppression of the hypothalamic and pituitary part of the axis. Assessment with short Synacthen tests may confirm adrenal failure (see Appendix 1, protocol 12).

The recommendation is that the dose of prednisolone is reduced very slowly (by 1 mg daily per month) once the patient is on 5 mg daily: thus, this should take at least 5 months.

Assessment of the HPA axis in this circumstance is difficult. Even 1 month after oral steroids have been discontinued, patients may fail a short Synacthen test (although they usually pass a long Synacthen test). ACTH does not have a role in treatment, as the defect lies in the hypothalamus and the pituitary rather than in the adrenal itself.

Reassessment of patients who have discontinued oral steroids 6 months previously shows that they will usually pass a short Synacthen test, even if they are on inhaled steroids.

Potencies of available steroids

The activity of steroids is dependent on many factors, including absorption, CBG affinity, hepatic metabolism and affinity for the glucocorticoid receptor. Synthetic steroids tend to be poorly bound to CBG and have a high affinity for the glucocorticoid receptor. Table 6.7 lists the comparative potencies of various steroid preparations.

Summary of steroid cover for surgery

- Minor procedure under local anaesthetic: usually no extra supplement required.
- Moderately stressful procedure (e.g. endoscopy/arteriography): hydrocortisone 100 mg intramuscularly/intravenously before procedure.

Table 6.7   Potencies of steroid preparations

Hormone	Glucocorticoid activity	Mineralocorticoid activity	Replacement dose (mg/day)
Hydrocortisone	1	1	15–30
Cortisone acetate	0.7	0.7	25–37.5
Prednisone	4	0.7	2.5–7.5
Methylprednisolone	5	0.5	
Dexamethasone	30	0	0.25–0.75
Fludrocortisone	10	400	0.05–0.2

- Major surgery: (1) Hydrocortisone 100 mg intravenously/intra-muscularly prior to induction of anaesthesia, continue 8 hourly for 24 hours. (2) If no complications, reduce dose to 25 mg 6-hourly for 24 hours; taper to maintenance dose over 3 to 5 days. (3) Increase to 400 mg/day if fever, hypotension or other problems; add fludrocortisone when patient resumes oral medication.

Pregnancy

Glucocorticoid and mineralocorticoid regimens are continued as usual, with occasional patients requiring increased glucocorticoid in the third trimester.

Labour is managed with intravenous saline and hydrocortisone 25 mg 6-hourly. This regimen is increased to 100 mg 6-hourly, during the delivery or if labour becomes complicated. In the postpartum period the dose can be tapered to maintenance within 3 days.

Addison's disease should be considered in any pregnant patient who presents with symptoms and signs of hyperemesis and electrolyte imbalance that does not improve with the usual measures.

Prognosis

Prior to the isolation and subsequent availability of glucocorticoids, Addison's disease was rapidly fatal within 2 years of diagnosis.

Since then, life expectancy has improved markedly and, with current regimens (including adequate medical therapy and education), it is similar to that of a normal population. The time of greatest risk is prior to diagnosis and, unfortunately, even today, the discovery is sometimes only made at postmortem examination.

Further Reading

Addison T. *On the Constitutional and Local Effects of Disease of the Supra-Renal Capsules.* London: Highley, 1855.

Betterle C, Greggio NA, Volpato M. Autoimmune polyglandular syndrome type 1. *J Clin Endocrinol Metab* 1998;**83**(4):1049–55.

Betterle C, Scalici C, Presotto F, *et al.* The natural history of adrenal function in autoimmune patients with adrenal autoantibodies. *J Endocrinol* 1988;**117**(3):467–75.

Betterle C, Volpato M, *et al.* Adrenal cortex and steroid 21-hydroxylase autoantibodies in children with organ-specific autoimmune diseases: markers of high progression to clinical Addison's disease. *J Clin Endocrinol Metab* 1997;**82**(3):939–42.

Bhatia E, Jain SK, Gupta RK, Pandey R. Tuberculous Addison's disease: lack of normalisation of adrenocortical function after antituberculous chemotherapy. *Clin Endocrinol (Oxf)* 1998;**48**(3):355–9.

Fallo F, Betterle C, Budano S, Lupia M, Boscaro M, Sonino N. Regression of cardiac abnormalities after replacement therapy in Addison's disease. *Eur J Endocrinol* 1999;**140**(5):425–8.

Ferreira JG, Borri ML, *et al.* Acute adrenal haemorrhage: diagnosis, treatment and follow-up. *Int Urol Nephrol* 1996;**28**(6):735–41.

Gebre-Medhin G, Husebye ES, *et al.* Oral dehydroepiandrosterone (DHEA) replacement therapy in women with Addison's disease. *Clin Endocrinol (Oxf)* 2000;**52**(6):775–80.

Jeffcoate W. Assessment of corticosteroid replacement therapy in adults with adrenal insufficiency. *Ann Clin Biochem* 1999;**36**(2):151–7.

Kaukinen K, Collin P, Mykkanen AH, Partanen J, Maki M, Salmi J. Celiac disease and autoimmune endocrinologic disorders. *Dig Dis Sci* 1999;**44**(7):1428–33.

Kendereski A, Micic D, Sumarac M *et al.* White Addison's disease: what is the possible cause? *J Endocrinol Invest* 1999;**22**(5):395–400.

Kong MF, Jeffcoate W. Eighty-six cases of Addison's disease. *Clin Endocrinol (Oxf)* 1994;**41**(6):757–61.

Laureti S, Casucci G, *et al.* X-linked adrenoleukodystrophy is a frequent cause of idiopathic Addison's disease in young adult male patients. *J Clin Endocrinol Metab* 1996;**81**(2):470–4.

McAulay V, Frier BM. Addison's disease in type 1 diabetes presenting with recurrent hypoglycaemia. *Postgrad Med J* 2000;**76**(894):230–2.

Maclaren NK, Riley WJ. Inherited susceptibility to autoimmune Addison's disease is linked to human leukocyte antigens-DR3 and/or DR4, except when associated with type-I autoimmune polyglandular syndrome. *J Clin Endocrinol Metab* 1986;**62**(3):455–9.

Orth DN, Kovacs WJ, DeBold CR. The Adrenal Cortex. In Wilson JD, Foster DW, eds. *Williams Textbook of Endocrinology* 8th edn. Philadelphia (PA): WB Saunders, 1992:9.505.

Parker LN, Levin ER, Lifrak ET. Evidence for adrenocortical adaptation to severe illness. *J Clin Endocrinol Metab* 1985;**60**(5):947–52.

Peacey SR, Guo CY, *et al.* Glucocorticoid replacement therapy: are patients overtreated and does it matter? *Clin Endocrinol* 1997;**46**(3):255–61.

Sadeghi-Nejad A, Senior B. Adrenoleukodystrophy presenting as Addison's disease in childhood. *N Eng J Med* 1990;**322**(1):13–16.

Seissler J, Schott M, Steinbrenner H, Peterson P, Scherbaum WA. Autoantibodies to adrenal cytochrome P450 antigens in isolated Addison's disease and autoimmune polyendocrine syndrome type II. *Exp Clin Endocrinol Diabetes* 1999;**107**(3):208–13.

Seminara SB, Oliveira LM, *et al.* Genetics of hypogonadotrophic hypogonadism. *J Endocrinol Invest* 2000;**23**(9):560–5.

Soderbergh A, Rorsman F, Halonen M *et al.* Autoantibodies against aromatic L-amino acid decarboxylase identifies a subgroup of patients with Addison's disease. *J Clin Endocrinol Metab* 2000;**85**(1):460–3.

Trainer PJ, Besser GM. *The Barts Endocrine Protocols.* London: Churchill Livingstone, 1995.

Zelissen PM, Bast EJ, Croughs RJ. Associated autoimmunity in Addison's disease. *J Autoimmun* 1995;**8**(1):121–30.

7

Congenital Adrenal Hyperplasia

Karim Meeran

Introduction

Congenital adrenal hyperplasia (CAH) is a group of inherited conditions caused by defective activity of one of the five enzymes involved in the synthesis of cortisol from cholesterol. The biochemical pathway of steroid synthesis (Figure 7.1) also applies to steroidogenesis in the ovary (see Chapter 8) and testis (see Chapter 9).

The term 'adrenal hyperplasia' refers to the tendency for the adrenals to become enlarged under the influence of excessive adrenocorticotrophic hormone (ACTH). Many of the enzymes that hydroxylate steroids are members of the cytochrome P450 family of enzymes: the nomenclature P450c21 refers to this, the carbon atom (c21) in the steroid molecule being the one that is hydroxylated by the enzyme.

The commonest form of CAH is caused by 21-hydroxylase deficiency, which results in high concentrations of substrate before the block (17-hydroxyprogesterone) and reduced concentrations of products after the block (11-deoxycortisol and cortisol). Since the same enzyme is active on the aldosterone synthesising pathway, there will be mineralocorticoid deficiency also.

The manifestations of each of the CAHs are thus due to both the excessive amount of some steroids and the deficiency of others. The degree to which these are clinically apparent depends on the residual activity of the relevant enzymes.

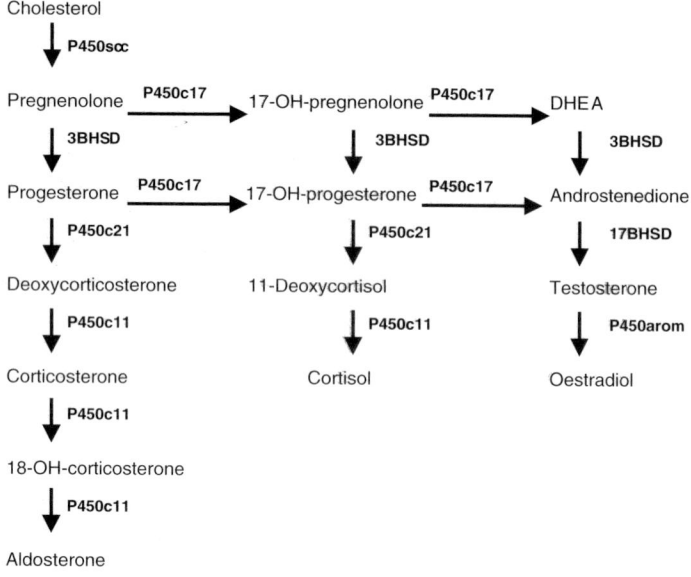

Figure 7.1 Steroid biosynthesis.

Complete 21-Hydroxylase (P450c21) Deficiency

Total ablation of this enzyme activity occurs due to deletion or a nonsense mutation in the *CYP21B* gene. This occurs in about 1:14,000 live births worldwide, with a predominance in some populations. These patients are unable to synthesise any glucocorticoid or mineralocorticoid, and so will present with a salt-losing (addisonian) crisis early, with hyponatraemia, hyperkalaemia and hypovolaemic shock. They are also exposed to increased concentrations of androgens *in utero*, and hence will be virilised. In genotypic girls, this may result in ambiguous genitalia. Occasionally, female neonates are thought to be boys.

Thus females, with ambiguous genitalia are at risk of an addisonian crisis, and should be kept in hospital. Electrolytes and a urine steroid profile should be measured.

Partial 21-Hydroxylase Deficiency (Simple Virilising CAH)

Rather that total ablation of the enzyme, here the enzyme activity is severely limited, to either between 1 and 2% of normal, or (at the milder end of the spectrum) to between 20 and 60% of normal. These children usually synthesise enough cortisol and aldosterone to prevent an addisonian crisis, and thus usually present with the manifestations of excess androgens. There are a large number of different mutations that result from unequal crossing over of the *CYP21B* gene (active normal gene) with a pseudogene (known as *CYP21A* or *CYP21P*). Thus, the phenotypic appearance of these individuals is variable, from severe virilisation to mild hirsutism.

Polycystic ovaries are a feature of several conditions, including CAH, Cushing's syndrome and the polycystic ovary syndrome (PCOS). The finding in a woman of a testosterone > 5 nmol/l should arouse suspicion that the aetiology may not be PCOS. The excess adrenal androgens result in some suppression of the gonadotrophins – luteinising hormone (LH) and follicle-stimulating hormone (FSH) – which can, in turn, lead to infertility in both males and females. The milder end of the spectrum (where the enzyme activity of 21-hydroxylase is between 20 and 60% of normal) may affect as many as 1% of the general population who present with mild hirsutism if female, or may not have any clinical phenotype in males.

The serum concentration of 17-hydroxyprogesterone may be only marginally raised, or in the normal range. Thus, a dynamic test may be required to confirm the diagnosis. It is important to carry out this test in the early follicular phase, when progesterone levels are low. In patients with irregular cycles, measuring a serum progesterone at the same time as the 17-hydroxyprogesterone can avoid any doubt. If this is raised to >5 nmol/l, this is suspicious of possible CAH. A short Synacthen test with measurement of both cortisol and 17-hydroxyprogesterone should be carried out in this circumstance. Individuals with CAH may fail to have an adequate rise in cortisol (peak < 550 nmol/l) with a generous concentration of 17-hydroxyprogesterone.

In a hirsute woman, the differential diagnosis includes an adrenal or ovarian tumour, Cushing's syndrome and polycystic ovarian disease. Suppression of the androgens with dexamethasone excludes an autonomous steroid-producing tumour, and the stimulation test above (short Synacthen test) confirms or excludes CAH. Management of the hirsute woman is covered more fully in Chapter 8.

11β-Hydroxylase (P450c11) Deficiency

It is important to note that the precursor deoxycorticosterone (on the pathway to aldosterone) is a mineralocorticoid receptor agonist, and can thus result in sodium retention, hypokalaemia, volume expansion, suppressed plasma renin activity (PRA) and hypertension (see Chapter 22). This hypertension is often absent in young children, so it is important to distinguish 21-hydroxylase deficiency (common) from 11-hydroxylase deficiency. One of the commonest pitfalls is an apparent salt-losing crisis in one of these children, who have an intercurrent illness such as gastroenteritis. The label of 21-hydroxylase deficiency may stick for several years until hypertension becomes apparent years later. Measuring 11-deoxycortisol (compound S) levels are helpful, as these are raised in 11-hydroxylase deficiency but are low in both forms of 21-hydroxylase deficiency. Both conditions result in high levels of 17-hydroxyprogesterone levels, and hence virilisation. Treatment with replacement hydrocortisone usually results in resolution of the hypertension by suppressing deoxycorticosterone production.

The plasma concentration of the intermediates reflects the intra-adrenal levels poorly, so that levels of 17-OHP in the plasma are often higher than 11-deoxycortisol levels even in patients with 11-hydroxylase deficiency.

17α-Hydroxylase (P450c17) Deficiency

This enzyme deficiency results in a deficiency of sex steroids (and hence androgens), so that there is incomplete development of the external genitalia in both sexes. In males there is incomplete development of the external genitalia and, in females, oestrogen deficiency results in failure to develop secondary sexual characteristics at the age of puberty. Thus, teenagers may present with apparent delayed puberty and have no evidence of secondary sexual characteristics. The same enzyme is expressed in the gonads, so that no androgens can be produced either by the gonads or by the adrenals.

In addition, shunting of pregnenolone into the mineralocorticoid pathway results in excess 11-deoxycorticosterone and aldosterone, both of which are mineralocorticoid receptor agonists. This results in hypertension with hypokalaemic alkalosis, similar to that in 11-hydroxylase deficiency, but without the effects of excess androgens. Biochemically, these individuals may be confused with individuals with Conn's syndrome with bilateral adrenal hyperplasia.

3β-Hydroxysteroid Dehydrogenase Deficiency

This enzyme is responsible for the conversion of Δ_5 to Δ_4 steroids, where Δ refers to the position of the double bond in the steroid molecule. Thus, Δ_5 3β-hydroxysteroids (pregnenolone, 17-hydroxypregnenolone and dehydroepiandrosterone (DHEA)) are converted to Δ_4 3-ketosteroids (progesterone, 17-hydroxyprogesterone and androstenedione). There is deficiency of cortisol, excess pregnenolone (which is ineffective as a mineralocorticoid) and excess DHEA, which is only weakly androgenic. Thus, there is ambiguity of both genotypic males and females.

These individuals often present with salt wasting, and are thought to have classical 21-hydroxylase deficiency. However, puberty may be delayed, resulting in the diagnosis being revisited.

P450scc (20,22-Desmolase) Deficiency

This enzyme catalyses the initial reaction for steroid synthesis from cholesterol. This is an extremely rare condition, with only 30 cases reported worldwide. Complete deficiency will result in global adrenocortical failure, with salt wasting.

A summary of the clinical features of the deficiencies is presented in Table 7.1. Box 7.1 presents what the specialist registrar

---

**Box 7.1   What to do when presented with a
neonate or child with ambiguous genitalia**

Endocrine SPRs may be contacted for advice shortly after a neonate is born with ambiguous genitalia. Proceed as follows:

1. Warn the obstetricians and paediatricians that the child is at risk of an addisonian crisis and must not be sent home
2. Examine the neonate, looking in particular for features of hypotension
3. Examine the genitalia to confirm that they are ambiguous
4. Arrange for electrolytes to be checked urgently and make sure the samples are sent immediately. Also take blood for steroids, including cortisol, 17-hydroxyprogesterone and 11-deoxycortisol (compound S). A serum sample will be adequate for these, as steroids are stable. A spot urine should be sent for a urinary steroid profile. A blood sample should also be sent for an adrenocorticotrophic hormone (ACTH) level at the same time. This must be sent urgently as, unlike steroids, ACTH is unstable and thus needs to get to your laboratory urgently

(Continued)

Box 7.1　contd

5.　There is no excuse for an addisonian crisis occurring and hydrocortisone should be administered as soon as possible

6.　Arrange a buccal smear to be examined for Barr bodies. If one is present, this confirms that the child is 46XX, and the child has therefore been virilised, causing the ambiguity. If there is no Barr body (unlikely), then the child may be 46XY and has been feminised

Table 7.1　Clinical features of steroid enzyme deficiencies

Enzyme deficiency	Virilisation/ambiguity	Salt loss	Blood pressure
21 complete	XX virilised/ambiguous XY precocious (not ambiguous)	May have adrenal salt-losing crisis	Low
21 partial	XX virilised/ambiguous XY precocious (not ambiguous)	Mild	Normal
11-Hydroxylase deficiency	XX virilised/ambiguous XY precocious (not ambiguous)	None	High blood pressure with hypokalaemia
17-Hydroxylase deficiency	Failure of normal sexual development. Males may appear ambiguous because of lack of development. Females may present with apparent pubertal failure	None	High blood pressure with hypokalaemia
3β-Hydroxysteroid dehydrogenase deficiency	Ambiguity in both directions with hypospadias in males (testosterone deficiency) and clitoromegaly in females (DHEA excess)	May have adrenal salt-losing crisis	Low

DHEA = dehydroepiandrosterone.

A summary of the clinical features of the deficiencies is presented in Table 7.1. Box 7.1 presents what the specialist registrar should do when faced with the clinical problem of ambiguous genitalia.

Prenatal Diagnosis

CAH is autosomal recessive. The gene for 21-hydroxylase is on chromosome 6, whereas that for 11-hydroxylase is on chromosome 8.

In families with one affected individual, there is thus a 25% risk of subsequent pregnancies being affected. The critical time to prevent ambiguous female genitalia is to suppress androgens at least between weeks 5 and 13 of pregnancy. This can be carried out by administration of dexamethasone to the mother as soon as she misses her first period. This is clearly too early to have any form of prenatal diagnosis, and will only be of benefit to those who are XX, preventing ambiguity. Ideally, affected females and their partners should have genetic counselling before conception.

Treatment

All the forms of CAH discussed above require hydrocortisone replacement. In neonates, the dose used is discussed in Chapter 24. The aims of treatment are not only to replace the missing glucocorticoid but also to suppress ACTH and, hence, the excessive androgens. The dosing and timing of glucocorticoid replacement is controversial, because some paediatricians use long-acting glucocorticoids at night (e.g. dexamethasone 0.5 mg *nocte*) to maximally suppress ACTH and androgen production, with approximately 0.2 mg in the morning. This is obviously the *REVERSE* of the usual circadian rhythm, but is justified on the grounds of inhibiting virilisation or hisutism. This may result in Cushing's syndrome. The relative potencies of the various glucocorticoids are given in Table 6.7.

A more physiological replacement is that used in patients with adrenal or pituitary failure. This treatment requires approximately 10 mg hydrocortisone first thing in the morning, with 5 mg at noon and a further 5 mg at about 6 p.m. This gives patients a normal replacement, but may not adequately suppress androgens, and may thus have an impact on the rate of progression of puberty. Whereas adrenal androgens are not responsible for puberty, they can induce true precocious puberty, by 'priming' the hypothalamo–pituitary–gonadal axis.

Rather than using excess glucocorticoid to suppress virilisation, some authors have suggested the use of anti-androgens. A few severely affected patients have been subjected to adrenalectomy to remove the source of excess androgens, and are then given hydrocortisone in standard doses for replacement, as in the treatment of Addison's disease.

Further Reading

New MI, Lorenzen F, Lerner AJ *et al*. Genotyping steroid 21-hydroxylase deficiency: hormonal reference data. *J Clin Endocrinol Metab* 1983;**57**:320–6.

Savage MO. Congenital adrenal hyperplasia. *Clin Endocrinol Metab* 1985;**14**:893–909.

Speiser PW, White PC. Congenital adrenal hyperplasia due to steroid 21-hydroxylase deficiency. *Clin Endocrinol* 1998;**49**:411–17.

8

Reproductive Endocrinology

Andrew Rodin

The Menstrual Cycle

The normal menstrual cycle is a complex feedback system, consisting of stimulatory and inhibitory hormone signals that result in the release of a single mature oocyte. A variety of factors contribute to the regulation of this process, including hormones, paracrine and autocrine factors.

The first day of menses represents the first day of the cycle. The follicular phase begins with the onset of menses and ends on the day of the luteinising hormone (LH) surge. The luteal phase begins on the day of the LH surge and ends at the onset of the next menses.

The average adult menstrual cycle lasts 28 days, with approximately 14 days in the follicular phase and 14 days in the luteal phase. There is relatively little cycle variability among women between the ages of 20 and 40, but there is more cycle variability for the first 5–7 years after menarche and for the last 10 years before complete cessation of menses. Women in their 40s tend to have slightly shorter cycles. Changes in cycle length are primarily due to changes in the follicular phase, with the luteal phase remaining relatively constant.

Evaluation of the menstrual cycle and timing of ovulation

The methods of menstrual cycle evaluation are given in Table 8.1.

Table 8.1   Methods of menstrual cycle evaluation

- Menstrual cycle charting
- Basal body temperature monitoring
- Measurement of follicle size
- Measurement of the serum progesterone concentration
- Detection of the LH surge

LH = luteinising hormone.

Menstrual cycle charting

- Simple and inexpensive.
- The patient records the onset and cessation of menses for several months in succession.
- The patient should also note symptoms, which can be a useful clinical indicator of normal reproductive hormone cycling, including an increase in thin cervical mucus secretions at mid-cycle and premenstrual changes, such as menstrual cramps, breast tenderness and appetite or mood changes.

Basal body temperature monitoring

- Progesterone released from the corpus luteum at the time of ovulation has potent effects on the hypothalamus, one of which is to increase body temperature. Daily temperature monitoring can therefore be used to reflect progesterone production and hence previous ovulation.
- The woman takes her temperature every morning while she is still in the basal state. An approximately 0.5°F (0.3°C) rise in body temperature can be detected in the luteal phase of the menstrual cycle compared to the follicular phase. In a normal cycle, the temperature rise begins 1 or 2 days after the LH surge and persists for at least 10 days. The subsequent fall in basal body temperature can be used as an indicator of the onset of menses.

Measurement of follicle size

- Follicle tracking using ultrasound is used to detect the preovulatory follicle, which is usually more than 18 mm in diameter.

Serum progesterone concentration

- Another simple test is measurement of the serum progesterone level in the mid-luteal phase 18 to 24 days after the onset of menses. A progesterone concentration above 30 nmol/l suggests that ovulation has occurred in that cycle.

Detection of the LH surge

- Measurement of LH in mid-cycle using urine strip tests can be used to detect the LH surge.

Premenstrual Syndrome

The premenstrual syndrome (PMS) is characterised by the presence of both physical and behavioural symptoms that occur repetitively in the second half of the menstrual cycle. Symptoms of the premenstrual syndrome are given in Table 8.2. Other common symptoms include acne, oversensitivity to environmental stimuli, anger, easy crying and gastrointestinal upset. Hot flushes, heart palpitations and dizziness occur in 15–20% of patients.

Diagnosis

The diagnosis of PMS depends upon a variety of criteria including:

- symptoms of PMS
- the timing with which these symptoms occur
- the severity of the symptoms
- the absence of hormone or drug ingestion
- the absence of other medical conditions which could cause these symptoms.

Table 8.2   Symptoms of the premenstrual cycle

	Symptoms	Prevalence
Physical	Abdominal bloating	90%
	Breast tenderness	>50%
	Headaches	>50%
Behavioural	Extreme sense of fatigue	>90%
	Tension	>80%
	Irritability	>80%
	Labile mood	>80%
	Depressed mood	>80%
	Increased appetite	70%
	Forgetfulness	>50%
	Difficulty concentrating	>50%

Differential diagnosis

The differential diagnosis of premenstrual syndrome includes:

- psychiatric disorders
- perimenopause.

In women with PMS, the concurrent incidence of affective disorder is approximately 50%. Women who present with PMS have a much higher incidence of previous depression and are thought to be at greater risk for depression in the future. Women with PMS consume more alcohol than women without PMS.

Treatment of premenstrual syndrome

A large number of therapies have been used in PMS. They can be classified according to their effectiveness (Table 8.3).

The overall response rate to treatment with fluoxetine at a daily dose of 20 mg is 60–75% and the beneficial response is maintained for many years. Higher doses cause more side effects while not providing more benefit. The most common reasons for failure to continue the treatment are headache, anxiety and nausea, the combined incidence of which is approximately 15%.

'Medical oophorectomy' with a gonadotrophin-releasing hormone (GnRH) agonist, such as leuprorelin, is beneficial in PMS although the physical symptoms may be more responsive than mood symptoms. Furthermore, side effects (particularly those related to hypo-oestrogenism) may limit the use of these drugs for long-term therapy. However, symptom relief is maintained by the addition of oestrogen/progestogen replacement, without a negative impact on endometrial histology, bone density or lipid profiles.

Table 8.3   Effectiveness of premenopausal therapies

Efffective	Possibly effective	Ineffective
Fluoxetine	Oral contraceptives	Progesterone
Sertraline	Exercise and relaxation	Tricyclic antidepressants
Nefazodone	techniques	Monoamine oxidase
GnRH agonist	Diuretics	inhibitors
GnRH agonist +		Lithium
'add-back' therapy		Diet and vitamin
Danazol		supplements

GnRH = gonadotrophin-releasing hormone.

Danazol inhibits pituitary gonadotrophin secretion and, when given in sufficient doses to inhibit ovulation, is an effective therapy for PMS. However, the androgenic side effects of danazol limit its use to patients who fail to respond adequately to other therapies.

A protocol for the clinical management of PMS

1. Establish the diagnosis:

    *   presence of typical symptoms
    *   symptom-free during the follicular phase.

2. If there is no socioeconomic dysfunction, consider exercise and relaxation therapy first. Use drug treatment if these therapies do not provide relief.

3. In PMS with socioeconomic dysfunction, start on treatment immediately with fluoxetine 20 mg/day.

4. If there are significant side effects from fluoxetine, try either a lower starting dose or a second selective serotonin re-uptake inhibitor (SSRI) such as sertraline.

5. Patients who do not respond to SSRIs are candidates for ovulation suppression agents. A GnRH agonist, such as leuprorelin (3.75 mg every 4 weeks) is preferable to danazol because of the more favourable side-effect profile. In patients who respond well to GnRH agonists, therapy may be extended beyond 6 months with 'add-back' oestrogen/progestogen therapy.

Amenorrhoea

Amenorrhoea (absence of menses) can be a transient, intermittent or permanent condition resulting from dysfunction of the hypothalamus, pituitary, ovaries, uterus or vagina. It is classified as either primary (absence of menarche by age 16) or secondary (absence of menses for more than three cycle intervals or 6 months in women who previously had menses).

Causes of amenorrhoea due to abnormalities in the hypothalamic–pituitary–ovarian axis are given in Table 8.4.

Primary Amenorrhoea

Causes

Primary amenorrhoea is usually the result of a genetic or anatomical abnormality. However, most causes of secondary amenorrhoea

Table 8.4   Amenorrhea due to abnormalities in the hypothalamic–pituitary–ovarian axis

Abnormality	Causes
Hypothalamic dysfunction	• Functional – weight loss, eating disorders, exercise, stress, severe or prolonged illness • Congenital GnRH deficiency • Inflammatory or infiltrative diseases • Tumours, e.g. craniopharyngioma • Pituitary stalk damage • Cranial irradiation • Brain injury – trauma, haemorrhage, hydrocephalus • Syndromes – Prader–Willi, Laurence–Moon–Biedl
Pituitary dysfunction	• Hyperprolactinaemia • Other pituitary tumours – acromegaly, Cushing's syndrome • Other tumours – meningioma, glioma, germinoma • Empty sella syndrome • Pituitary infarct or apoplexy
Ovarian dysfunction	• Ovarian failure – spontaneous, premature, surgical • Polycystic ovary syndrome
Other	• Hyperthyroidism • Hypothyroidism • Exogenous androgen use

GnRH = gonadotrophin-releasing hormone.

can present as primary amenorrhoea. The most common causes are given in Table 8.5.

Congenital anatomical abnormalities

Menses cannot occur without an intact uterus, endometrium, cervix, cervical os and vaginal opening.

Imperforate hymen. An imperforate hymen may be associated with cyclical pelvic pain and a perirectal mass from sequestration of blood (haematocolpos). This condition is diagnosed by physical examination and is easily corrected with surgery.

Transverse vaginal septum. One or more transverse vaginal septa can occur at any level between the hymenal ring and the cervix.

Table 8.5 Causes of primary amenorrhoea

Chromosomal abnormalities causing gonadal dysgenesis	45%
Physiological delay of puberty	20%
Müllerian agenesis	15%
Transverse vaginal septum or imperforate hymen	5%
Absent production of gonadotrophin-releasing hormone (GnRH)	5%
Anorexia nervosa	2%
Hypopituitarism	2%
Other causes: prolactinoma, craniopharyngioma, hypothyroidism, ovarian failure, and adrenal disease	1%

After menarche, the clinical picture is similar to that associated with an imperforate hymen.

Abnormal müllerian development

Mayer–Rokitansky–Küster–Hauser syndrome is characterised by agenesis or partial agenesis of the müllerian structures (fallopian tubes, uterus and upper-third of vagina) in 46XX women.

Androgen insensitivity syndrome (testicular feminisation) is an X-linked recessive disorder in which 46XY individuals are resistant to testosterone due to a defect in the androgen receptor. The phenotype is often voluptuously feminine. The external genitalia are typically female in appearance, but testes may be palpable in the labia or inguinal area. The testes make müllerian inhibiting substance which causes regression of all müllerian structures. Breast development occurs at puberty but pubic and axillary hair is sparse. The diagnosis of this disorder is based upon the absence of the upper vagina, uterus and fallopian tubes on physical examination and pelvic ultrasonography, serum testosterone levels in the male range and a male 46XY karyotype. The testes should be surgically excised after puberty because of the increased risk (2–5%) of developing testicular cancer after age 25.

Vanishing testes syndrome occurs in 46XY individuals who appear to be normal females. The gonads apparently fail to develop in this disorder, and the resulting phenotype depends upon when the failure occurred. Early failure prior to testicular development (before about 8 weeks of gestation) is associated with streak-like inactive gonads that never produce testosterone, oestrogen or müllerian inhibiting substance. This results in feminisation of both the internal and external genitalia and gonadal failure. A later onset of testicular failure results in variable abnormalities. The diagnosis of the vanishing testes syndrome is made from the findings of gonadal failure, lack of progression through puberty and elevated serum follicle-stimulating hormone (FSH) and LH concentrations in the presence of a male karyotype. Since the risk of developing a gonadal tumour (gonadoblastoma or dysgerminoma) is of the order of 30%, early removal of testicular remnants is recommended.

Ovarian abnormalities

The main ovarian causes of primary amenorrhoea are ovarian failure due to chromosomal abnormalities, primarily Turner's syndrome, and polycystic ovary syndrome (PCOS).

Turner's syndrome. Women with Turner's syndrome usually have a 45X0 karyotype. Amenorrhoea occurs because the ovaries are replaced with fibrous tissue and do not produce significant amounts of oestrogen. The external genitalia, uterus and fallopian tubes develop normally until puberty but then oestrogen-dependent maturation fails to occur. Oestrogen and cyclical progesterone replacement at puberty will result in normal pubertal development: growth of pubic and axillary hair; breast growth; cyclical vaginal bleeding; and growth and maturation of the uterus and external genitalia. Some women have a mosaic karyotype (45X0/46XX). They may have amenorrhoea but, in some cases, there is spontaneous menstruation and pregnancy may occur. Partial deletions and structural rearrangements of the X chromosome can also result in primary or secondary amenorrhoea and the Turner phenotype. In addition, some cases of gonadal dysgenesis result from autosomal recessive inheritance (46XX gonadal dysgenesis), but these cases lack the somatic features of Turner's syndrome.

Polycystic ovary syndrome. Typically, the menstrual disturbances in PCOS have a peripubertal onset. Some women may present with primary amenorrhoea, but more commonly there is a normal or slightly delayed menarche followed by irregular cycles or secondary amenorrhoea.

Other causes of ovarian failure. Autoimmune ovarian failure and chemotherapy or radiation-induced ovarian failure may present as primary amenorrhoea but more commonly present as secondary amenorrhoea.

Hypothalamic and pituitary disease

A common cause of primary amenorrhoea is functional hypothalamic amenorrhoea. Less commonly, tumours and infiltrative lesions of the hypothalamus or pituitary can result in amenorrhoea. These are covered in Chapter 2.

Congenital GnRH deficiency. Primary amenorrhoea can be due to congenital GnRH deficiency. This syndrome is called idiopathic hypogonadotrophic hypogonadism or, if it is associated with anosmia, Kallmann's syndrome. Affected women have apulsatile and low levels of serum gonadotrophins due to the absence of hypothalamic GnRH. Congenital GnRH deficiency can be inherited as an autosomal dominant, autosomal recessive or X-linked condition, but more than two-thirds of cases are sporadic.

Constitutional delay of puberty. Constitutional delay is characterised by both delayed adrenarche and gonadarche, and is often difficult to distinguish clinically from congenital GnRH deficiency. Girls with constitutional delay go on to have completely normal pubertal development.

Hypothalamic amenorrhoea. Functional hypothalamic amenorrhoea (FHA) is characterised by abnormal hypothalamic GnRH secretion, leading to altered gonadotrophin secretion. Serum LH levels are low or normal and serum oestradiol is low. Serum FSH levels are often in the normal range, with a high FSH to LH ratio that is similar to the pattern seen in prepubertal girls. Multiple factors may contribute to the pathogenesis of FHA, including eating disorders such as anorexia nervosa, exercise and stress. Both weight loss below a certain target level (approximately 10% below ideal body weight) and exercise are associated with amenorrhoea. There is, however, marked variability between subjects in the degree of weight loss or exercise required to induce amenorrhoea. Most cases of amenorrhoea associated with exercise are also accompanied by weight loss or a severe decrease in percentage body fat.

Hyperprolactinaemia. Hyperprolactinaemia is a rare cause of primary amenorrhoea. It is associated with galactorrhoea in 50 to 80% of cases.

Other infiltrative diseases of the hypothalamus and pituitary. These can result in reduced GnRH release, low or normal serum gonadotrophin concentrations and amenorrhoea. These include craniopharyngioma, germinoma, Langerhans cell histiocytosis, sarcoidosis and haemochromatosis. These are more fully covered in Chapters 1 and 2.

Diagnostic evaluation

Key points in the history of primary amenorrhoea are given in Table 8.6.

Key points in the examination of primary amenorrhoea are given in Table 8.7.

Table 8.6   History of primary amenorrhoea

History	Interpretation
Lack of pubertal development	Suggests ovarian or pituitary failure or chromosomal abnormality
Family history of delayed or absent puberty	Suggests genetic disorder
Short stature	May indicate Turner's syndrome or hypothalamic–pituitary disease
Poor neonatal/childhood health	Neonatal crisis might suggest congenital adrenal hyperplasia. Poor health may be a manifestation of hypothalamic–pituitary disease
Symptoms of hyperandrogenism or virilisation	Consider ovarian or adrenal causes of androgen excess
Recent stress, illness, change in weight, diet, eating behaviour or exercise	Might suggest functional hypothalamic amenorrhoea
Systemic disease, e.g. sarcoidosis	May cause hypothalamic amenorrhoea
Galactorrhoea	Consider causes of hyperprolactinaemia
Visual field defects, headaches, fatigue, polyuria, polydipsia	Consider hypothalamic–pituitary disease

Table 8.7   Examination of primary amenorrhoea

Examination	
Evaluation of pubertal development	Current height, weight and arm span (normal arm span for adults is within 5 cm of height) and an evaluation of the woman's growth chart
Assessment of breast development	By Tanner staging
Genital examination	To assess clitoral size, pubertal hair development, intactness of the hymen, depth of the vagina, and presence of a cervix, uterus and ovaries
Examination of the skin	To look for hirsutism, acne, striae, increased pigmentation, vitiligo, acanthosis nigricans
Features of Turner's syndrome	Low hair line, webbed neck, shield chest, widely spaced nipples, hypertension with radio-femoral pulse delay

Figure 8.1 summarises the investigative pathways to exclude
congenital abnormalities as a cause for primary amenorrohea.

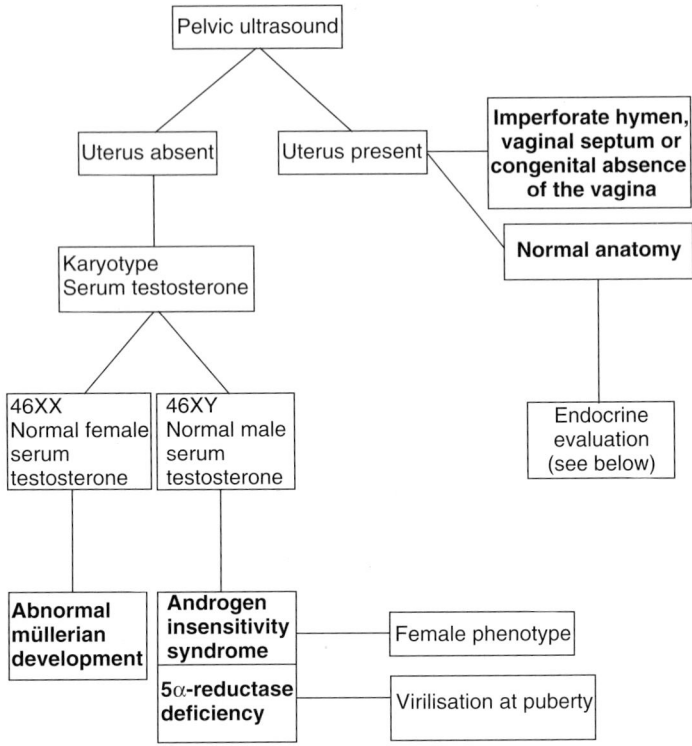

Figure 8.1   Investigations in primary amenorrohea to exclude
congenital anatomical causes.

Figure 8.2 summarises an approach to the endocrine assessment of women with primary amenorrohea.

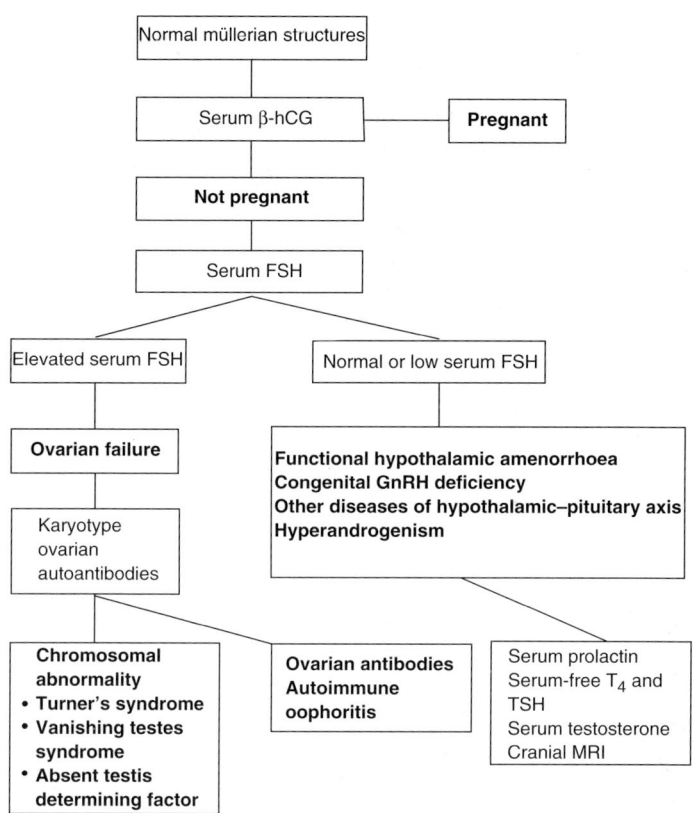

Figure 8.2   A stepwise approach to the endocrine evaluation of women with primary amenorrohea.

Secondary Amenorrhoea

Secondary amenorrhoea is defined as the absence of menses for more than three cycle intervals or 6 months in women who previously had menses. The menstrual cycle is susceptible to outside influences and so a single missed period is rarely significant.

Causes of secondary amenorrhoea

Pregnancy is the most common cause of secondary amenorrhoea. After excluding pregnancy, the most common causes of secondary amenorrhoea are

- ovarian disease (40%)
- hypothalamic dysfunction (35%)
- pituitary disease (19%)
- uterine disease (5%)
- other (1%).

Ovarian disease

Polycystic ovary syndrome (PCOS) accounts for approximately 20% of cases of amenorrhoea. The excess androgens in this disorder can come from the ovaries and/or the adrenal glands. Diagnostic criteria include hyperandrogenism and oligomenorrhea or amenorrhoea. In PCOS, hyperandrogenism is usually manifested clinically as acne and/or hirsutism and chemically as an elevation in the serum concentration of at least one androgen. Important features are its peripubertal onset and worsening with weight gain. In women with a short history, later onset of symptoms or evidence of virilisation, other diagnoses, such as ovarian or adrenal tumours and late-onset congenital adrenal hyperplasia, should be considered.

Ovarian failure usually occurs at approximately 50 years of age during the course of normal menopause but occurs before age 40 in approximately 5% of amenorrhoeic women. This syndrome is called premature menopause or premature ovarian failure. Premature ovarian failure can be idiopathic, or associated with autoimmune ovarian destruction, chromosomal abnormalities, radiation therapy or chemotherapy.

The lack of ovarian function leads to oestrogen deficiency, endometrial atrophy and the absence of menstruation. The perimenopausal period may be characterised by a waxing and waning clinical course with intermittent follicular development, oestradiol production and menstrual bleeding. Loss of the negative feedback effect of oestradiol on the hypothalamus and pituitary results in elevated serum FSH. This will distinguish ovarian failure from hypothalamic amenorrhoea in which the serum FSH concentration is low or normal.

Hypothalamic dysfunction

One of the most common types of secondary amenorrhoea is FHA. By definition, this excludes pathological disease. Although rare, infiltrative diseases of the hypothalamus can cause secondary amenorrhoea.

FHA is characterised by a decrease in GnRH pulse frequency and amplitude as a result of one or more of the following: low body weight; low body fat; poor nutrition; stress; or strenuous exercise. A small percentage of patients with FHA have no obvious precipitating factor for their amenorrhoea.

Weight loss to approximately 10% below ideal body weight and exercise are associated with amenorrhoea. There is, however, marked inter-patient variability in the degree of weight loss or exercise required to induce amenorrhoea. Most cases of amenorrhoea associated with exercise are also associated with weight loss, and normal cycles may be maintained if caloric intake is sufficient to match the energy expenditure. Diet and body composition are also important. Severe restriction of fat consumption and decreased body fat mass are associated with amenorrhoea. Emotional stress and stress induced by illness are additional causes of hypothalamic amenorrhoea.

Infiltrative lesions of the hypothalamus (e.g. lymphoma, Langerhans cell histiocytosis or sarcoidosis) can result in diminished GnRH secretion, low or normal serum gonadotrophin levels and amenorrhoea. Haemochromatosis should also be considered if there is an appropriate family history or if the patient has other suggestive manifestations such as bronzed skin, diabetes mellitus or otherwise unexplained heart or liver disease. However, these conditions are rare compared with FHA.

Pituitary disease

A prolactin-secreting pituitary tumour is responsible for almost 20% of cases of secondary amenorrhoea and is the most common pituitary cause (90%). Hyperprolactinaemia has a similar presentation to FHA but there is the additional finding of galactorrhoea in 50–80%

of women. The empty sella syndrome, hypothyroidism and other types of pituitary tumours account for the majority of the remaining cases of pituitary origin.

Uterine disease

Asherman's syndrome is the only uterine cause of secondary amenorrhoea. It results from scarring of the endometrial lining, which is usually secondary to postpartum haemorrhage or endometrial infection followed by instrumentation such as a dilatation and curettage. This condition prevents the normal build-up and shedding of endometrial cells, leading to absent menses.

Clinical evaluation

The clinical evaluation of secondary amenorrhoea is given in Table 8.8.

Management of amenorrhoea

Aims

- To correct the underlying pathology, if possible.
- To help the woman to achieve fertility if desired.
- To prevent complications of the disease process.

Counselling. All women with amenorrhoea should be counselled regarding its cause, treatment and their reproductive potential.

Surgery. This is often required in patients with either congenital anatomical lesions or Y chromosome material. For example, surgical correction of a vaginal outlet obstruction is necessary before menarche, or as soon as the diagnosis is made after menarche, to allow passage of menstrual blood. In those patients with a Y chromosome, gonadectomy should be performed to prevent the development of gonadal neoplasia. However, this should be delayed until after puberty in patients with complete androgen insensitivity syndrome. These patients have a normal pubertal growth spurt and feminise at the time of expected puberty. Tumours do not usually develop until after this time. Treatment of Asherman's syndrome consists of hysteroscopic lysis of adhesions followed by oestrogen administration to stimulate regrowth of endometrial tissue.

Table 8.8   Clinical evaluation of secondary amenorrhoea

History	• Symptoms of pregnancy
	• Recent stress; change in weight, diet or exercise habits; or illness that might result in hypothalamic amenorrhoea
	• Drugs: oral contraceptives; androgenic drugs like danazol or high-dose progestogens; drugs that increase serum prolactin, including metoclopramide and antipsychotic drugs
	• Symptoms of other hypothalamic–pituitary disease, including headaches, visual field defects, fatigue, or polyuria and polydipsia
	• Symptoms of oestrogen deficiency, including hot flushes, vaginal dryness, poor sleep, or decreased libido
	• Galactorrhoea (suggestive of excess prolactin) or hirsutism, acne and a history of irregular menses (suggestive of hyperandrogenism as in PCOS)
	• Obstetric catastrophe, severe bleeding, dilatation and curettage, or endometritis or other infection
Physical examination	• Measurement of height and weight
	• Signs of other illnesses and evidence of cachexia
	• Signs of oestrogen deficiency – skin, breasts, and genital tissues
	• Galactorrhoea
	• Skin – hirsutism, acne, striae, acanthosis nigricans, vitiligo, thinness, and bruising
Basic laboratory testing	Serum hCG, LH, FSH, prolactin, testosterone, free T_4/TSH
Further evaluation	Depends on initial findings but might include:
	1. Pelvic ultrasonography
	2. MRI of pituitary and hypothalamus
	3. Serum DHEAS and tests to exclude Cushing's syndrome and/or non-classic congenital adrenal hyperplasia
	4. CT of adrenal glands
	5. Ovarian and other organ-specific autoantibodies
	6. Karyotype
	7. Serum ferritin, angiotensin-converting enzyme
	8. Evaluation for Asherman's syndrome – The endometrium is primed with oral conjugated oestrogens (2.5 mg daily for 35 days) and medroxyprogesterone (10 mg daily for days 26 to 35). Failure to bleed after this suggests significant endometrial scarring. Hysterography or hysteroscopy is then performed.

CT = computed tomography, DHEAS = dehydroepiandrosterone sulphate, FSH = follicle-stimulating hormone, hCG = human chorionic gonadotrophin, LH = luteinising hormone, MRI = magnetic resonance imaging, PCOS = polycystic ovary syndrome, T_4 = thyroxine, TSH = thyroid-stimulating hormone.

Ovarian failure. Women with ovarian failure should be started on hormone replacement therapy after appropriate counselling on the benefits and risks of such treatment.

Polycystic ovary syndrome. In this condition, amenorrhoea may result in endometrial hyperplasia. Hyperandrogenism may result in menstrual disturbance, hirsutism, acne and infertility, and the treatment used depends on the clinical problems in each case.

Functional hypothalamic amenorrhoea. This can usually be reversed by weight gain, reduction in the intensity of exercise or by resolution of illness or emotional stress. For those who remain amenorrhoeic, oestrogen–progestogen replacement therapy should be used to prevent osteoporosis and heart disease. If pregnancy is desired, women with FHA can be treated with exogenous gonadotrophins or pulsatile GnRH if necessary.

Irreversible hypothalamic or pituitary dysfunction. Amenorrhoea due to pituitary or hypothalamic disease that is not reversible (e.g. congenital GnRH deficiency) is treated with oestrogen–progestogen replacement. For women who want to become pregnant, either exogenous gonadotrophins or, in the case of hypothalamic disease, pulsatile GnRH can be given.

Polycystic Ovary Syndrome

Polycystic ovary syndrome is an important cause of both menstrual irregularity and androgen excess in women.

Classically, PCOS is associated with hirsutism, irregular menstrual cycles, obesity and typical ovarian morphology. For other hyperandrogenic women, however, there has been considerable controversy about the diagnostic criteria (Table 8.9).

The diagnosis does not depend on the results of biochemical tests or pelvic ultrasonography and the presence of polycystic ovarian morphology alone is insufficient to make the diagnosis of PCOS in women who have regular menstrual cycles or are not hyperandrogenic. Women with other known causes of hyperandrogenism, such

Table 8.9 Diagnostic criteria for PCOS

Menstrual irregularity and
Evidence of hyperandrogenism
    Clinical: hirsutism, acne, frontal balding, or
    Biochemical: increased serum androgens

as congenital adrenal hyperplasia, androgen-secreting tumours, Cushing's syndrome and hyperprolactinaemia, are excluded.

Clinical manifestations

In addition to menstrual dysfunction and hyperandrogenism, women with PCOS may have hypothalamic–pituitary abnormalities, poly-cystic ovaries on pelvic ultrasonography, infertility, obesity and insulin resistance. A familial pattern occurs in some cases.

Menstrual dysfunction

The menstrual dysfunction of PCOS can be manifested in several different ways. The most common problem is anovulation and erratic menstruation. Most women with PCOS have an adequate amount of biologically active oestrogen since androgens can be converted to oestrogens peripherally in the absence of normal ovarian function. Thus, women with PCOS may have constant mitogenic stimulation of the endometrium, leading to endometrial hyperplasia, intermittent breakthrough bleeding and dysfunctional uterine bleeding. The constant mitogenic stimulation increases the risk of endometrial cancer in amenorrhoeic women with PCOS.

Typically, the onset of menstrual disturbances in PCOS has a peripubertal onset. Affected women may have a normal or slightly delayed menarche followed by irregular cycles. Other women may have apparently regular cycles at first and subsequently develop menstrual irregularity in association with weight gain. Many obese women with PCOS resume more regular menstrual cycles after relatively small amounts of weight loss.

Hyperandrogenism

In PCOS, hyperandrogenism may be manifested clinically by hir-sutism or acne, or less often, by male pattern balding. Women with PCOS are not virilised (possession of mature masculine somatic characteristics). Depending upon the androgen measured and the technique employed, between 50 and 90% of women with PCOS have elevated serum androgen levels. The excess androgens can be derived from the ovary and/or the adrenal cortex.

Hypothalamic–pituitary abnormalities

Many women with PCOS have abnormalities of hypothalamic–pituitary function in their reproductive axis. Women with PCOS may have increased serum LH levels and also have increased LH pulse frequency and amplitude. Serum FSH levels may be normal or low in PCOS, leading to an elevated LH/FSH ratio compared to normally cycling young women in the early follicular phase. Some women (7%) with PCOS have mildly elevated serum prolactin levels of uncertain significance.

Typical ovarian morphology on ultrasonography

Polycystic ovaries have a classical appearance. The original description was by Stein and Leventhal. They described their findings at laparotomy of enlarged multicystic ovaries with thickened, glistening, pearly-white capsules. Histologically, there is a thickened and sclerotic cortex which gives the appearance of a capsule on gross examination, and it has been proposed that this change forms an impenetrable barrier which prevents ovulation. There are multiple, peripherally located, small preantral and antral follicles which are generally atretic, and the volume of stroma is increased.

With high-resolution transvaginal ultrasonography (Box 8.1), the histological findings can be corroborated noninvasively. Between 80 and 100% of women with PCOS have a classical ultrasound appearance. Ovarian volume is increased and there are many (at least 8–10 in each ovary), small (2–8 mm) follicles arranged peripherally around an increased amount of stroma.

Box 8.1   Ultrasound has been used to demonstrate polycystic ovaries in:

92% of women with idiopathic hirsutism
87% of women with oligomenorrhoea
26% of women with amenorrhoea
22% of women in the adult population

Infertility

Infertility was included in the original description of PCOS by Stein and Leventhal. Most women with PCOS ovulate intermittently and may therefore take longer to conceive or may have fewer children. However, some women with PCOS do have infertility. As well as anovulation, other factors appear to be important, including an increased early miscarriage rate in PCOS. This is associated with high serum LH levels, but the mechanism is poorly understood.

Obesity, insulin resistance and diabetes

Obesity is associated with insulin resistance and at least one-half of women with PCOS are obese. Insulin resistance and hyperinsulinaemia are also important in the pathogenesis of PCOS and this is independent of obesity. Acanthosis nigricans is seen on the neck and in the axillae of insulin-resistant women with PCOS. Up to 45% of obese women with PCOS have either impaired glucose tolerance (35%) or type 2 diabetes mellitus (10%) by age 40. In addition to their underlying insulin resistance, women with PCOS who have a family history of type 2 diabetes have a concurrent impairment of insulin secretion that may put them at increased risk for overt diabetes. The familial nature of PCOS has led to investigations of possible genetic linkages of this disorder to type 2 diabetes. A unique defect in serine phosphorylation of the insulin receptor that results in decreased activation of the insulin receptor has been identified in about 50% of women with PCOS. The relevance of this abnormality is not clear, but serine phosphorylation of P450c17 may also be involved in the regulation of adrenal androgen synthesis. Familial PCOS has also been linked to an insulin regulatory locus on chromosome 11.

Predisposition to coronary heart disease

The presence of obesity and insulin resistance may predispose women with PCOS to coronary heart disease. Amongst women undergoing coronary angiography, 42% were found to have polycystic ovaries and this was associated with hirsutism, lower levels of high-density lipoprotein (HDL) cholesterol, and higher concentrations of free testosterone, triglycerides and C-peptide. The women with polycystic ovaries had more extensive coronary disease than those with normal ovaries. Furthermore, in women who had undergone ovarian wedge resection for PCOS 22–33 years earlier, the risk of developing a myocardial infarction was increased seven-fold.

Biochemical abnormalities

The biochemical abnormalities found in PCOS are shown in Table 8.10.

Table 8.10   Biochemical abnormalities in polycystic ovary syndrome

Biochemical parameter	Typical change
Serum total testosterone	Increased
Serum sex hormone-binding globulin	Decreased
Serum free testosterone	Increased
Serum oestradiol	Normal
Serum oestrone	Normal
Serum LH	Normal / increased
Serum FSH	Normal / decreased
Serum prolactin	Normal / slightly increased
Fasting blood glucose	Normal / impaired / diabetic

FSH = follicle-stimulating hormone; LH = luteinising hormone.

Clinical evaluation of women with menstrual irregularity and hirsutism is shown in Table 8.11.

Differential diagnosis

The vast majority of patients with menstrual irregularity and hirsutism will have PCOS. The diagnosis is suggested by the history and findings on physical examination. The main purpose of laboratory investigations is to exclude other rarer possibilities (Table 8.12).

The main diagnostic question is how to identify the small proportion of women who have other causes for their hyperandrogenism (Table 8.13).

Further investigations

Clinical suspicion (e.g. rapidly progressive hirsutism in a previously well woman) of an alternative diagnosis and/or a serum testosterone concentration above 5 nmol/l should prompt further investigations (Table 8.14).

Management of PCOS

Treatment should be tailored to the needs of the individual patient. Before planning treatment, the issue of fertility should be discussed with the patient, since – if she wishes to become pregnant – this will have a major influence on the choice of therapy. In those women who are obese, most, if not all, of the features of PCOS can be improved by weight reduction and probably also by drugs that decrease insulin resistance and therefore secretion.

Table 8.11   Clinical evaluation of women with menstrual irregularity and hirsutism

Assessment	Observations
History	• Menstrual irregularity, typically from menarche • Hirsutism and/or acne • Frontal balding • Weight gain • Infertility
Examination	• Height, weight, waist circumference or body mass index • Hirsutism (Ferriman and Gallwey score) • Acne • Virilisation (frontotemporal balding, clitoromegaly, increased muscle mass, deepening of voice, breast atrophy) • Acanthosis nigricans • Blood pressure
Initial investigations	• Serum testosterone • Serum LH • Serum FSH • Serum prolactin • Serum TSH • Fasting blood glucose • Fasting blood lipids

FSH = follicle-stimulating hormone, LH = luteinising hormone, TSH = thyroid-stimulating hormone.

Table 8.12   Other causes of hyperandrogenism

Late-onset congenital adrenal hyperplasia
Ovarian and adrenal tumours
Cushing's syndrome
Drugs (testosterone, anabolic steroids, danazol, androgenic progestogens)
Hyperprolactinaemia

Table 8.13   Clinical pointers to a rare cause for hyperandrogenism

Abrupt onset
Short duration
Sudden, progressive worsening of hirsutism
Onset in 3rd decade of life or later, rather than near puberty
Symptoms or signs of virilisation

Table 8.14 **Further investigations of hyperandrogenism**

Possible diagnosis	Further investigations
Late-onset congenital adrenal hyperplasia	• Serum 17-hydroxyprogesterone-basal and 60 min after tetracosactide (Synacthen) 250 µg IM • Urinary steroid profiling
Cushing's syndrome	• 24-hour urinary free cortisol or low-dose dexamethasone suppression test
Adrenal androgen-secreting tumour	• Serum DHEAS • CT abdomen
Ovarian androgen-secreting tumour	• Transvaginal ultrasonography

CT = computed tomography, DHEAS = dehydroepiandrosterone sulphate, IM = intramuscularly.

Metabolic effects

Treatment that reduces insulin resistance and therefore diminishes insulin secretion can have beneficial effects, including a reduction in ovarian androgen secretion that may reduce hair growth and restore menstrual regularity and fertility.

Weight reduction, increased aerobic exercise and stopping smoking result in increased insulin sensitivity. The most extensively studied of these factors is weight reduction: loss of more than 5% of body weight has been shown to restore regular menstrual cycles, improve fertility and decrease hirsutism.

Oral contraceptives have long-term benefits on insulin resistance in women with PCOS. Glucose intolerance, hyperinsulinaemia and serum free testosterone levels are reduced. Metformin can reduce insulin resistance and hyperinsulinaemia in women with PCOS and may also reduce ovarian androgen production (and serum free testosterone concentrations) and restore normal menstrual cyclicity. Thiazolidinediones and d-chiro-inositol also increase insulin sensitivity in women with PCOS and are also likely to prove useful, alone or in combination therapy.

Metformin has been used in the treatment of type 2 diabetes for many years. It is relatively well tolerated and is not known to have teratogenic effects. However, toxicology studies to show that metformin is safe in pregnancy have not been performed. Gastrointestinal side effects (anorexia, nausea, vomiting, diarrhoea) are common initially but can be minimised by taking metformin with or after food and by increasing the dose gradually. As yet, there are not good data for the use of metfomin in non-diabetic women; many of the benefits may be related to the reduction in weight rather than metformin. Metformin is probably most effective in obese patients and, at present, it is recommended that the dose be increased from 500 mg daily to 850 mg three times a day over 12 weeks. If side effects occur, the patient should revert to the maximum tolerated dose. The effectiveness of this treatment should be assessed after 6 months. If there has been no response at this stage, treatment should be discontinued. In patients who respond well, treatment with metformin can be continued but should be reviewed regularly. There are no data from long-term use of metformin in PCOS yet.

Menstrual irregularity

The most common method of providing regular periods is the use of a combined oral contraceptive. This therapy also inhibits ovarian androgen production (by inhibiting gonadotrophin secretion) and raises sex hormone-binding globulin (SHBG) production, so that the serum free testosterone concentration falls. Absence of pregnancy should be confirmed before oral contraceptive therapy is commenced. If the woman has not had a menstrual period for 6 or more weeks, withdrawal bleeding should be induced by administration of a progestogen, such as medroxyprogesterone acetate (Provera), 5–10 mg daily for 10 days. Oral contraceptive pills vary in their oestrogen and progestogen content and it may be necessary to try different preparations to find the best one for an individual woman. In general, a preparation with the lowest oestrogen and progestogen content which gives good cycle control and minimal side effects is chosen.

Hirsutism and acne

Hirsutism can be treated by removal of hair by plucking, shaving, depilatory creams, waxing, electrolysis or laser. Drug treatments can improve acne, reduce the rate of hair growth and make hairs that grow finer and less pigmented. Whereas acne often improves within 6–8 weeks, improvement in hirsutism may take many months.

The most commonly used treatment is co-cyprindiol (Dianette), which is a combined oral contraceptive containing 35 µg ethinyl-oestradiol and 2 mg cyproterone acetate.

If this is ineffective, cyproterone acetate (25–50 mg daily from day 1 to day 10 of the cycle) can be added. Common side effects of cyproterone acetate include weight gain, lethargy, headache and mood change.

Spironolactone also acts as an anti-androgen. It can be used without a contraceptive pill, but may cause irregular or heavy menstrual bleeding. The dose is 50–100 mg twice daily.

Flutamide (starting dose 125–250 mg twice daily) is an effective anti-androgen. Its use is limited by the risk of hepatic side effects, including occasional fatalities.

Finasteride is a 5α-reductase inhibitor, blocking the conversion of testosterone to the more potent androgen, dihydrotestosterone. It is as effective as spironolactone and is not associated with significant side effects in women. The dose is 5 mg daily (although 1 mg is probably just as effective).

Other treatments for acne include oral antibiotics and isotretinoin, which is prescribed by dermatologists.

Infertility

Approximately 80% of women with PCOS ovulate in response to clomiphene, but only about 50% become pregnant. The starting dose of clomiphene is 50 mg daily on days 2 to 6 of the cycle. Ovulation should be assessed by measurement of the serum progesterone concentration in the mid-luteal phase. If ovulation does not occur, the dose of clomiphene can be increased to 100 mg from day 2 to 6 of the cycle. Most women who are going to respond will do so within the first 3 cycles. Clomiphene treatment should not be continued for longer than 6 cycles because of a possible increased risk of ovarian cancer. Clomiphene therapy increases the risk of twin pregnancy from 1 in 80 to about 1 in 20. Other side effects include abdominal discomfort, dizziness, hot flushes, breast discomfort, visual disturbance and ovarian hyperstimulation. Metformin may have a role in ovulation induction in obese women with PCOS, either given alone or in combination with clomiphene. If used in this way, metformin should be discontinued when ovulation is confirmed.

A number of other methods are available to induce ovulation in those who do not respond to clomiphene:

- *Conventional gonadotrophin therapy.* The combination of gonadotrophins and human chorionic gonadotrophin (hCG) results in a high ovulation rate and a cumulative pregnancy rate of 50–70%. There is a multiple gestation rate of about 30% and a risk of ovarian hyperstimulation.

- *Pulsatile GnRH therapy.* Ovulation rates are 40–60% in women with PCOS. The advantage is that most ovulatory cycles are monofollicular. Ovulation rates can be increased (to 76%) by pretreatment with a GnRH agonist for 6–8 weeks before starting pulsatile GnRH therapy.
- *Combined GnRH agonist–gonadotrophin therapy.* Treatment with GnRH agonists has been used to decrease the levels of endogenous LH prior to commencing exogenous gonadotrophin therapy. In women with PCOS, this does not appear to confer any clinical advantages over conventional gonadotrophin therapy.
- *Low-dose gonadotrophin therapy.* This is the preferred medical treatment. A low starting dose of gonadotrophins is used and small stepwise increases encourage monofollicular development. The risks of multiple gestation and hyperstimulation are reduced. Ovulation rates are of the order of 70% and the pregnancy rate is 55%.

In the past, wedge resection of the ovaries was a standard treatment for infertility in women with PCOS. This procedure has been replaced by laparoscopic ovarian laser electrocautery. Ovulatory cycles can be restored for many months and can thus prevent the need for fertility drugs.

Hirsutism

Definition

Hirsutism is the development of androgen-dependent terminal body hair in a woman in places in which terminal hair is normally not found. Terminal body hairs are the thick, dark, pigmented hairs normally seen in men on the face, chest, abdomen and back. There are differences in female body hair in different geographical populations and a woman's definition of hirsutism may differ depending upon her ethnic background and upon her subjective view of normal body hair distribution.

Nearly all hirsute women have an increased production rate of androgens, usually testosterone, but the increase may not be sufficient to raise the serum testosterone concentration above the normal range. Another important factor is increased conversion of testosterone to dihydrotestosterone in peripheral tissue, including hair follicles.

There are two conditions characterised by generalised hair growth that do not represent true hirsutism:

1. Androgen-independent hair, which is the soft, vellus unpigmented hair that covers the entire body. In infants, this hair is called lanugo.
2. Hypertrichosis refers to diffusely increased total body hair. This is usually caused by drugs such as phenytoin, penicillamine, diazoxide, minoxidil and cyclosporin. Hypertrichosis can also occur in some systemic illnesses, such as hypothyroidism, anorexia nervosa, malnutrition, porphyria and dermatomyositis.

Epidemiology

The overall prevalence of hirsutism is unknown. In a classic study of 430 British women aged 15–64 years attending a general medical clinic, no woman had terminal hair on the upper back or upper abdomen, 10% had hair on the chest, 22% had hair on the chin, and 49% had hair on the upper lip. However, in most of the women who had hair in any of these regions, there were rarely more than a few scattered hairs.

Causes of hirsutism

Hirsutism is caused by increased androgen production by the ovaries or adrenal glands, or by increased target organ production of androgen (Table 8.15).

The vast majority of cases are due to idiopathic hirsutism or PCOS.

Idiopathic hirsutism

The diagnosis of idiopathic hirsutism is one of exclusion. It applies to women with hirsutism and no other clinical abnormalities. There

Table 8.15　Causes of hirsutism

Idiopathic hirsutism
Polycystic ovary syndrome (PCOS)
Congenital adrenal hyperplasia
Virilising ovarian tumour
Virilising adrenal tumour
Acromegaly
Prolactinoma
Drugs

is no menstrual irregularity and no other identifiable cause of their hirsutism. Serum androgen levels are usually normal or only mildly elevated. The distinction between idiopathic hirsutism and PCOS may be one of degree.

Polycystic ovary syndrome

PCOS is the most common cause of androgen excess in women. There is evidence of hyperandrogenism and menstrual irregularity. The androgen excess in women with PCOS usually becomes evident about the time of puberty or soon after, because androgen production is increased by both puberty (increased ovarian steroid production) and adrenarche (increased adrenal androgen production).

Hyperprolactinaemia

Some women with hirsutism have hyperprolactinaemia, but whether it alone can cause hirsutism is not clear. The elevation in serum prolactin is associated with increased serum dehydroepiandrosterone sulphate (DHEAS) concentrations. However, the underlying problem in many of these women is probably PCOS, with the hyperprolactinaemia being caused by the increase in the serum oestrone concentration that occurs in women with this disorder. DHEAS is such a weak androgen that the hirsutism associated with hyperprolactinaemia is probably due more to the ovarian hyperandrogenism of PCOS rather than any effect of hyperprolactinaemia itself.

Drugs

Danazol, testosterone, anabolic steroids and androgenic progestogens can cause hirsutism.

Congenital adrenal hyperplasia

Excess adrenal androgen production, driven by adrenocorticotrophic hormone (ACTH), is a key feature of most forms of congenital adrenal hyperplasia. These disorders may be recognised at birth or in early infancy, but late-onset or non-classical forms occur. The prevalence of late-onset congenital adrenal hyperplasia among hirsute women has varied from 1 to 15% in different studies. Affected women present peripubertally with hirsutism and menstrual disturbance. Most cases are due to 21-hydroxylase (P450c21) deficiency (see Chapter 7).

Hyperthecosis

Hyperthecosis is an ovarian disorder that is characterised by increased production of testosterone by luteinised thecal cells in the stroma, leading to increased serum testosterone concentrations. It is unclear whether hyperthecosis is a distinct disorder or part of the spectrum of PCOS. The clinical history is usually one of gradual onset of hirsutism and other manifestations of androgen excess.

Ovarian tumours

Hirsutism caused by androgen-secreting tumours is most likely to start later and progress more rapidly than in PCOS. Most women have serum testosterone concentrations above 5 nmol/l, and often much higher, so that affected women become virilised. These tumours can be identified by transvaginal ultrasonography. Androgen-secreting tumours constitute only 5% of all ovarian tumours. Histologically, they are Sertoli–Leydig cell tumours (arrhenoblastoma), granulosa-theca cell tumours and hilus cell tumours

Adrenal tumours

Adrenal tumours are a rare cause of androgen excess. Some are adrenal adenomas that secrete mostly testosterone, but most are carcinomas that often secrete not only androgens but also cortisol. Thus, the clinical picture is of a woman who becomes virilised and has Cushing's syndrome. DHEAS is produced almost exclusively by the adrenal glands. An unequivocally elevated serum DHEAS value is suggestive of an adrenal carcinoma but some adrenal carcinomas lose the ability to sulphate DHEA, so that a normal serum DHEAS value does not exclude the diagnosis.

Severe insulin resistance

Women with severe insulin resistance and marked hyperinsulin-aemia often have hirsutism. The marked hyperinsulinaemia causes ovarian hyperandrogenism, possibly through an action on the theca cell receptors for insulin-like growth factor-1 (IGF-1). Insulin also decreases the serum SHBG concentration, thereby increasing the serum free testosterone. There are a number of syndromes of severe insulin resistance, including genetic defects of the insulin receptor, the production of antibodies to the insulin receptor and several syndromes of lipoatrophy and lipodystrophy.

Clinical evaluation

History

The most important clinical information is the time course of symptoms and whether or not the woman is virilised. The age at onset, the rate of progression and any change with any treatment or with fluctuations in weight should be determined (Table 8.16). A later age of onset, progressively worsening symptoms or a rapid rate of progression suggest the possibility of an ovarian or adrenal tumour, but could be caused by responses to previous treatments or changes in weight.

Physical examination

The physical examination (Table 8.17) provides information about the extent of hirsutism and, sometimes, about its cause.

Table 8.16 History of hirsutism

History	Information required
Menstrual history	• Age at menarche • Regularity of menstrual cycles • Pregnancies • Oral contraceptive use
Cutaneous manifestations of hyperandrogenism	• Hirsutism • Acne • Frontal balding
Virilisation	• Change in body shape; fat distribution, breast size • Deepening of the voice
Breasts	• Galactorrhoea
Weight history	• Weight gain
Drug history	• Danazol, androgenic progestogens, testosterone, anabolic steroids
Family history	• History of hirsutism, acne, menstrual disorders, infertility, obesity, diabetes, early cardiovascular disease

Table 8.17   **Physical examination of hirsutism**

Examination	Observations
Hirsutism	• Extent and distribution of terminal hair should be determined. The Ferriman and Gallwey scoring system assesses 9 areas (upper lip, chin, upper arms, upper back, lower back, front of chest, upper abdomen, lower abdomen and upper thighs) and each area is scored from 0 to 4. A Ferriman and Gallwey score of 8 or more is abnormal
Other signs of androgen excess	• Acne, seborrhoea, temporal balding
Evidence of virilisation	• Deep voice, android body shape, frontal balding • Clitoromegaly – this can be determined on the basis of clitoral length (>10 mm) or an increased clitoral index (length × width >35 mm^2)
Body habitus	• Shape, weight and BMI • Body fat distribution
Breasts	• Galactorrhoea
Other skin signs	• Acanthosis nigricans • Striae • Thin skin • Bruising
Blood pressure	• Hypertension
Abdominal and pelvic examination	• May reveal mass lesions

BMI = body mass index.

Initial investigations

The clinical picture (Table 8.18 and Box 8.2) will determine the initial strategy for investigations in women with hirsutism.

> ### Box 8.2   Further evaluation is necessary in premenopausal women with:
>
> • A serum testosterone concentration greater than 5 nmol/l
> • Signs of virilisation

Table 8.18   Clinical picture of hirsutism

Clinical picture	Initial investigations
Long-standing hirsutism	Serum testosterone
Long-standing hirsutism and irregular menstrual cycles	Serum testosterone, LH, FSH, prolactin
Short history of hirsutism or progressive hirsutism	Serum testosterone, DHEAS

DHEAS = dehydroepiandrosterone sulphate, FSH = follicle-stimulating hormone, LH = luteinising hormone.

Further investigations

Further investigations (Table 8.19) are planned according to clinical suspicion and the results of the preliminary investigations.

In some women with hirsutism and a high serum testosterone concentration, computed tomography (CT) scanning does not identify an adrenal tumour and pelvic ultrasonography fails to locate an ovarian tumour. These patients may have a small ovarian tumour (especially a hilus-cell tumour) that is too small to be detected by pelvic ultrasonography. Laparoscopy or laparotomy should be considered in this situation. An alternative approach which may be

Table 8.19   Further investigations in hirsutism

Indication	Next investigations
Hirsutism ± virilisation Serum testosterone >5 nmol/l Serum DHEAS normal	Transvaginal ultrasonography to look for an ovarian tumour
Hirsutism ± virilisation Serum testosterone >5 nmol/l Serum DHEAS elevated	CT abdomen to look for an adrenal tumour
Early onset hirsutism Serum testosterone >5 nmol/l	Short Synacthen test to measure serum 17-hydroxyprogesterone response or urine steroid profiling to test for congenital adrenal hyperplasia
Clinical features of Cushing's syndrome	Overnight low-dose dexamethasone suppression test or 24-hour urine cortisol

CT = computed tomography, DHEAS = dehydroepiandrosterone sulphate.

used to localise the site of excessive testosterone production is to use ovarian and adrenal venous sampling in anticipation of surgical exploration.

Oral Contraceptives

There are two types of oral contraceptive pills: combination pills that contain both oestrogen and progestogen, and the progestogen-only pill (also referred to as the 'mini-pill').

Combined oral contraceptives (COC) are the most effective preparations for general use and also have non-contraceptive benefits. Furthermore, the decrease in both oestrogen and progestogen content in the so-called second-generation COC led to a reduction in both side effects and cardiovascular complications. Healthy, non-smoking women can take the COC until the menopause if they wish.

Oral progesterone-only contraceptives may offer a suitable alternative when oestrogens are contraindicated, including patients with a history of venous thromboembolism or a predisposition to venous thrombosis. They have a higher failure rate than COC preparations. Menstrual irregularities are more common but tend to resolve with long-term treatment.

Efficacy of contraception with COC

When taken properly, COC are a very effective form of contraception. Although the theoretical failure rate is 0.1%, the actual failure rate is 2–3% due primarily to missed pills or failure to resume therapy after the 7-day pill-free interval.

Mechanisms of contraceptive action

The most important action for providing contraception is oestrogen-induced inhibition of the mid-cycle surge of gonadotrophin secretion so that ovulation does not occur. COC also suppress gonadotrophin secretion during the follicular phase of the cycle, thereby preventing follicular maturation. However, a substantial proportion of women do develop follicles while taking a COC that contains 30 or 35 µg of ethinyloestradiol. This highlights the importance of preventing the mid-cycle surge of gonadotrophin secretion. Other oestrogen-mediated mechanisms of action include suppression of ovarian steroid production, due to suppression of gonadotrophin secretion, and a possible reduction in responsiveness of the pituitary to GnRH.

Progestogen-related mechanisms also may contribute to the contraceptive effect. These include:

- actions on the endometrium, rendering it less suitable for implantation
- alterations in cervical mucus, which becomes less easily penetrable by sperm
- impairment of normal tubal motility and peristalsis.

Non-contraceptive benefits of COC

Non-contraceptive benefits of COC treatment include:

- avoidance of dysmenorrhoea
- less iron deficiency anaemia
- less premenstrual syndrome
- less benign breast disease
- protection against endometrial and ovarian cancer
- protection against pelvic inflammatory disease.

Other uses of COC

Apart from their contraceptive role, COC are useful in the treatment of a number of conditions (Box 8.3).

Box 8.3 Combined oral contraceptives are useful in the treatment of:

Hyperandrogenism (idiopathic hirsutism and PCOS)
Dysmenorrhoea
Menorrhagia
Other menstrual disorders such as hypothalamic amenorrhoea
Primary hypogonadism
Premenstrual syndrome (possibly beneficial)

PCOS = polycystic ovary syndrome.

The beneficial effects of COC in women with hyperandrogenism are mediated by:

- An increase in the serum SHBG concentration, which results in a decrease in serum free androgen concentrations.
- Inhibition of gonadotrophin secretion, which results in a decrease in ovarian androgen secretion.

- Inhibition of adrenal androgen secretion. The mechanism of this action is not well understood. It may occur through an elevation in the serum cortisol-binding globulin (CBG) concentration, which results in an increase in the serum free cortisol concentration which, in turn, inhibits pituitary ACTH secretion.

Contraindications

There are a number of absolute and relative contraindications to the use of COC. The absolute contraindications are:

- pregnancy
- personal history of venous or arterial thrombosis
- severe or multiple risk factors for arterial disease or venous thromboembolism
- heart disease associated with pulmonary hypertension or risk of embolus
- severe migraine, migraine with typical focal aura and migraine treated with ergot derivatives
- transient cerebral ischaemic attacks
- liver disease, including disorders of hepatic excretion (e.g. Dubin–Johnson or Rotor's syndromes), infective hepatitis (until liver function returns to normal)
- systemic lupus erythematosus
- porphyria
- liver adenoma
- gallstones
- evacuation of hydatidiform mole (until gonadotrophin levels return to normal)
- history of haemolytic-uraemic syndrome
- history during pregnancy of pruritus, cholestatic jaundice, chorea or deterioration of otosclerosis, pemphigoid gestationis
- breast or genital tract cacinoma
- undiagnosed vaginal bleeding
- breast feeding (until weaning or for 6 months after birth).

Choice of COC

The preparation with the lowest oestrogen and progestogen content that gives good cycle control and minimal side effects in the individual woman is chosen. The oestrogen content ranges from 20 to 50 µg. Low-strength preparations (containing 20 µg ethinyloestradiol) are suitable for overweight or older women, providing there are no specific contraindications. The standard strength COC contain 30 or 35 µg or 30–40 µg ethinyloestradiol in phased preparations. High-strength preparations (containing 50 µg ethinyloestradiol or 50 µg mestranol) provide greater contraceptive security but with an increased risk of side effects. Their use is mainly in situations of reduced bioavailability, such as long-term use of enzyme-inducing antiepileptic drugs.

The androgenic activity of progestogens increases the side effects and metabolic complications of COC. Newer progestogens including norgestimate, desogestrel and gestodene are 19-nortestosterone derivatives, but they have some structural modifications that lower their androgenic activity. Although they bind to the androgen receptor, the affinity is low, and they have little effect on serum SHBG concentrations (which are lowered by androgens and raised by oestrogens). The COC containing these newer progestogens (the third-generation COC) have less of an effect on carbohydrate and lipid metabolism and are more effective in reducing acne and hirsutism in hyperandrogenic women. They are therefore a good option for women who have difficulty tolerating or have metabolic complications with an older COC.

Risks and side effects associated with COC

Side effects

Early side effects of COC. These include bloating, nausea, breast tenderness, and mood changes. They may be troublesome enough to lead to discontinuation of the COC, but these side effects usually subside in several months. Weight gain is not a consistent finding with low-dose pills.

Breakthrough bleeding. This is the most common side effect of COC. Its occurrence does not indicate a decrease in contraceptive efficacy but reflects tissue breakdown as the endometrium adjusts to a new thin state in which it is fragile and atrophic. Breakthrough bleeding was less of a problem when the oestrogen content of COC was high, because oestrogen stabilises the endometrium. The frequency of bleeding is independent of the type of progestogen, and is increased in women who smoke cigarettes, probably due to the accelerated metabolism of oestrogen caused by smoking. If pills are missed, this results in an increase in breakthrough bleeding as well as a decrease in contraceptive efficacy. If breakthrough bleeding persists after three cycles, additional oestrogen should be given for one or two cycles to stabilise the endometrium. If the bleeding does not stop, investigations to exclude structural causes for the bleeding, such as uterine fibroids or polyps, should be performed.

Amenorrhoea. Amenorrhoea occurs in 5–10% of cycles while taking a COC; it also results from the development of an atrophic endometrium. This is usually dealt with by changing the COC preparation to one containing more oestrogen. Amenorrhoea after stopping the COC should be investigated in the same way as any other case of amenorrhoea.

Risks

Cardiovascular disease. Early high-dose COC use was associated with an increase in cardiovascular morbidity and mortality. However, the reduction in oestrogen content to 30 or 35 µg of ethinyloestradiol has increased safety substantially. There is no evidence that standard strength COC increase the risk of cardiovascular disease in women under the age of 30 years or in non-smoking women without other risk factors.

Coronary heart disease. There is no increase in mortality of women currently taking a COC, with the exception of women over the age 35 years who smoke. Any increased risk of myocardial infarction (thought to be related to a thrombotic mechanism rather than the development of atherosclerotic plaques) is also confined to older women who smoke. Heavy smokers (15 or more cigarettes per day) are at particularly high risk as compared with light smokers (fewer than 15 cigarettes per day). Furthermore, women who have taken a COC in the past are not at increased risk of coronary heart disease later in life. Third-generation COC (those containing desogestrel, norgestimate or gestodene) may be associated with a lower incidence of coronary heart disease than older preparations. COC should not be prescribed for women over age 35 years who smoke. For younger women, the benefits of COC appear to outweigh the risks of smoking, as long as there is no family history of thromboembolic disease.

Hypertension. COC use frequently causes a mild elevation in blood pressure, and hypertension can occur. The relative risk of hypertension compared with women who have never used COC is 1.8 for current users and 1.2 for previous users.

Stroke. The link between stroke and COC use has been controversial. Many older studies suggesting this association were done with

COC containing high doses of oestrogen. Several studies have addressed the effect of COC containing less than 50 μg of ethinyl-oestradiol on stroke risk with conflicting results. There may be an excess stroke risk in women who use standard strength COC, but this is small and is even less in women who do not smoke or have hypertension. The absolute risk of stroke in young women is, in any case, very low (11.3 cases per 100,000 patients per year).

Carbohydrate and lipid metabolism. Abnormal glucose tolerance tests were fairly common in women taking high-dose COC, but few women developed diabetes. Women taking standard strength COC have normal glucose tolerance, but these pills do cause mild insulin resistance. The effect of COC on serum lipids depends upon the oestrogen dose and the androgenicity of the progestogen. In general, serum triglyceride concentrations rise slightly, but there are no consistent changes in serum high-density (HDL) or low-density lipoprotein (LDL) cholesterol concentrations. The oestrogen component of COC increases serum triglycerides and HDL cholesterol concentrations, and lowers serum LDL cholesterol concentrations. These favourable effects may contribute to the beneficial effect of oestrogen on cardiovascular risk. The progestogen usually increases serum LDL cholesterol and lowers serum HDL cholesterol concentrations, particularly the androgenic progestogens such as levonorgestrel. The newer progestogens, such as desogestrel, tend to raise serum HDL cholesterol and lower LDL cholesterol concentrations.

Venous thromboembolism. The use of COC is associated with an increased risk of venous thromboembolic disease but the risk is considerably smaller than that associated with pregnancy. In all cases, the risk of venous thromboembolism increases with age and in the presence of other risk factors for venous thromboembolism, such as obesity. The incidence of venous thromboembolism in healthy non-pregnant women who are not taking a COC is about 5 cases per 100,000 women per year. In women taking a COC containing a second-generation progestogen (e.g. levonorgestrel), the incidence of venous thromboembolism is increased to about 15 cases per 100,000 women per year. The risk of thromboembolism may be higher with the third-generation progestogens, desogestrel and gestodene. The incidence has been estimated to be about 25 per 100,000 women per year. In pregnant women, there are about 60 cases of venous thromboembolism per 100,000 pregnancies. The choice of COC should be made according to clinical need, with these relative risks having been discussed with the woman.

Breast cancer. There is a small increase in the risk of having breast cancer diagnosed in women taking the COC. This relative risk may be explained by earlier diagnosis. In women on COC who are found to have breast cancer, the cancer is more likely to be confined to the breast at the time of diagnosis. The age at which the COC is stopped is the most important factor, rather than the duration of use. There is a gradual decline in the risk after stopping the COC and there is no excess risk by 10 years. This small increase in the risk of breast cancer has to balanced against the benefits of the COC, including protective effects against ovarian and endometrial cancer.

Infertility

Infertility is defined as a failure to conceive after 1 year of unprotected intercourse. It may be primary, in a woman who has never conceived, or secondary. Normally, the maximum conception rate per ovulation is about 25–30%. After 6 months, the cumulative conception rate is about 60% and, after 1 year, it is 85%. Thus, up to 15% of couples experience infertility. The woman's age is the most important factor determining normal fertility. Conception rates after the age of 35 years are half those before the age of 25 years.

Causes of infertility

Male factors alone are responsible in about 30%, and are contributory in a further 20%, of infertile couples. Ovulatory disorders can be identified in the woman in 18–25% of infertile couples, tubal disease is found in about 20%, and a cervical factor is identified in about 5%. Infertility remains unexplained in approximately 20% of infertile couples.

    The endocrinologist's main contribution is in the diagnosis and management of anovulation.

Causes of anovulation

Hypogonadotrophic hypogonadal anovulation (hypothalamic amenorrhoea). This group accounts for 5–10% of anovulatory women. Affected women usually have amenorrhoea. They have low or low–normal serum FSH concentrations and low serum oestradiol concentrations due to decreased hypothalamic secretion of GnRH (e.g. FHA and Kallmann's syndrome), or pituitary unresponsiveness to GnRH (hypopituitarism).

Normogonadotrophic normoestrogenic anovulation. Women with normogonadotrophic normoestrogenic anovulation constitute the largest group of anovulatory women (60–85% of cases). These women may secrete normal amounts of gonadotrophins and oestrogens. However, FSH secretion during the follicular phase of the cycle is subnormal. This group includes women with PCOS. Some ovulate occasionally, especially those with oligomenorrhoea.

Hypergonadotrophic hypoestrogenic anovulation. This accounts for 10–30% of cases of anovulation. The primary causes are premature ovarian failure (absence of ovarian follicles due to early menopause) and ovarian resistance. Ovarian function ceases in 1% of women before the age of 40 years. In most, the follicles are exhausted for unknown reasons. In the resistant ovary syndrome, follicles remain but are unresponsive to FSH stimulation. Most of these women have amenorrhoea and, usually, they do not respond to medical therapy for anovulation. They are best treated by in-vitro fertilisation of donor oocytes.

Hyperprolactinaemic anovulation. Hyperprolactinaemia accounts for 5–10% of women with anovulation. These women are anovulatory because hyperprolactinaemia inhibits gonadotrophin and, therefore, oestrogen secretion. They may have regular anovulatory cycles, but most have oligomenorrhoea or amenorrhoea. Serum gonadotrophin concentrations are usually normal (see Chapter 5).

Induction of ovulation

Table 8.20 summarises the methods used to induce ovulation

Anti-oestrogen therapy

The mechanism of action of anti-oestrogens is not clear. They are thought to occupy oestrogen receptors in the hypothalamus and pituitary, thereby blocking the negative feedback action of oestradiol. Thus, serum FSH concentration rises, resulting in stimulation of follicle growth and follicular oestradiol production.

Clomiphene is most effective in normogonadotrophic anovulatory women. The usual starting dose of clomiphene is 50 mg/day from day 2 to day 6 after the onset of spontaneous or progesterone-induced menstrual bleeding. If ovulation does not occur, the dose should be increased in the next cycle to 100 mg/day for 5 days. If ovulation occurs, the same can be continued. Most women respond to clomiphene within six cycles at doses no greater than

Table 8.20   Methods used to induce ovulation

Treatment

Anti-oestrogens
- Clomiphene
- Tamoxifen

Exogenous gonadotrophins
- Human menopausal gonadotrophins
- Follitropin
- Chorionic gonadotrophin

Pulsatile GnRH

Suppression of hyperprolactinaemia
- Bromocriptine
- Cabergoline
- Quinagolide

GnRH = gonadotrophin-releasing hormone.

100 mg/day, but higher doses (200 mg/day) may be successful in some women. In obese, anovulatory women with PCOS, metformin or metformin with clomiphene may be effective in inducing ovulatory cycles. Tamoxifen, like clomiphene, is an anti-oestrogen capable of inducing ovulation. The usual starting dosage is 20 mg daily given for 5 days.

A menstrual calendar should be kept. A rise in the mid-luteal phase serum progesterone concentration (usually measured around day 21) is a useful marker of ovulation. Approximately 80% of appropriately selected normogonadotrophic anovulatory women ovulate after three cycles of clomiphene. Pregnancy rates are lower at 56%. Younger age and presenting with amenorrhoea (as opposed to oligomenorrhoea) appear to improve the likelihood of pregnancy once clomiphene-induced ovulation has occurred. After 6 months of treatment, the pregnancy rate per cycle falls substantially despite regular ovulation. In addition, pregnancy rates are lower in women who ovulate only after receiving higher doses of clomiphene. The risk of twin pregnancy is increased to about 1 in 20 clomiphene-induced pregnancies and the risk of the ovarian hyperstimulation syndrome is less than 1%.

Gonadotrophin therapy (Box 8.4)

Gonadotrophins extracted from the urine of postmenopausal women (human menopausal gonadotrophins, hMGs) have played a major role in ovulation induction therapy since 1961. The ratio of LH to FSH bioactivity in hMG is 1:1. Later, purified and highly purified urinary FSH became available and, since 1996, recombinant human FSH has been available.

The aim of ovulation induction with exogenous gonadotrophins is the formation of a single dominant follicle. To achieve this, specific treatment and monitoring protocols are needed.

Box 8.4   Indications for gonadotrophin therapy in anovulatory women

- Normogonadotrophic anovulatory women who have not ovulated or conceived with clomiphene treatment
- Hypogonadotrophic anovulatory women with hypopituitarism or hypothalamic amenorrhoea

---

Standard protocol.   In the standard gonadotrophin protocol, the starting dose of FSH is 150 units/day. When a pre-ovulatory follicle has developed, ovulation is induced using hCG. However, this regimen is associated with a multiple pregnancy rate of up to 36% and ovarian hyperstimulation occurs in up to 14% of treatment cycles.

Low-dose, step-up protocol.   In this protocol, the initial subcutaneous or intramuscular dose of FSH is 37.5–75 units/day. The dose is increased only if, after 14 days, there has been no response. If necessary, the dose is increased by 37.5 units/day at weekly intervals up to a maximum of 225 units/day. Ovulation is induced using hCG. This approach minimises the risk of excessive stimulation and therefore the risk of development of multiple follicles.

Low-dose, step-down protocol.   The low-dose step-down protocol mimics more closely the physiology of normal cycles. Treatment with FSH (150 units/day) is started shortly after spontaneous or progesterone-induced bleeding and continued until a dominant follicle (> 10 mm in diameter) is seen on transvaginal/ultrasonography. The dose is then decreased to 112.5 units/day for 3 days and then to 75 units/day. This is continued until hCG is administered to induce ovulation.

Cycle monitoring.   The ovarian response to gonadotrophin therapy is monitored using transvaginal ultrasonography to measure follicular diameter. Scans are usually performed every 2 or 3 days: hCG (10,000 units intramuscularly) is given when at least one follicle measures more than 18 mm in diameter. If more than three follicles larger than 16 mm are present, stimulation is stopped, hCG is withheld, and the use of barrier contraception is advised in order to prevent multiple pregnancies and ovarian hyperstimulation.

Outcomes. Using the low-dose, step-up protocol, rates of ovulation of 72% and pregnancy rates of 45% have been obtained. Multiple follicular development and ovarian hyperstimulation are less common than with the standard protocol, and pregnancy rates are similar. With the step-down protocol, the duration of treatment and total gonadotrophin dosage is reduced compared with the low-dose, step-up protocol and unifollicular development is more frequently achieved.

Pulsatile GnRH therapy (Box 8.5)

Pulsatile administration of GnRH stimulates the production of endogenous FSH and LH. GnRH is administered subcutaneously using a pump. A pulse interval of 90 min is used, with an initial dose of 15 μg per pulse. Pulsatile GnRH administration may be discontinued after ovulation, and the corpus luteum supported by hCG. Ovulation rates of 90% and pregnancy rates of 80% have been reported in women treated with pulsatile GnRH.

Box 8.5 Indication for pulsatile gonadotrophin-releasing hormone therapy in anovulatory women

Women with hypogonadotrophic hypogonadal anovulation who have normal pituitary function

---

Dopamine agonists (Box 8.6)

Dopamine agonists inhibit prolactin release from the pituitary. Bromocriptine, the first dopamine agonist drug to prove effective in the treatment of hyperprolactinaemia, remains in widespread use. Newer drugs, such as cabergoline, bind more specifically to dopamine D2 receptors on the lactotroph cells.

Bromocriptine therapy is started with 1.25 mg at night with food and the dose is gradually increased every few days to a usual dose of 2.5 mg three times a day. Further dosage adjustments are made until the serum prolactin concentration is normalised. Cabergoline treatment is started at 0.5 mg/week and the dose is increased at monthly intervals according to the serum prolactin response. Following correction of hyperprolactinaemia, approximately 80% of women will ovulate and pregnancy rates of 70–80% can be achieved. In a woman with a macroprolactinoma, treatment is usually continued during pregnancy but, in other cases, treatment is usually stopped once pregnancy is confirmed.

Box 8.6   Indication for dopamine agonist therapy in anovulatory women

Women with hyperprolactinaemic anovulation in whom the underlying cause (e.g. drug-induced) cannot be reversed

---

Menopause

Diagnosis

Menopause is defined as the cessation of menstrual periods in women that occurs at about age 50 years. A clinical diagnosis of menopause is made by the presence of amenorrhoea for 12 months, together with the occurrence of symptoms of menopause such as hot flushes. The pathognomonic endocrine finding is a high serum FSH concentration. The rise in serum LH begins after the rise in serum FSH and is less marked.

Changes occurring in the perimenopause

Perimenopause is a period of 2–8 years preceding menopause and the year after the last menstrual period. It is characterised by normal ovulatory cycles interspersed with anovulatory cycles of varying length so that menses become irregular. Heavy breakthrough bleeding, termed dysfunctional uterine bleeding, can occur during longer periods of anovulation. Thus, vaginal bleeding becomes unpredictable in both timing and amount. In addition, some women complain of hot flushes and vaginal dryness. The waxing and waning of ovarian function of the perimenopausal period can last for several years, with extended periods of oestrogen deficiency and increased gonadotrophin secretion followed by occasional follicular development, oestradiol production and apparently normal gonadotrophin secretion.

Chronic anovulation and progesterone deficiency in this transition period may lead to long periods of unopposed oestrogen exposure and therefore endometrial hyperplasia.

Irregular bleeding and menopausal symptoms during this perimenopausal transition may be treated by standard oestrogen–progestogen replacement therapy. However, because of the waxing and waning of ovarian function, which may include intermittent ovulation, some women still require contraception during this period.

In women with no symptoms of oestrogen deficiency but with dysfunctional uterine bleeding who smoke or have other reasons to avoid oestrogen replacement, monthly withdrawal bleeding can be induced with a progestogen such as medroxyprogesterone acetate (5–10 mg daily for 10–14 days per month).

Changes occurring in the menopause

Menopause is secondary to a genetically programmed loss of ovarian follicles. The age of menopause is reduced by about 2 years in women who smoke. There is also a tendency for women who have never had children and for those with more regular cycles to have an earlier menopause. With the cessation of ovarian follicular activity, menstrual periods stop and ovarian oestrogen production declines. Serum gonadotrophin concentrations increase. Serum FSH rises more than LH, probably due to the withdrawal of steroid negative feedback and cessation of inhibin production by ovarian follicles.

Hot flushes are the most common acute change during menopause, occurring in 75% of women. They are centrally mediated and are self-limited, ending within 5 years in 50–75% of women. Typically, a hot flush begins as a sudden sensation of heat in the face and upper chest and this rapidly becomes generalised. The sensation of heat lasts for a few minutes and is often associated with profuse perspiration and occasionally palpitations. Often, the flush is followed by chills and shivering. Hot flushes usually occur several times per day but this may vary from once or twice a day to as often as once per hour during the day and night. Treatment is with oestrogen replacement, or clonidine if this is not possible.

Table 8.21 summarises problems that are commonly associated with the menopause.

Table 8.21   Menopausal problems

Vasomotor changes
- Hot flushes
- Palpitations
- Sleep disturbance
- Headache

Neuropsychiatric changes
- Fatigue
- Irritability
- Depression
- Difficulty concentrating

Urogenital changes
- Decreased sexual function
- Vaginal dryness and dyspareunia
- Urinary incontinence
- Recurrent urinary tract infections

Skin changes
- Increased ageing and wrinkling of the skin

Bone changes
- Osteoporosis and fracture

Cardiovascular changes
- Altered lipid metabolism: increased serum total cholesterol, increased LDL, decreased HDL
- Increased incidence of coronary heart disease

HDL = high-density lipoprotein, LDL = low-density lipoprotein.

Benefits and risks of oestrogen replacement therapy

Oestrogen therapy in postmenopausal women has several beneficial effects as well as potentially serious risks (Table 8.22).

The decision to treat a postmenopausal woman with oestrogen should be based on assessment of the benefits and risks for that woman and discussion with her. Short-term oestrogen replacement therapy is indicated for relief of menopausal symptoms and long-term therapy for prevention of osteoporosis and coronary heart disease. Whether given short or long term, oestrogen can be given alone, as oestrogen with cyclical progestogen, and as continuous oestrogen and progestogen.

Vaginal atrophy may respond to a short course of vaginal oestrogen preparation given for only a few weeks and repeated if necessary.

Table 8.22   Benefits and risks of hormone replacement therapy

Benefits of HRT	Risks of HRT
Abolition of hot flushes and other symptoms of vasomotor instability	Increased risk of venous thromboembolism
Alleviation of genitourinary symptoms	Increased risk of breast cancer
Reduction of cardiovascular risk factors	Increased risk of endometrial carcinoma (eliminated by intermittent or continuous progestogen therapy)
Reduction of coronary heart disease mordidity and mortality	Increased risk of gall bladder disease
Prevention and treatment of osteoporosis	
Cosmetic effects	

Vasomotor symptoms require systemic oestrogen replacement for at least 1 year. Women who have an early menopause (before age 45 years) are at increased risk of osteoporosis, and hormone replacement therapy (HRT) should be recommended at least until the age of 50.

The decision about whether or not to embark on long-term HRT requires a careful assessment of the risks and benefits, including risk factors for osteoporosis. In menopausal women without a uterus, long-term HRT is almost certainly beneficial overall, since they do not need progestogen therapy. In women with a uterus, the need for administration of a progestogen may lessen the cardiovascular benefits of oestrogen replacement. Furthermore, use of HRT is associated with an increased risk of breast cancer. This increased risk is related to the duration of HRT, and the excess risk disappears within about 5 years of stopping treatment. The increased risk in women who have short-term HRT is very small. However, after 10 years of treatment, the risk is more appreciable and the need to continue HRT beyond 10 years needs careful evaluation.

Further Reading

Jeffcoate W. The treatment of women with hirsutism. *Clin Endocr* 1993;**39:**143–50.

Franks S. Polycystic ovary syndrome. *N Engl J Med* 1995;**333:**853–61.

Toozs-Hobson P, Cardozo L. Hormone replacement therapy for all? Universal prescription is desirable. *Br Med J* 1996;**313**:350–2.

Conn JJ, Jacobs HS. Managing hirsutism in gynaecological practice. *Br J Obstet Gynaecol* 1998;**105**:687–96.

The initial investigation and management of the infertile couple – evidence-based clinical guidelines No. 2. *RCOG* 1998.

The management of infertility in secondary care – evidence-based clinical guidelines No. 3. *RCOG* 1998.

The management of infertility in tertiary care – evidence-based clinical guidelines No. 6. *RCOG* 2000.

Kyei-Mensah AA, Jacobs HS. The investigation of female infertility. *Clin Endocrinol* 1995;**43**:251–5.

Godsland IA, Winkler U, Lidegaard O, Crook D. Occlusive vascular diseases in oral contraceptive users: epidemiology, pathology and mechanisms. *Drugs* 2000;**60**:721–869.

9

Male Hypogonadism

Pierre-Marc Gilles Bouloux

Introduction

Male hypogonadism describes the conglomeration of symptoms and signs secondary to androgen deficiency (AD). Clinical manifestations of hypogonadism depend upon the time of onset of the androgen deficiency. When AD occurs *in utero*, it manifests as ambiguous or abnormal development of the external genitalia (male pseudohermaphroditism) in the neonatal male; in adolescence it presents as delayed puberty, whereas in adulthood presentations with impotence, loss of libido and infertility may predominate. In order to understand the causes of AD, an understanding of the normal functioning of the hypothalamo–pituitary–testicular (HPT) axis, testosterone metabolism and the effects of testosterone on androgen-dependent tissues is essential.

Regulation of the HPT axis

The central control of the HPT axis is within the mediobasal hypothalamus, where GnRH (gonadotrophin-releasing hormone) neurones, some 2000 in number, receive neuronal signals from extrahypothalamic sites as well as the hypothalamus. There is no discrete GnRH-containing nucleus: rather, GnRH neurones are dispersed within the mediobasal hypothalamus, and are interconnected. The perikarya send axons which abut the median eminence portal vessels where the decapeptide GnRH is secreted in a pulsatile manner (pulse frequency 60–90 min in adulthood). In the pituitary, GnRH stimulates gonadotrophs, stimulating synthesis and pulsatile release of the gonadotrophins LH (luteinising hormone) and FSH (follicle-stimulating hormone) from the gonadotroph cells. The mediobasal hypothalamic GnRH pulse generator possesses intrinsic pulse-generating capability. However, GnRH neuronal activity is also under the influence of negative feedback effects of gonadal steroids, and by neuronal and paracrine input from extrahypothalamic and hypothalamic structures. Several neurotransmitters and neuropeptides appear able to modulate GnRH release both directly and indirectly: they include catecholamines, serotonin, γ-aminobutyric acid (GABA), opioid peptides, substance P, and corticotrophin-releasing hormone (CRH), neuropeptide Y (NPY), and possibly leptin. In particular, opioid peptides suppress GnRH release, an effect reversed by the specific opioid antagonist naloxone.

Both LH and FSH are therefore released in a pulsatile manner as a consequence of pulsatile GnRH neurosecretion. Gonadotrophs exposed to a continuous GnRH stimulus rapidly desensitise, as seen in clinical practice with the application of superactive analogues, which downregulate the GnRH receptors and make the gonadotrophs refractory to GnRH stimulation. Whereas LH pulses are readily observed, FSH pulses are less readily discernible due to its longer half-life. The peak and trough values of LH are as much as 50% above and below the mean concentration – the amplitude of pulses are greatest in primary testicular failure and lowest in hypothalamic hypogonadism. The pulsatile pattern of LH is increased at the onset of puberty, and is maximal after the onset of clinical puberty, whereas in adulthood, pulsatility is maintained throughout the day with no diurnal variation.

Testosterone is the main gonadal steroid affecting negative feedback of LH secretion, although its actions may in part be mediated through aromatisation to oestradiol in the hypothalamus. GnRH cells appear devoid of oestrogen receptors, and the negative feedback effect is therefore indirect. FSH secretion is under the predominant effect of the Sertoli cell product inhibin A. Thus, in males, an elevated FSH level indicates Sertoli/germ cell damage.

Regulation of testicular steroidogenesis

The glycoprotein LH acts on a specific LH receptor expressed on the Leydig cells of the testes, and stimulates steroidogenesis via a cyclic adenosine monophosphate (cAMP)-mediated pathway. The LH receptor possesses a large extracellular domain and seven transmembrane segments; LH receptor occupancy stimulates a signal transduction event which initiates a cascade whereby the parent compound cholesterol is progressively hydrolysed to various androgenic steroids. Steroidogenesis is covered in Chapter 7.

Testosterone metabolism

Testosterone is metabolised irreversibly to dihydrotestosterone (DHT) in peripheral target tissues such as prostate and hair follicles through the action of the NADPH-dependent non-P450 enzyme 5α-reductase, located on the endoplasmic reticulum and nuclear membrane. Conversion of androstenedione and testosterone to DHT by these two tissues accounts for virtually all of the DHT produced in man (300 µg/day). DHT is metabolised to 3-androstanediol glucuronide. In the periphery, testosterone can also be aromatised to oestradiol, with only 25% circulating oestradiol in man being secreted from the testes. Being lipid soluble, testosterone is transported in the bloodstream to androgen-responsive tissues tightly bound to sex hormone-binding globulin SHBG (44%) and loosely to albumin (54%); only 2–3% testosterone is free and bioavailable. The liver-derived glycoprotein SHBG comprises a mixture of variously sized subunits. It has a single high-affinity binding site for both androgens and oestrogens and is regulated by several factors (Table 9.1)

SHBG has two binding sites – one for steroids, the other for cell membrane recognition. Androgens such as testosterone enter the cytoplasm, where they interact with the androgen receptor (AR), a member of the steroid receptor family of nuclear transcriptional factors, whose action depends on ligand binding. Upon binding of androgen, the AR loses its inhibitory proteins such as hsp90; there

Table 9.1 Regulators of sex hormone-binding globulin (SHBG) production

Increased SHBG	Decreased SHBG
Oestrogens	Androgens
T4 and T3	Obesity
Phenytoin	Hirsutism, PCOS
Ageing in men	Prolactin and GH excess
Anorexia nervosa	Progestogens, glucocorticoids
Prepuberty	Menopause

GH = growth hormone, PCOS = polycystic ovary syndrome, T_3 = triidothyronine, T_4 = thyroxine.

is an increase in receptor phosphorylation and then a conformational change that converts it to an active DNA-binding state. After translocation to the cell nucleus, the androgen–testosterone complex undergoes dimerisation and binding to the hormone responsive element enhancer sequence in the promoter region of a target gene. In the presence of appropriate cofactors (e.g. AR specific cofactor ARA-70), the dimer then alters the rate of transcription of target genes. AR is found throughout the mammalian tissues, attesting to the diverse effects of androgens not only in development and maintenance of sexual function but also in other sexually dimorphic processes ranging from modulation of immune function to development of neural tissues.

Defective function of the AR leads to the syndromes of androgen insensitivity, the archetypal hormone resistance disorder. As a consequence of impaired negative feedback on LH secretion, testosterone is secreted in increased amounts from the testes, but tissues are refractory to the effects of androgens. Over 200 mutations have been described in the androgen receptor, causing a variety of severity of phenotype from complete (e.g. testicular feminisation) to partial androgen insensitivity (sexual ambiguity).

Role of AR in fetal sexual differentiation

Normal sexual development begins with the establishment of genetic sex at fertilisation, followed by *sexual determination* (gonadal development) and *sexual differentiation* (genital development). Although possessing bipotential gonadal tissue for the first 6 weeks of gestation, *SRY* gene expression from the Y chromosome then occurs and interactions with other autosomal and X chromosome loci initiate testes development. The developing testes secrete the Sertoli cell glycoprotein müllerian inhibiting hormone (MIH), which causes müllerian duct regression at 6–8 weeks' gestation. Testosterone production, under the influence of human chorionic gonadotrophin (hCG), stimulates wolffian duct development, with subsequent development into epididymes, vasa deferentia and seminal vesicles between week 9 and week 13. Fetal Leydig cells begin to secrete testosterone around 8 weeks. Development of the prostate, the prostatic urethra from the urogenital sinus and the masculinisation of the external genital primordia – the genital tubercle, urethral folds and labioscrotal swellings – also occur between 9 and 13 weeks' gestation, but require the more potent androgen DHT, the result of local testosterone metabolism by the type 2 5α-reductase enzyme in these tissues. DHT has a ×10-fold increased affinity for the AR.

Disorders Causing Male Hypogonadism

The causes of AD can broadly be classified as those originating from primary testicular dysfunction, disturbances of hypothalamo–pituitary function and those conditions caused by resistance to the effects of testosterone.

The clinical features of AD are critically influenced by its age of onset (Table 9.2). When occurring in fetal life, defective masculinisation of the genitals occurs, leading to intersexual states, ranging from testicular feminisation at one extreme, to hypospadias, micropenis and cryptorchidism. Prepubertal onset leads to eunuchoidism, whereby continued growth of long bones (growth hormone (GH)-related) due to delay in epiphyseal closure and failure of androgen-dependent vertebral growth leads to arm span greater than height, and heel–pubis exceeding crown–pubis by more than 5 cm. Postpubertal hypogonadism leads to loss of libido,

Table 9.2   Clinical features of androgen deficiency

Intrauterine	Prepubertal	Postpubertal
Inadequate masculinisation	Infantile penis	Decreased density of secondary sexual hair
Cryptorchidism	Scanty/absent pubic hair	Reduced shaving frequency
Hypospadias	Small testes, prostate	Reduced morning erections
Micropenis	Underdeveloped muscles	Loss of libido, impotence
Intersexual states	Female fat distribution	Atrophic prostate
	Gynaecomastia	Tiredness, muscle bulk ⇓
	Euneuchoid proportions	Gynaecomastia
	Osteoporosis	Dry smooth wrinkled skin
	Dry smooth skin	Normal voice
	Scanty axillary, body and facial hair	Normal body proportions
	Absence of temporal recession	Mild anaemia
	High pitch unbroken voice	Low bone density
	Mild anaemia	Lethargy, irritability
	Short stature	
	Delayed bone age	

impotence, decreased secondary sexual hair (facial, axillary, corporal, pubic), muscle atrophy, anaemia, decreased bone density and possibly diminished visuospatial skills.

Endocrine Investigation of Hypogonadism

In most cases, a blood sample should be drawn at 09.00 for testosterone and LS/FSH levels. High gonadotrophins associated with low testosterone levels are diagnostic of primary gonadal failure. Low testosterone levels with an inappropriately low LH/FSH level are indicative of hypothalamo–pituitary disease. A serum prolactin level should be performed if hypogonadotrophic hypogonadism (HH) is found. In acquired HH, a normal serum iron and TIBC will exclude haemochromatosis. Full anterior pituitary evaluation – basal thyroid-stimulating hormone (TSH), fT_4, 09.00 cortisol, IgF1/GH – is indicated if there is a suspicion of a hypothalamo–pituitary lesion.The presence of diabetes insipidus strongly suggests the presence of a hypothalamic lesion (e.g. glioma, germinoma, sarcoidosis, histiocytosis).

Free testosterone measurement

Free or non-SHBG bound testosterone represents the majority of circulating biologically active androgen and is particularly useful in conditions where the SHBG concentration is abnormal, for example in ageing men (free testosterone is frequently low despite normal total testosterone), and in obese individuals where, because of low SHBG levels, normal free testosterone levels may be present in the presence of low total testosterone. SHBG levels are therefore useful in deriving an estimate of the free testosterone concentrations.

Plasma DHT levels

These are only of value in patients suspected of having 5α-reductase deficiency. Diagnosis is usually confirmed by the family history and genital skin fibroblast studies.

Chromosomal analysis

These are of value in patients with suspected primary testicular failure due to Klinefelter's syndrome (XXY karyotype), where they have a prognostic value for fertility.

Androgen receptor studies

Molecular techniques are of greatest value in diagnosis of disorders of AR. SSCP (single-strand conformation polymorphism analysis) and polymerase chain reaction (PCR) sequencing strategies have been used to demonstrate gene rearrangements, deletions, premature termination codons and single nucleotide substitutions of the AR gene. Skin fibroblast culture is occasionally useful for precise characterisation of the associated functional defects.

Seminal analysis

This is clearly important where the presentation is with infertility.

Dynamic hormone tests in evaluation of hypothalamo–pituitary disease

GnRH test

This tests the gonadotroph readily releasable LH/FSH pool. It is usually given in a 100 μg dose and LH/FSH measured at 0, 30 and 60 min. It is of limited value clinically. Typically, patients with GnRH deficiency have a poor LH/FSH response to the 100 μg GnRH test, but in the presence of an intact gonadotroph population, may begin to release LH/FSH with a second larger (500 μg) dose of GnRH.

hCG stimulation test

This is a test of Leydig cell function, which can be stimulated by a single high dose of intramuscular hCG (2000–5000 IU), leading to a peak in testosterone levels after 72–96 hours. Patients with Leydig cell dysfunction will not respond to hCG with increased testosterone production. Its major use is in children with cryptorchidism, when an increase in testosterone after hCG administration indicates that the testes are present, distinguishing them from boys with anorchidism.

Pulsatile LH/FSH sampling

This can delineate patterns of abnormal gonadotrophin secretion but should be considered a research tool.

Imaging of the hypothalamo–pituitary region

In patients with hypogonadotrophic hypogonadism with evidence of other pituitary hormone deficiencies, magnetic resonance imaging

(MRI) examination of the hypothalamo–pituitary region gives the best spatial anatomo–pathological resolution. MRI is essential for ruling out structural lesions of this region, and may confirm a diagnosis of Kallmann's syndrome, where olfactory bulbs and olfactory sulci are characteristically absent.

Disorders Associated with Hypogonadism
(Table 9.3)

Hypothalamo–pituitary disorders, congenital

Isolated gonadotrophin deficiency

This may be isolated (idiopathic hypogonadotrophic hypogonadism or IHH) or associated with anosmia (Kallmann's syndrome). Males are more commonly affected than females, and height tends to be normal for age, tall adult height being achieved if the patients are untreated. There is delayed bone age, a normal adrenarche, and, when severe, boys will present with undescended testes, and some with micropenis. Many will present with delayed puberty when the distinction with simple pubertal delay may pose difficulties. Absent LH pulsatility in nocturnal studies in IHH may distinguish this condition from simple pubertal delay. Evidence of other pituitary hormone involvement should be sought, and MRI performed to exclude a structural lesion of the hypothalamo–pituitary region.

Kallmann's syndrome may be sporadic or familial (particularly X-linked) and is the most common form of IHH with delayed puberty. Anosmia or hyposmia due to agenesis or hypoplasia of the olfactory lobes is associated with GnRH deficiency. Males are affected six times more commonly than females. The magnitude of GnRH deficiency correlates with testicular volume. Associated, though inconstant defects include cleft lip (autosomal/sporadic forms), imperfect facial fusion, seizure disorders, short fourth metacarpals, pes cavus, neurosensory hearing loss, cerebellar ataxia, unilateral or bilateral renal agenesis (X-linked forms) and mirror movements of the upper extremities (X-linked form). Fewer than 10% of patients have a normal MRI scan. In Kallmann's syndrome, fetal GnRH neurones fail to migrate from the olfactory placode into the hypothalamus, presumably because the migratory pathway is interrupted by a developmental defect affecting olfactory bulb histogenesis.

Table 9.3   Causes of hypogonadism

Hypothalamo–pituitary	*Congenital*
	Isolated GnRH deficiency
	Kallmann's syndrome
	Prader–Willi syndrome
	Laurence–Moon–Biedl syndrome
	Fertile eunuch syndrome
	PROP 1 gene defect
	HESX1 gene defect (pituitary hypoplasia)
	Gordon–Holmes ataxia
	Acquired
	Trauma (stalk section)
	Post surgery, irradiation
	Infiltrative disorders: sarcoidosis, tuberculosis
	Fungal infection, haemochromatosis
	Pituitary infarction, carotid aneurysm
	Pituitary adenoma, germinoma, glioma
	Craniopharyngioma
	Malnutrition, anorexia nervosa, depression
	Systemic disease (chronic liver disease)
	Chronic renal failure
	Lymphocytic hypophysitis
	Hyperprolactinaemia (prolactinoma, drug-induced hypothyroidism)
	GnRH antagonist, superactive GnRH agonists
Testicular	Chromosomal defects (Klinefelter's syndrome)
	Biosynthetic defects of testosterone synthesis
	Androgen resistance
	Torsion of the testes
	Testicular irradiation, orchitis
	Androgen antagonists (cyproterone acetate, spironolactone, cimetidine, flutamide)

GnRH receptor mutations

A number of autosomally recessive genetic forms of HH have been described where there were either homozygous or compound heterozygous loss of function mutations of the GnRH receptor.

Defects of DAX-1 gene

This uncommon X-linked disturbance of adrenocortical formation is caused by a defect in the *DAX-1* gene (dosage–sensitive sex reversal hypoplasia congenita gene). It is characterised by severe glucocorticoid and mineralocorticoid deficiency and, at puberty, androgen deficiency. There is evidence for both hypothalamic GnRH deficiency and a reduced gonadotroph pituitary pool in this condition.

Isolated LH deficiency (fertile eunuch syndrome)

This is associated with deficient testosterone production, which responds to the administration of hCG and variable degrees of spermatogenesis. It is rarely associated with a defect in the gene encoding the LHβ subunit.

PROP1 and HESX1 defects

These autosomal recessive conditions are associated with multiple pituitary hormonal deficiencies due to developmental defect of the pituitary.

HH associated with other syndromes

Prader–Willi syndrome. This is a syndrome of early-onset childhood hyperphagia, massive obesity and carbohydrate intolerance, infantile hypotonia lethargy, short stature by 15 years of age and emotional instability. There is a characteristic facies, with almond-shaped eyes, triangular mouth and narrow bifrontal diameter. Patients have delayed puberty and hypothalamic hypogonadism, despite a tendency to early adrenarche. Affected boys have micropenis and cryptorchidism. Patients have an abnormality in the long arm of chromosome 15q11-q13.

Laurence–Moon and Bardet–Biedl syndromes. Both are autosomal recessive disorders associated with hypothalamic hypogonadism and retinitis pigmentosa. In the Laurence–Moon syndrome, spastic paraplegia is present, whereas in the Bardet–Biedl syndrome, polydactyly and obesity are present.

Acquired forms of gonadotrophin deficiency

Functional gonadotrophin deficiency

Chronic systemic disease and malnutrition (as in anorexia nervosa) is associated with reversible gonadotrophin deficiency. These include such disorders as Crohn's disease, cystic fibrosis, thalassaemia major (transfusion haemosiderosis with gonadotroph damage), chronic renal failure and Cushing's syndrome.

Excessive exercise

This may be associated with diminished LH pulsatility and functional hypogonadism (testosterone levels down to 3–4 nmol/l) that is reversible upon stopping excessive training programmes.

Pituitary–hypothalamic disorders

A large number of pituitary lesions are associated with HH. By the time HH is present, patients are usually GH-deficient, and progressive pituitary lesions then lead to TSH, adrenocorticotrophic hormone (ACTH) and finally prolactin deficiency.

Tumours include craniopharyngioma, pituitary adenoma and, importantly, prolactinoma. Cranial irradiation, haemochromatosis (usually associated with selective gonadotroph damage), infiltrative disorders such as sarcoidosis, tuberculosis and histiocytosis X may damage the hypothalamo–pituitary axis and be associated with HH.

Patients with HH and clinical suspicion of pituitary lesions should have their visual fields carefully charted, a full anterior and posterior pituitary hormonal evaluation, as well as MRI imaging.

Hyperprolactinaemia has a large number of causes (see Chapter 3), and the mechanism of hyperprolactinaemic hypogonadism is complex. High prolactin inhibits the GnRH pulse generator, and interferes with the gonadal effects of the gonadotrophins. Prolactin-secreting tumours, in addition, may damage the gonadotroph population of the anterior pituitary, causing gonadotrophin deficiency. Dopamine agonists such as bromocriptine and cabergoline will suppress hyperprolactinaemia, often restoring normal HPT relationships, as well as shrinking prolactinomas.

Primary testicular failure

Klinefelter's syndrome

This occurs in 1 in 1000 newborn males, and has a wide range of clinical features, ranging from marked feminisation to full virilisation. Small firm testes are a constant feature. Histologically, the tubules are severely affected by hyalinisation and infertility is the invariable rule. Very rarely, small foci of spermatogenesis are found histologically, and these are usually in XY/XXY mosaics. It is not usually diagnosed prepubertally, although eunuchoidism may be present from an early age. Feminine fat contours may occur together with gynaecomastia and diminished secondary sexual hair on the face and body. FSH levels are invariably grossly elevated, but LH levels may range from normal adult levels to elevated. Seminiferous tubules are grossly atrophic and, histologically, Leydig cells give the illusory appearance of being hyperplastic. Testosterone levels, which may be at the lower end of the normal adult reference range in the 2nd and 3rd decades then tend to fall off rapidly. SHBG levels are raised, as are oestradiol levels, and the oestradiol : testosterone ratio is raised. Osteoporosis is present, patients are of tall stature, and there is a 20-fold increase in the incidence of breast cancer.

Dystrophia myotonica

This is an autosomal dominant condition characterised by frontal balding, mental retardation, cataracts and primary gonadal failure, associated with raised FSH levels and variable Leydig cell failure.

Acquired causes of primary testicular failure

Trauma, torsion of the testes, irradiation damage, infections (e.g. mumps), inflammation and infiltrations (e.g. leukaemia) may affect the testes and compromise testicular function and testosterone secretion. Several drugs can cause hypogonadism. They include spironolactone and ketoconazole and the antiandrogens flutamide and cyproterone acetate. Cimetidine is an antiandrogen and may cause gynaecomastia.

Renal failure is commonly associated with testicular failure affecting both spermatogenesis and testosterone production, with raised gonadotrophins.

Treatment of Male Hypogonadism

Induction of puberty

Patients aged 12–13 with delayed puberty, irrespective of aetiology, who are psychologically disadvantaged, should be considered for therapeutic induction of puberty. Similarly, patients with constitutional growth and pubertal delay should be viewed as having a transient form of hypogonadism with relative GH deficiency and should be treated, with the proviso that low doses of testosterone are used (this should not cause premature fusion of the epiphyses and reduction of growth potential). The aim of treatment is to respect the normal cadence of puberty and maintain the patient's development in line with that of his peers, stimulating linear growth, avoiding the long-term consequence of underaccretion of peak bone mass and preventing the adverse psychological seque-lae of delayed maturation. A well-established regimen consists of giving 50 mg testosterone enanthate every 4–6 weeks in the first year, and then increasing to 100 mg, 4 weekly, in the second year, and 200–250 mg, 4 weekly, in the third year. Alternatively, testos-terone undecanoate given at a dose of 40 mg on alternate days for the first year, 40 mg daily in the second year and 80 mg, twice a day, in the third year may be acceptable. The drug must be taken with food to facilitate absorption. Serial monitoring of bone age at 6–12 monthly intervals is important in detecting inappropriate acceleration of skeletal maturation, thereby enabling better titration of replacement therapy. Properly titrated, such testosterone dosage regimens do not suppress endogenous gonadotrophin secretion in patients with simple pubertal delay, in whom serial measurement of testicular volume can be used as marker of underlying gonadotrophin (FSH) secretion. Puberty generally progresses off treatment when testicular volumes have reached around 8 ml.

Physiological replacement in the adult male

The cause of hypogonadism must be established prior to therapy and corrected when possible. For example, a patient with hypogonadism suffering from a prolactinoma will often resume normal HPT func-tion after normalisation of prolactin using a dopamine agonist. Medical treatment of other pituitary tumours is usually not possible, and surgery will be indicated. Occasionally, debulking of a func-tionless pituitary tumour is associated with relief of a stalk effect and normalisation of HPT activity. The more frequent scenario is that the patient is left with long-term HH. In patients with hypothalamic disease and associated GnRH deficiency, pulsatile subcutaneous or intravenous GnRH 25–100 ng/kg/pulse at 90 min intervals will restore normal pulsatile gonadotrophin secretion with normalisation of testosterone levels and resumption of spermatogenesis. Treatment is usually of prolonged duration (up to 12–18 months). Thrice-weekly intramuscular gonadotrophins (e.g. recombinant FSH 225 IU intramuscularly × 3 weekly and hCG 2000 IU × 2 weekly) for 12 to 18 months is similarly effective. However, although these treatments will restore testicular volumes into the normal range and initiate spermatogenesis, they are costly and inconvenient to administer and should only be used in patients seeking fertility. Both regimens may take up to 2 years to achieve adequate spermatogenesis, and thus, once effective, consideration should be given to storing several samples of frozen sperm for any future attempts at pregnancy.

Testosterone replacement therapy (TRT)

The major goal of testosterone therapy is to replace testosterone levels to as close a physiological concentration as possible, enabling androgen-dependent functions to be induced or restored, using the safest delivery methods possible. Naturally occurring molecules are preferred to synthetic preparations, to guarantee the broad spectrum of testosterone effects. Testosterone owes its specific biological activity to the keto group in position 3, the double bond in position 4 and the hydroxy group in position 17 of the basic androstane structure. For therapeutic use, chemical modification of the molecule is required, usually by way of esterification in position 17. Subsequent esterase activity will release the native testosterone molecule.

Oral preparations

Native testosterone is inactivated in the liver in about 10 min. In order to produce physiological levels, 400–600 mg testosterone must be given orally: i.e. about × 100 the amount produced by the human testes per day.

Testosterone undecanoate

Esterification in the 17-α position by undecanoic acid allows absorption of the molecule by the lymphatic channels, thereby largely avoiding the first pass effect into the liver. Absorption is thus enhanced if the patient takes the drug with a fatty meal. One 40 mg capsule contains 25 mg testosterone, and peak serum levels are reached about 2–6 hours after ingestion, such that 2–4 capsules are required daily using multiple dosing regimens. Because of modest increases in serum testosterone levels, as well as short-lived peaks and trough levels between doses, testosterone undecanoate is best suited to patients with residual capacity to secrete testosterone such as Klinefelter's syndrome, or for patients in whom intramuscular preparations are not suitable (e.g. patients on warfarin therapy). Metabolism of testosterone undecanoate by intestinal 5α-reductase activity generates a high DHT : testosterone ratio. Thus, plasma DHT estimation may be useful to monitor such patients.

Methyl testosterone and fluoxymesterone

These are 17α-derivatives, the methyl group protecting the molecule from being metabolised in the liver. Fluoxymesterone contains a fluoride atom in addition to an additional hydroxy group. However, they are associated with a transaminitis, occasional cholestasis and peliosis hepatis, and therefore these preparations should be considered obsolete.

Mesterolone

This is derived from the 5α-reduced testosterone metabolite dihydrotestosterone, and is likewise not subject to hepatic metabolism following oral administration. As a DHT derivative, it can only compensate for DHT-dependent functions and not for the immediate effects of testosterone or those following aromatisation of the molecule. It is therefore not suitable for replacement therapy in hypogonadism.

Intramuscular preparations

When esterified with an aliphatic side chain in the 17 position, the duration of action of testosterone is prolonged, depending on the length and structure of the side chain. The propionate ester has the shortest half-life; the phenylpropionate ester has a longer half-life and the isocaproate ester a longer half-life still. When combined (in doses of 20 mg/ml propionate, 40 mg/ml phenylpropionate and 40 mg/ml isocaproate: Sustanon 100), they theoretically give the most physiological testosterone pharmacokinetic profile when given by weekly intramuscular injections in adults. Testosterone enanthate (Primoteston Depot 250 mg/ml intramuscularly 3 weekly) has a terminal half-life of 4.5 days, but as pharmacokinetics studies show, supraphysiological peaks are achieved, and are maintained for several days followed by a logarithmic decline to below the starting levels by day 12. Repeated injections therefore generate a saw-tooth effect, patients frequently complaining of a 'high' (well-being, sexual activity, mood) lasting about 1 week after injection followed by a low before the next injection is due.

Transdermal testosterone preparations

Daily physiological testosterone production rate is around 6 mg in the adult. Scrotal skin, because of its high blood supply and relatively thin stratum corneum, facilitates transscrotal testosterone absorption, which enables physiological testosterone levels to be achieved with a single daily scrotal patch application. The TTS Testoderm (*Testoderm*: Ferring Pharmaceuticals) system consists of a 40 or 60 cm^2 polymer membrane loaded with 10 or 15 mg natural testosterone. The membrane is applied once a day in the morning, and since the preparation does not contain an enhancer, skin irritations are unusual. The scrotum must be rid of hair to enable maximal absorption, and because of high scrotal 5α-reductase activity, DHT : testosterone ratios, like oral testosterone undecanoate (Restandol) are elevated.

The *Andropatch* system is presented as a 2.5 or 5 mg patch system with alcohol as an excipient, and is applied at night-time to intact clean and dry skin on the back, abdomen, upper arms or thighs; the application site is changed every 24 hours. The dose is adjusted to 2.5–7.5 mg acccording to morning testosterone levels. Local reactions total some 10%, and the patch should not be applied to pressure points (bony prominences) or the scrotum. Local skin reactions usually respond to mild topical steroid application.

Virormone (Ferring) is a non-alcohol-containing system that delivers approximately 5 mg percutaneously per 24 hours. It is applied to the arm, back or upper buttocks every 24 hours. The testosterone level is measured on the fourth day 2–4 hours after patch application, and the dose is increased to two patches if necessary.

Testosterone pellets

Testosterone implants are among the oldest testosterone preparations, consisting of pure testosterone moulded into cylindrical forms of 12 mm length and 4.5 mm diameter. Each implant is 200 mg, and is usually implanted through a 0.5–1 cm incision under local anaesthetic under the abdominal skin or the buttock. The dose range is 600 mg to 1 g, and testosterone levels reach a peak within 1 month and slowly decline over the next 4–6 months. There is a 5% extrusion rate with implants. Most patients require six monthly applications and find this treatment modality particularly convenient.

Choice of TRT

Intramuscular testosterone esters, testosterone implants, oral testosterone undecanoate and transdermal preparations may all be used for TRT, the choice depending very much on patient preference. Testosterone implants tend to be reserved as maintenance treatment in young adults already having been initiated on intramuscular or oral preparations. Many patients respond well to testosterone esters every three weeks, although the 'saw-tooth' serum testosterone characteristics are less with weekly i.m. injections. Peak and trough testosterone estimations help to identify the 10% or so patient who clear the drug rapidly, and who would benefit from dosage increase.

Monitoring TRT in hypogonadism (Table 9.4)

In general, well-being and activity are good parameters for checking effectiveness of replacement. Libido, and sexual thoughts and fantasies, improve and nightly and morning erections improve in frequency, as does the volume of ejaculate at orgasm. Muscle mass and strength increase in hypogonadal men on testosterone, and body weight increases by about 5%, with a relatively greater increase in muscle mass. Secondary sexual hair improves, and shaving frequency increases. Sebum production increases, and hair becomes greasier. Bone density improves.

Complications of androgen replacement therapy

Complications of androgen replacement therapy include acne, transient priapism, gynaecomastia, fluid retention, slight increases

Table 9.4   Criteria for monitoring testosterone replacement therapy

Psychological and sexual responses	General well-being Intellectual and physical activity Mood, libido Frequency of morning erections Sexual activity, fantasies
Somatic effects	Body weight, proportions, growth Muscle mass and strength Fat and hair distribution Sebum production Deepening of the voice
Laboratory parameters	Testosterone, SHBG, LH/FSH Lipids, liver function tests Haematocrit, PSA
Prostate	Ejaculatory volume, prostate size Prostate size (digital or ultrasonic examination)
Bones	Bone density

FSH = follicle-stimulating hormone, LH = luteinising hormone,
PSA = prostate-specific antigen, SHBG = sex hormone-binding globulin.

in haematocrit and sleep apnoea. Those at risk are obese older men with thick necks and high upper airways resistance identified by a high haematocrit and a propensity to snore. Such side effects are not generally seen with standard replacement therapies, and are most frequently seen with abuses of androgens: for example, as part of performance-enhancing regimens.

In the ageing male, transdermal preparations are preferable, and since they are associated with more physiological blood levels, they are less likely to promote prostatic enlargement. Physiological TRT does not enlarge the prostate volume over the normal range. However, any ageing male on TRT should, as a precaution, be submitted to a periodic digital or ultrasonic examination of the prostate and/or an annual prostate-specific antigen (PSA) estimation.

Further Reading

Bagatell CJ, Heimann JR, Rivier JE, Bremner WJ. Effects of endogenous testosterone and oestradiol on sexual behaviour in normal young men. *J Clin Endocrinol Metab* 1994;**78**:711–16.

Davidson JM, Camargo CA, Smith ER. Effects of androgens on sexual behaviour in hypogonadal man. *J Clin Endocrinol Metab* 1979;**48**:955–8.

Handelsman DJ, Conway AJ, Boylan LM. Pharmacokinetics and pharmacodynamics of testosterone pellets in man. *J Clin Endocrinol Metab* 1990;**71**:216–22.

Nieschlag E. Testosterone replacement therapy: something old, something new (commentary). *Clin Endocrinol (Oxf)* 1996;**45**:261–2.

Prader A. Delayed adolescence. *J Clin Endocrinol Metab* 1975;**4**:143–55.

Stuart S, Howards MD. Treatment of male infertility. *New Engl J Med* 1995;**332**:312–17.

World Health Organization – Nieslag E, Wang CH, Handelsman DJ, *et al.* (eds), *Guidelines for the Use of Androgens.* Geneva: WHO, 1992.

10

Hyperthyroidism

Anthony D Toft

Introduction

Hyperthyroidism or thyrotoxicosis is the clinical syndrome resulting from excessive secretion of the thyroid hormones, thyroxine
(T_4) and/or triiodothyronine (T_3). The prevalence in the community
is of the order of 1%, most commonly affecting middle-aged and
elderly women. The causes are shown in Table 10.1, with Graves'
disease and nodular goitre accounting for about 90% of cases; conditions such as struma ovarii and choriocarcinoma are so rare that
they may not be encountered by an endocrinologist during his or
her professional career. On the other hand, iodine-induced hyperthyroidism is becoming more common with the increasing use of
the antidysrhythmic agent amiodarone, and may be seen in epidemic form during iodine prophylaxis programmes in areas of
endemic goitre.

Clinical Features

The classical symptoms of thyroid hormone excess and those
which are less common and may not immediately raise the possibility of hyperthyroidism are shown in Table 10.2. There is great
individual variation in the dominant features: heat intolerance
and sweating may be attributed to the menopause and pruritus
results in referral to a dermatologist; angina may occur in the
absence of significant coronary artery disease. Older patients may
present with atrial fibrillation or cardiac failure, others with
apathy and generalised muscle weakness, and in some the combination of anorexia and weight loss raises a suspicion of gastric
carcinoma.

Table 10.1   Causes of hyperthyroidism and their relative frequencies in a series of over 2000 patients presenting to the Endocrine Clinic, Royal Infirmary, Edinburgh, during a 10-year period

Cause	Frequency (%)
Graves' disease	72
Multinodular goitre	15
Toxic adenoma	5
Thyroiditis	
Subacute (de Quervain's)	2
Postpartum	2
Iodine-induced	
e.g. amiodarone and 'herbal' medicines	2.5
Extrathyroidal sources of thyroid hormone excess	
Factitious hyperthyroidism	0.2
Struma ovarii	–
TSH-induced	
Pituitary tumour	0.2
Choriocarcinoma and hydatidiform mole[a]	–
Gestational hyperthyroidism[a]	1
Follicular carcinoma ± metastases	0.1

[a] Due to intrinsic thyroid-stimulating activity of human chorionic gonadotrophin (hCG).

Establishing the diagnosis of hyperthyroidism
(Table 10.3)

Although the diagnosis may be clinically apparent, it is important to seek confirmation by one or more tests of thyroid function as treatment involves long-term antithyroid drugs or destruction of the gland with iodine-131 or surgery.

Serum TSH

Using the currently sensitive third-generation assays, serum thyroid-stimulating hormone (TSH) concentrations are less than 0.05 mU/l in hyperthyroidism. A detectable concentration excludes hyperthyroidism with the rare exceptions of a TSH-secreting pituitary tumour or thyroid hormone resistance, when serum TSH may be normal or

Table 10.2   Symptoms of hyperthyroidism

Classical	Less common
Weight loss	Pruritus
Increased appetite	Ankle oedema, in absence of cardiac
Heat intolerance	failure[b]
Breathlessness on exertion	Angina[c]
Palpitations	Exacerbation of asthma
Tremor	Increased insulin requirements in
Insomnia	patients with diabetes mellitus
Irritability	Diarrhoea
Emotional lability	Anorexia and vomiting
Restlessness	Apathy
Poor concentration	Impotence
Hyperdefaecation[a]	Infertility
Proximal muscle weakness	Gynaecomastia
Amenorrhoea/oligomenorrhoea	Periodic paralysis[d]

[a] Usually 2–3 formed, but softer than usual, stools daily.
[b] In part due to reversal to day : night ratio of urinary sodium excretion.
[c] May be due to coronary artery spasm in the absence of significant coronary atheroma.
[d] Especially ethnic Cantonese.

elevated. A low concentration is not specific for hyperthyroidism but is frequently observed in patients with significant non-thyroidal illness, nodular goitre or in those receiving thyroxine or amiodarone therapy. Following treatment of hyperthyroidism, a low serum TSH concentration may be recorded for 6–8 weeks after restoration of thyroid hormone concentrations to normal due to delayed recovery of the thyrotrophs, previously suppressed by high circulating T_3 and T_4. Indeed, it is possible to record low thyroid hormone concentrations and low TSH in the early weeks and months after treatment of thyrotoxicosis, and in this situation T_4 is a better predictor of impending hypothyroidism than TSH.

A low serum TSH concentration is not specific for hyperthyroidism.

Serum T_3 and T_4

Most laboratories measure the metabolically active free thyroid hormones, and both will be elevated in 98% of patients with hyperthyroidism, uncomplicated by non-thyroidal illness. In 'T₃ thyrotoxicosis', serum T_3 is raised but T_4 normal, although usually in the upper part of the reference range. This form of hyperthyroidism is most commonly found in patients with nodular goitre, in those who have relapsed following thyroid surgery and in areas of relative iodine deficiency. Total T_3 and T_4 measurements are less affected by non-thyroidal illness, but have the disadvantage of mirroring changes in the concentration of thyroxine-binding proteins; elevated values are recorded in pregnancy and in those taking oestrogens or raloxifene, and low concentrations in patients with hypoproteinaemia.

Ideally, if a diagnosis of hyperthyroidism is suspected, serum T_3, T_4 and TSH concentrations should be measured. However, many laboratories use TSH as a screening test, measuring T_3 and/or T_4 if the result is low.

Establishing the cause of hyperthyroidism

Although the cause of hyperthyroidism may be evident clinically in a patient with the typical features of Graves' disease or a large multinodular goitre, many patients with thyrotoxicosis have no palpable thyroid enlargement, ophthalmopathy or dermopathy. It is important to determine the cause of hyperthyroidism, as this may influence therapy.

TSH-receptor antibody (TRAb)

This is present in the serum of over 90% of patients with Graves' disease, and may become positive for the first time following treatment of hyperthyroidism with iodine-131. Measurement of TRAb is useful in distinguishing between hyperthyroidism due to Graves' disease and that due to postpartum thyroiditis when it is not detectable. It is not used routinely in the investigation of thyrotoxicosis.

Isotope scanning

Imaging of the thyroid 20–30 min after intravenous ^{99m}Tc will distinguish between a solitary toxic adenoma and the diffuse uptake of Graves' disease in a patient with no goitre. In some older patients with Graves' disease and raised TRAb concentrations, isotope scanning may show a nodular pattern of distribution.

Isotope uptake test

The ability of the thyroid to concentrate either iodine-131 or ^{99m}Tc was useful in the past as a test of thyroid function, elevated values being found in hyperthyroidism. These tests are now of value in determining the cause of hyperthyroidism in those forms in which the uptake is negligible – namely, postpartum thyroiditis, de Quervain's thyroiditis, thyrotoxicosis factitia, and that which is iodine-induced.

Graves' Disease

Graves' disease is distinguished clinically from other types of hyperthyroidism by the presence of a diffuse goitre over which there may be a bruit, ophthalmopathy and rarely pretibial myxoedema. One or more of these features may be absent, particularly in the elderly, and it is well recognised that the ophthalmopathy and dermopathy may present for the first time months or even years after successful treatment of the hyperthyroidism. Graves' disease can occur at any age but is rare before puberty and most common in the 35–55 age group. There is often a family history of auto-immune thyroid disease or of one or more of the other organ-specific autoimmune disorders, such as type 1 diabetes mellitus, pernicious anaemia, Addison's disease, premature ovarian failure and myasthenia gravis. The aetiology and other features of Graves' disease are covered in Chapter 11.

The natural history of the hyperthyroidism of Graves' disease is shown in Figure 10.1. It is the minority of patients (30%) who experience a single episode of hyperthyroidism, lasting several months, followed by prolonged remission and in some by the onset of thyroid failure 10–20 years later. The majority have continuous hyperthyroidism or a relapsing and remitting course over many years.

Which treatment for Graves' thyrotoxicosis?

Each of the treatments of the hyperthyroidism of Graves' disease – antithyroid drugs, surgery and radioactive iodine – is effective but none is perfect. Although a course of antithyroid drugs would be indicated for those patients destined to have a single episode of hyperthyroidism, it has not proved possible to predict the natural history with any degree of accuracy, and treatment remains empirical. The choice depends upon the prejudices of the physician and, increasingly, of the patient, and upon local circumstances, such as the availability of an experienced thyroid surgeon.

On a group basis, small goitre, low serum concentration of TRAb and increasing age favour remission after a course of antithyroid drugs, whereas the risk of relapse in a young male with

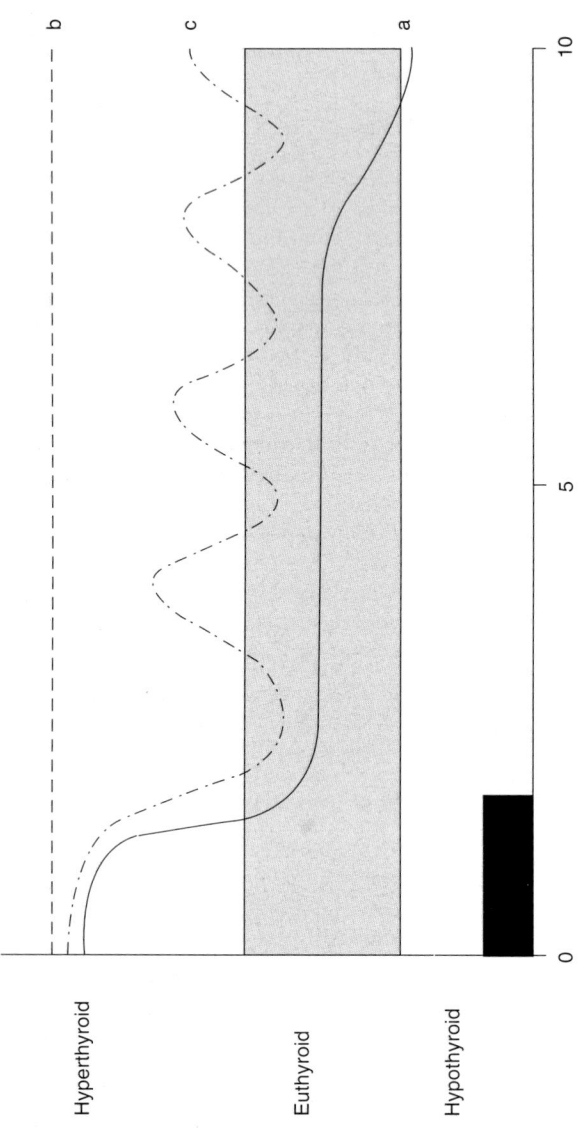

Figure 10.1 The natural history of the hyperthyroidism of Graves' disease. It is the minority who have a single short-lived episode of hyperthyroidism lasting a few months only (a). The majority have either a continuous (b) or relapsing and remitting course (c) over many years. The solid block indicates the normal duration of antithyroid therapy.

severe hyperthyroidism and a large vascular goitre is so great that most would advocate surgery as the primary treatment. Standard practice in Europe has been that the initial treatment of most patients under 40–45 years of age is with an antithyroid drug, with a recommendation for surgery should relapse occur. In the United States, however, iodine-131 therapy is not restricted to older patients and the use of antithyroid drugs and surgery is relatively uncommon.

Antithyroid drugs

The most effective and commonly used antithyroid drugs are the thionamides, carbimazole and its active metabolite, methimazole (not available in the UK). These drugs act by inhibiting the synthesis of thyroid hormones, principally by interfering with the iodination of tyrosine. There is also some evidence for an immunosuppressive action which is of doubtful clinical significance, except perhaps in the management of patients with ophthalmopathy. The other thionamide, propylthiouracil, is in addition a potent inhibitor of type I outer ring deiodinase and inhibits T_4 to T_3 conversion acutely. There is no evidence that this effect is of any clinical relevance. Propylthiouracil tends to be reserved for those patients who have developed an adverse reaction (such as rash) to carbimazole or methimazole.

Antithyroid drugs have no significant influence on the natural history of the hyperthyroidism of Graves' disease.

Duration of therapy

The conventional period of antithyroid drug therapy of 12–24 months is best viewed as a compromise by which those destined to have a single short-lived episode of hyperthyroidism are identified and primary destructive therapy with iodine-131 or by surgery avoided. The majority of patients, however, relapse usually within the first 2 years. More prolonged antithyroid drug therapy, continuous or intermittent, is not usually favoured by physician or patient as the gain, in terms of increased remission rate, is small. Long-term treatment with antithyroid drugs is, however, appropriate in patients with underlying autonomous thyroid function (Graves' disease or nodular goitre) in whom hyperthyroidism has been precipitated by amiodarone and in whom chronic treatment with the antidysrhythmic agent is planned.

Indefinite treatment with carbimazole may also be appropriate in the elderly and infirm patient who may also be incontinent of urine and in whom iodine-131 therapy is either logistically difficult or may be hazardous for the carers.

Dosage

Carbimazole is available as 5 mg and 20 mg tablets. The initial dose is 40–45 mg daily for 3–4 weeks, reducing to 30 mg for a further 3–4 weeks, with further adjustments on the basis of measurement of serum concentrations of T_3, T_4 and TSH, until a maintenance dose of 5–15 mg daily is achieved, usually within 3–4 months. Patients begin to feel an improvement at 10–14 days. Once daily dosage is appropriate for all but the most severely thyrotoxic, who benefit from being given carbimazole 20 mg twice daily or 15 mg three times daily. Initial changes in drug dosage should be based on thyroid hormone concentrations due to the delay in recovery of thyrotroph function. After 10–12 weeks, TSH is the best guide to the dose of carbimazole, high and low concentrations indicating excessive and inadequate therapy, respectively. In patients with mild hyperthyroidism both symptomatically and biochemically – e.g. TSH less than 0.05 mU/l, free thyroxine (fT_4) = 30 pmol/l, free triiodothyronine (fT_3) = 9 pmol/l – a starting dose of carbimazole of 20 mg daily is indicated.

The appropriate dose of propylthiouracil is 10 times that of carbimazole.

'Block and replace' therapy

In this regime, carbimazole is continued in the high dosage of 40–60 mg/day after the patient is euthyroid, and hypothyroidism avoided in the long term by adding thyroxine in a dose of 100–150 μg/day. The dose of thyroxine, but not of carbimazole, is adjusted to maintain serum TSH within the lower part of the reference range. This combination therapy has long been thought to be beneficial in patients with significant ophthalmopathy, presumably as a result of avoiding hypothyroidism and possibly also as a consequence of the immunosuppressive action of high-dose carbimazole. It is also useful in those with 'brittle' hyperthyroidism, fluctuating between over- and undertreatment with antithyroid drugs despite good compliance and supervision and now known to be due to changing concentrations and activities of TRAb.

Remission rates are not improved by block and replace therapy.

Table 10.3   Different patterns of thyroid hormone concentrations that may be associated with a low serum thyroid-stimulating hormone (TSH)

TSH (mU/l) (0.15–3.5)	fT$_4$ (pmol/l) (10–26)	fT$_3$ (pmol/l) (3.5–7.5)	Diagnosis
< 0.05	60	12.0	Hyperthyroidism
< 0.05	24	10.0	T$_3$ thyrotoxicosis
< 0.05	20	6.2	Subclinical hyperthyroidism, usually in the presence of nodular goitre
< 0.05	34	4.0	Non-thyroidal illness
< 0.05	50	2.8	Amiodarone therapy
< 0.05	8	4.0	Four months following iodine-131 therapy; hypothyroid with raised TSH 2 months later
< 0.05	26	5.5	Thyroxine therapy

fT$_3$ = free triiodothyronine; fT$_4$ = free thyroxine.

Adverse reactions

The adverse effects of antithyroid drugs (Table 10.4) can occur at any time but almost always within 3–6 weeks of starting treatment.

Table 10.4   Adverse effects of antithyroid drugs

Agranulocytosis (0.2–0.5%)

Rash, usually urticarial and may be associated with migratory polyarthritis (1–2%)

Nausea
Loss of taste   } May be self-limiting and not necessarily an
Headache   indication for change of drug
Hair loss

Cholestatic jaundice
ANCA-positive vasculitis } Exceptionally rare
Lupus-like syndrome
Nephrotic syndrome

There is some cross-sensitivity between carbimazole and propyl-thiouracil. Although it is common practice to change to the alternative antithyroid drug in the event of a minor adverse reaction, such as a skin rash, most would regard the development of agranulocytosis as an absolute contraindication to further drug therapy.

Agranulocytosis. This is the most serious adverse reaction but fortunately only affects 0.2–0.5% of patients. It is characterised by fever, systemic upset, oropharyngeal bacterial infection and a granulocyte count of less than $0.1–0.25 \times 10^9/l$. The onset is sudden and the consensus is that there is no purpose in routine monitoring of the white blood cell count. Patients should simply be instructed to contact their medical practitioner immediately in the event of developing a sore throat or mouth ulceration. After stopping antithyroid drug therapy the white blood count returns to normal within 1–3 weeks, during which time the affected patients should be isolated initially and treated with broad-spectrum antibiotics. Recovery of white blood cell count may be hastened by the use of granulocyte colony-stimulating factor. If agranulocytosis (neutrophyl count < 0.1) occurs with any thionamide, some would not use the other thionamides because there is some risk of agranulocytosis as a class effect of that medication; other would feel it is safe to use the other thionamides as this risk is small. If both thionamides are contraindicated (because of the unit policy regarding avoiding thionamides if there has been any reaction, or because of allergy to both thionamides), then one needs to consider definitive therapy. One could precede the radioactive iodine or surgery with beta-blockade (some would also advocate the use of lithium carbonate 400 mg twice a day).

Mild leucopenia with a relative lymphocytosis is common in Graves' disease and is not a contraindication to antithyroid drugs.

β-adrenoreceptor blocking drugs

These drugs are used in conjunction with thionamides partly to relieve symptoms and also to reduce the risk of atrial fibrillation. Typically, propranolol is used at 80–240 mg/day. Nadolol is a useful once daily non-selective β-blocker, whereas esmolol is useful perioperatively, given intravenously titrated against heart rate.

Surgery

The indications for thyroid surgery for Graves' disease are shown in Table 10.5. The optimum time for operation in a pregnant patient is around 20 weeks' gestation. An additional indication would be if

Table 10.5   Indications for thyroid surgery for Graves' disease

- Relapse after course of antithyroid drugs
- Severe hyperthyroidism and large vascular goitre
- Uncontrolled hyperthyroidism during pregnancy
- Poor compliance with antithyroid drugs
- Adverse reaction to both carbimazole and propylthiouracil

a patient planned to spend a significant period in a remote part of the world with a poorly developed health care system, as of all the therapies for the hyperthyroidism of Graves' disease, surgery provides the best chance of a tablet-free existence.

Preparation for surgery

Standard practice. When the patient is euthyroid, a date for surgery is arranged, and potassium iodide (60 mg three times a day) substituted for the antithyroid drug 10–14 days prior to operation. The iodine maintains euthyroidism and reduces the vascularity of the gland.

Alternative regime. In patients with mild to moderate hyperthyroidism where there are domestic or business reasons for urgent surgery, it is safe to use a combination of propranolol (Inderal-LA), 160 mg/day, and potassium iodide (60 mg three times a day) for a period of 10 days. This regimen results in thyroid hormone concentrations reaching near normal values, and is also useful in patients who are allergic to both carbimazole and propylthiouracil.

Poorly compliant patients. These patients are usually in their late teens or early twenties, some of whom are poorly compliant because of fear of weight gain. It may be necessary to admit to hospital for 10 days prior to surgery to ensure that a combination of carbimazole (60 mg/day), propanolol (160 mg/day) and potassium iodide (60 mg three times a day) is taken under supervision. This should result in a sufficient reduction in thyroid hormone concentrations to ensure safe anaesthesia and surgery.

Complications of surgery

Haemorrhage. Bleeding into the wound during the evening of the operation is the most serious complication which, if unrecognised, may result in asphyxia and death. It is a surgical emergency that requires immediate return to the operating theatre and reopening of the wound.

Hypocalcaemia. This presents with circumoral paraesthesia and tingling of the fingers and occasional tetany; it develops 12–18 hours after surgery, affects 10% of patients and is usually temporary. It responds to 10 ml of 10% calcium gluconate intravenously. Hypocalcaemia persisting beyond 48 hours is usually a sign of permanent hypoparathyroidism; 1% of patients develop permanent hypoparathyroidism and treatment is with One-Alpha (1α-hydroxycholecalciferol), 1–3 μg/day, indefinitely.

Vocal cord palsy. Damage to a recurrent laryngeal nerve is rare (1%). Much more common are minor voice changes due to transection of the superior laryngeal nerve. This is not an issue for the majority of patients, but surgery is relatively contraindicated for those who depend upon their voice for a living, e.g. opera singers.

Keloid scarring. This is unpredictable but is most common in the young and in African or African-Caribbean ethnic groups.

Outcome

The results of surgery for Graves' disease are shown in Table 10.6. Temporary hypothyroidism occurs in 25% of patients, such that serum T_4 is low and TSH is as high as 100 mU/l at 3 months. If no treatment is given, serum T_4, if not TSH, will be normal at 6 months (Table 10.7). If patients are symptomatic at 3 months, thyroxine in a dose of 75 μg daily should be prescribed and thyroid function reassessed at 6 months. Hypothyroidism persisting beyond 6 months should be considered permanent. With time, the proportion of patients remaining euthyroid following subtotal thyroidectomy diminishes, as, patients become hypothyroid, which reflects the natural history of Graves' disease. Late recurrence of hyperthyroidism, even 20–40 years after apparently successful surgery, is well recognised.

Table 10.6   Expected outcome of thyroid surgery for Graves' disease by an experienced surgeon

	1 year (%)	10 years (%)
Euthyroid[a]	80	50
Hypothyroid	15	40
Hyperthyroid	5	10

[a] A variable proportion of patients will have subclinical hypothyroidism, which is increasingly treated with thyroxine, rather than awaiting the development of overt hypothyroidism and the possible loss to follow-up.

Table 10.7   Temporary hypothyroidism following subtotal thyroidectomy for Graves' disease. At no point was thyroxine therapy given

Hormone	Time (months)							
	1	2	3	4	5	6	9	12
fT_4 (pmol/l)	8	6	6	15	16	20	22	21
TSH (mU/l)	< 0.05	23	40	22	12	8.2	3.4	1.8

fT_4 = free thyroxine, TSH = thyroid-stimulating hormone.

Iodine-131 therapy

Iodine-131 therapy is contraindicated in pregnancy or in *men or women* planning pregnancy for the next 4 months. There is no evidence for teratogenicity, although the number of children born to mothers previously treated with iodine-131, is still relatively small. After 40 years of extensive use of iodine-131, there is no good evidence for increased cancer rates in those organs receiving maximum irradiation – i.e. thyroid, stomach and oesophagus, and bladder – and the risk of leukaemia is infinitesimally small. However, theoretically, the risk of radiation-induced cancer increases with time after exposure and most endocrinologists try to avoid iodine-131 therapy in patients under 30 years of age. Furthermore, a significant proportion of patients will not countenance any form of irradiation therapy, particularly as other modalities are available and given the recommendation that they should avoid close contact with young children for up to 12 days following a standard dose of 400 MBq iodine-131.

Mode of action

Like elemental iodine, iodine-131 is avidly concentrated by the thyroid follicular cells, which are subsequently killed, giving rise to the high initial rate of hypothyroidism. Other cells may still function but are unable to divide in the future. It is this sterilisation of the infrequently dividing follicular cells coupled with the ultimate autoimmune-mediated thyroid failure of many patients with Graves' disease that is responsible for the continuing annual incidence of hypothyroidism of 2% after the first year.

Dosage

All attempts to calculate a dose of iodine-131 that will ensure cure of hyperthyroidism without a high incidence of hypothyroidism have failed. Equally, it is not possible to guarantee hypothyroidism by using higher than average doses. It is, therefore, increasingly common to prescribe a standard dose of 400 MBq iodine-131 (approximately 11 mCi) to all patients with Graves' disease.

Follow-up

Patients should be reviewed at 2 months, 4 months, 6 months, 12 months and annually thereafter with, ideally, measurement of T_3, T_4 and TSH; some would see patients even more frequently, such as 3-weekly, immediately after iodine. If there is no significant fall in thyroid hormone concentrations at 2 months, and certainly if hyperthyroidism persists at 4 months, a further dose of iodine-131 should be given. As in patients following subtotal thyroidectomy, hypothyroidism occurring in the early months may be temporary (25%); and, if thyroxine therapy is needed for symptomatic relief, a dose of 50–75 μg/day should be given. Only at a later date should any decision for thyroxine replacement be made. If, while taking thyroxine, TSH is elevated at 6 months, hypothyroidism is permanent and the dose of thyroxine is increased accordingly. If TSH is normal or suppressed at this stage, thyroxine should be stopped and thyroid function reassessed after a further 4–6 weeks. Achieving the correct dose of thyroxine may be difficult initially due to the presence of TRAb and therefore an autonomous thyroid remnant, although insufficient on its own to maintain euthyroidism (Figure 10.2). Patients with temporary hypothyroidism in the first few months following iodine-131 may, of course, develop permanent thyroid failure at a later date.

Temporary hypothyroidism occurs in a significant proportion of patients within the first 6 months after surgery or radioactive iodine therapy for Graves' disease and may even be followed by recurrent hyperthyroidism.

Outcome

Figures will vary from centre to centre but a typical outcome of radioactive iodine therapy of Graves' disease is shown in Table 10.8. Some 10% of patients will require a second dose of iodine-131 to induce euthyroidism and the occasional patient will respond after a

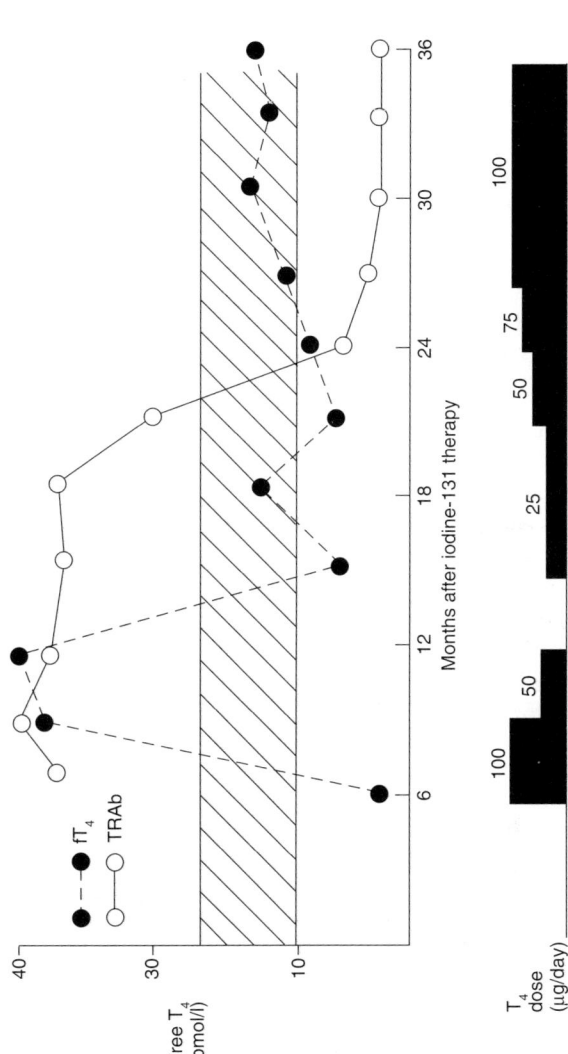

Figure 10.2 Difficulty in controlling hypothyroidism with thyroxine in the early stages after iodine-131 therapy for Graves' disease due to high concentrations of thyroid-stimulating hormone (TSH)-receptor antibody (TRAb), stimulating a thyroid remnant which, although functioning autonomously, is unable to maintain euthyroidism. As the antibody concentration declines, the dose of thyroxine necessary to restore serum thyroxine (T_4) and TSH increases.

Table 10.8   Expected outcome of iodine-131 therapy for Graves' disease, using a standard dose of 400 MBq

	1 year (%)	10 years (%)
Euthyroid	20	5
Hypothyroid	80	95
Hyperthyroid[a]	0	0

[a] 10% of patients require two or more doses of iodine-131 within the first year.

third dose. If hyperthyroidism persists, the gland should be considered resistant and treatment given with antithyroid drug therapy. This may be required for several years until the cumulative effect of the radioactive iodine and the underlying autoimmune process is evident.

Thyroxine requirements may increase with time following treatment of Graves' disease with radioactive iodine.

Carbimazole as an adjunctive therapy

Iodine-131 may take some 6–8 weeks to be effective, and during this latent period hyperthyroidism may be exacerbated with an increase in morbidity and even mortality in those with severe thyrotoxicosis and associated cardiovascular disorders. For this reason, it is reasonable not only to render the patient euthyroid before iodine-131 treatment but also to continue the antithyroid drug for 6 weeks after. In order not to interfere with the efficacy of iodine-131, the antithyroid drug is not given for some 48–96 hours before and after therapy. If this course of action is not taken, the thyroid gland is more resistant to the effects of iodine-131 and larger doses may be necessary. An added advantage of pretreatment with an antithyroid drug is that the patient is more likely to comprehend the various aspects of treatment when not in the agitated and unreceptive state of moderate to severe hyperthyroidism. The block and replace regimen may used following radioactive iodine for 4 months, then discontinued, in order to circumvent temporary hypothyroidism; this may be especially useful to avoid exacerbation of thyroid eye disease.

For patients with mild disease, a β-adrenoceptor antagonist, such as propranolol, 160 mg/day in slow release form (Inderal-LA), will provide symptomatic relief until the radioactive iodine is effective.

Contraindications to iodine-131 and caution with iodine-131

Absolute. Iodine-131 should not be given to patients who are or may be pregnant because of the risk of inducing fetal hypothyroidism after the 12th week, by which time the thyroid has developed. If lowering the age threshold for therapy, it is good practice to have a negative pregnancy test beforehand. Patients should be advised to avoid becoming pregnant for 4 months after iodine-131 treatment.

Relative. Of the three treatments for the hyperthyroidism of Graves' disease, iodine-131 is most often associated with deterioration in ophthalmopathy. This can be minimised in patients with mild to moderate disease by prednisolone in a dose of 30 mg/day for 4–6 weeks after treatment. The risk of significant worsening of eye disease is relatively small and must be balanced against that of high-dose steroids in a population which is predominantly female and menopausal or postmenopausal. Hypothyroidism is also a risk factor for deterioration of ophthalmopathy, and careful review of thyroid function and treatment with thyroxine if TSH is elevated is essential. Most endocrinologists will not treat patients with active severe thyroid eye disease with iodine-131, preferring to use block and replace therapy. Such patients would need an ophthalmic review.

Toxic Multinodular Goitre

Patients presenting with hyperthyroidism due to a multinodular goitre are usually over 60 years of age. Thyroid enlargement will have started as the diffuse soft goitre of young adulthood and there may be a history of treatment with iodine at this stage which will have been of no benefit. Whatever causes the thyroid enlargement persists and chronic stimulation of the gland leads to nodular hyperplasia over a period of some 20 years, resulting in a readily palpable and usually visible goitre. Concentrations of serum T_3 and T_4 are normal, although TSH may be suppressed (subclinical hyperthyroidism). Over the next 20 years or so the goitre continues to grow and the nodules which function autonomously reach a sufficient size and number to cause hyperthyroidism. Thyroxine therapy may have been given in the mistaken belief that it leads to goitre shrinkage or prevents recurrent growth after surgery, but it simply hastens the development of thyrotoxicosis.

Presentation

The hyperthyroidism of multinodular goitre is usually less severe than that of Graves' disease, and may be of the 'T$_3$ variety'. Typical results would be a serum fT$_4$ of 36 pmol/l and fT$_3$ of 9.0 pmol/l. As the hyperthyroidism is often of longer duration before it is recognised and affected patients are elderly, cardiovascular manifestations, such as atrial fibrillation, may predominate.

Treatment

Treatment with carbimazole would need to be continued indefinitely, as relapse is inevitable when the antithyroid drug is stopped. If there is significant mediastinal compression assessed clinically, by computed tomography (CT) scanning or measurement of flow volume loops, surgery is the treatment of choice, after rendering the patient euthyroid; otherwise, iodine-131 is indicated. Post-therapy hypothyroidism is unusual. Response may not be evident for some 3–4 months and doses as high as 1200 MBq may be necessary for patients with large goitres, in which case treatment must be given as an inpatient or the dose fractionated for outpatients.

Toxic Adenoma

For a hyperfunctioning follicular adenoma to cause hyperthyroidism, it is usually greater than 3 cm in diameter and palpable on careful examination of the neck. The diagnosis is confirmed by demonstrating ^{99m}Tc concentration exclusively within the nodule. Up to 50% of patients have 'T$_3$ thyrotoxicosis'. Treatment is by hemithyroidectomy in younger patients, or with iodine-131. As the suppressed inherently normal thyroid tissue receives little or no irradiation, subsequent hypothyroidism is less than 10% in most series. If thyroid isotope scanning were to be performed when the patient was euthyroid, a normal diffuse uptake would be demonstrated with no evidence of the adenoma.

Special Situations

Thyrotoxic crisis

Thyrotoxic crisis is the term given to an exacerbation of severe hyperthyroidism, usually unrecognised or inadequately treated and precipitated by intercurrent infection, surgery or iodine-131 therapy. Patients are agitated, often irrational, with pyrexia, tachycardia, chest pain and possibly cardiac failure. There may be vomiting. With earlier diagnosis and better management of hyperthyroidism, thyrotoxic crisis is fortunately extremely rare. Treatment is supportive with intravenous fluids, broad-spectrum antibiotics and β-adrenoceptor antagonists. New thyroid hormone synthesis is prevented by the administration of carbimazole (60 mg/day), but most important of all is the use of sodium ipodate (Oragrafin) or sodium iopanoate (Telepaque), which not only have an iodine effect in inhibiting preformed thyroid hormone release but also reduce T_4 to T_3 conversion by preventing outer-ring deiodination. Serum T_3 concentrations fall dramatically within 24 hours compared with 5–7 days following potassium iodide. The dose of these agents is 0.5–1.0 g/day and treatment should be continued for 10–14 days until carbimazole begins to take effect.

Subclinical hyperthyroidism

Subclinical hyperthyroidism is the term used to describe patients in whom serum TSH is suppressed but T_3 and T_4 concentrations are normal although usually in the upper part of their respective reference ranges. Prolonged subclinical hyperthyroidism as, for example, in patients with nodular goitre, is a risk factor for osteoporosis and for atrial fibrillation and is an indication for treatment rather than the expectant policy of the past.

Atrial fibrillation

A variety of atrial and ventricular tachycardias have been described in hyperthyroidism, but the commonest arrhythmia is atrial fibrillation: it is rare in patients under 40 years of age, unless there is severe long-standing thyrotoxicosis or coexistent structural heart disease. The prevalence increases with age, such that 50% of hyperthyroid males over the age of 60 are in atrial fibrillation at presentation. Atrial fibrillation is not necessarily accompanied by marked elevation of serum concentrations of T_3 and T_4 and may be associated with subclinical hyperthyroidism.

Sixty percent of patients with hyperthyroid atrial fibrillation will revert spontaneously to sinus rhythm within a few weeks of restoration of normal tests of thyroid function, and approximately half the remainder will respond to DC cardioversion, if serum TSH concentrations are normal or raised at the time of the procedure.

Hyperthyroid atrial fibrillation is typically resistant to digoxin, due to in part to an increase in renal clearance and the apparent volume of distribution of the drug, and it is often necessary to add a non-selective β-adrenoceptor antagonist to achieve adequate control.

Systemic embolisation, particularly cerebrovascular, is increased in hyperthyroid atrial fibrillation although the risk is difficult to quantify. Patients over 50 years of age with valvular or hypertensive heart disease appear to be at greatest risk. Whether younger patients with structurally normal hearts benefit from anticoagulants is not known, but a decision to withhold warfarin would be more secure if there were no evidence of atrial thrombus at transoesophageal echocardiography. As the development of a dense hemiplegia complicating a readily reversible metabolic disease is a clinical disaster, anticoagulation with warfarin (target INR 2–3:1) should be considered in all patients with hyperthyroid atrial fibrillation. Anticoagulant control may be difficult, because hyperthyroidism is associated with an increased sensitivity to warfarin.

Pseudohyperthyroidism

When thyroid function tests are measured in hospitalised patients with a variety of conditions it is not uncommon to record low serum TSH and raised fT_4 concentrations, raising the possible diagnosis of hyperthyroidism. If serum T_3 is unequivocally normal, the biochemical abnormality is due to non-thyroidal illness. However, from time to time, serum T_3 concentrations are equivocal and unless there are helpful clinical signs such as goitre or ophthalmopathy, it may be difficult to exclude the possibility of mild hyperthyroidism. Even after measurement of TRAb and isotope scanning, the diagnosis may remain in doubt. In this situation, a trial of carbimazole 20 mg/day for 2 months is a reasonable option.

Routine measurement of thyroid function in hospitalised patients with non-thyroidal illness should be discouraged, as results may be misinterpreted and inappropriate antithyroid therapy started.

Gestational hyperthyroidism

During the early weeks of pregnancy, serum TSH concentrations are undetectable in some 10% of women due to the weak thyrotrophic effect of human chorionic gonadotrophin (hCG). In most cases, thyroid hormone concentrations are in the upper part of the reference ranges and patients are asymptomatic. Hyperthyroidism may complicate hyperemesis gravidarum, particularly in Asian women, but there is not a good correlation between serum hCG concentrations and severity of biochemical disturbance. It may be necessary to treat the mother with an antithyroid drug for some 4–6 weeks, but not beyond the 12th week of gestation in order to avoid adversely affecting fetal thyroid function.

There is a rare familial condition of gestational hyperthyroidism. The woman becomes thyrotoxic in the first trimester for the course of her pregnancy, with resolution at delivery. The condition recurs in other pregnancies and may be seen in family members: there are none of the immune features of Graves' disease. This condition probably represents a high affinity of an abnormal TSH receptor for hCG.

Graves' disease in pregnancy

Maternal hyperthyroidism in pregnancy is usually due to Graves' disease: this is covered in Chapter 11.

If hyperthyroidism recurs after delivery, and is due to Graves' disease and not postpartum thyroiditis, and the mother wishes to breastfeed, propylthiouracil is the drug of choice as it is transferred to the milk one-tenth as well as carbimazole. Carbimazole will not affect thyroid function in the infant if a dose of less than 15 mg/day is employed.

Further Reading

Davies TF, Roti E, Braverman LE, DeGroot LJ. Thyroid controversy – stimulating antibodies. *J Clin Endocrinol Metab* 1998;**83**:3777–85.

Franklyn JA. The management of hyperthyroidism. *New Engl J Med* 1994;**330**:1731–8.

Franklyn JA, Sheppard M. Radioiodine for hyperthyroidism (editorial). *Br Med J* 1992;**305**:727–8

Perros P. Antithyroid drug treatment before radioiodine in patients with Graves' disease: soother or menace? *Clin Endocrinol* 2000;**53**:1–2.

Philippou G, McGregor AM. The aetiology of Graves' disease: What is the genetic contribution? *Clin Endocrinol* 1998;**48**:393–5.

Toft AD. Thyroxine suppression therapy in Graves' disease. *Ballière's Clin Endocrinol Metab* 1997;**11**:537–48.

Toft AD, Boon NA. Thyroid disease and the heart. *Heart* 2000;**84**:455–60.

Wiersinga WM, Prummel MF. An evidence-based approach to the treatment of Graves' ophthalmopathy. *Endocrinol Metab Clin N Am* 2000;**29**:297–319.

11

Graves' Disease

John H Lazarus and Kofi Obuobie

Graves' Disease – Natural History and Treatment

The autoimmune thyroid disease first described by Robert Graves and now called Graves' hyperthyroidism is characterised by hyperthyroidism, goitre and in some cases by ophthalmopathy, dermopathy and acropachy. Hyperthyroidism, the most common feature of Graves' disease, is due to the presence of stimulating antibodies against the thyroid-stimulating hormone (TSH) receptor, TSHR-Ab. The end result is diffuse thyroid growth and increased thyroid hormone synthesis. The prevalence in the UK population is about 2.2%, with an estimated annual incidence of 3 per 1000 population. There is a peak frequency in the fourth decade with a female preponderance of 7:1 to 10:1. There is often a family history of autoimmune thyroid disease or of one or more of the other organ-specific autoimmune disorders, such as type 1 diabetes mellitus, pernicious anaemia, Addison's disease, premature ovarian failure and myasthenia gravis. Patients with Graves' disease are at increased risk of developing these conditions.

Pathology and pathogenesis

The thyroid gland in patients with Graves' hyperthyroidism is characterised by follicular hyperplasia, patchy and predominantly T-cell infiltration with very few germinal centres.

The hyperthyroidism is due to the presence in the circulation of an antibody directed against the TSH receptor on the thyroid follicular cell. The antibody, known as the TSH-receptor antibody (TRAb), is unique in that once bound to its antigen it stimulates thyroid hormone production and probably also goitre formation. In some patients, there is a mixture of stimulating and blocking TRAb and, if their relative proportions fluctuate, patients may alternate between hypothyroidism and hyperthyroidism, resulting in difficulty in control with antithyroid drugs. Indeed, Graves' disease may occasionally develop for the first time in patients who have been hypothyroid and taking thyroxine for many years, presumably due to a switch in production from blocking to stimulating forms of TRAb. Patients with Graves' disease may also have thyroid peroxidase antibody associated killer T-cell-mediated thyrocyte damage. Therefore, patients may become hypothyroid for more than one reason.

It is clear from identical twin studies that there is a genetic predisposition to developing Graves' disease, but environmental factors (Table 11.1) are at least as important. What triggers the onset in genetically susceptible individuals is not clear but stress modulates the immune response and major life events, such as the death of a close relative, appear to be related to the onset of the hyperthyroidism of Graves' disease. There is also evidence for the presence of TSH receptors on the cell surfaces of bacteria such as *Yersinia enterocolitica* and certain strains of *Escherichia coli,* and the antibodies produced as a result of infection with these organisms may crossreact with thyroid follicular receptors. Iodine

Table 11.1 Aetiological factors in Graves' disease

Initiating event – unknown – proposed factors:
- *Infections*: There is molecular mimicry between *Yersinia enterocolitica*, some viruses and the TSH receptor
- *Stress*
- *Sex steroids*: The disease is more common in women, presumably mediated by more oestrogen and less testosterone
- *Genetic susceptibility*: There is a 60% concordance in monozygotic twins and the disease clusters within families
- *Smoking* is a recognised risk factor for Graves' disease, especially Graves' ophthalmopathy

Antigen is processed in antigen-presenting cell, e.g. macrophages. The complex of processed antigen and major histocompatibility class II molecules are then presented to CD4 helper T cells. These T cells are activated by the complex and in turn activate specific B-cell clones. These activated B lymphocytes in turn produce TSH (thyroid-stimulating hormone) receptor stimulating antibody.

Table 11.2   Features of thyroid-stimulating hormone (TSH) receptor antibodies in Graves' disease

- Primarily produced in the thyroid gland
- Bind to the extracellular domain of the TSH receptor
- Stimulatory in function – specific to Graves' disease
- Oligoclonal, IgG1 immunoglobulin
- Unique to humans
- Levels decline after thyroidectomy and antithyroid drugs
- Rise early after iodine-131 therapy – fall late
- Stimulate the synthesis of the sodium/iodide symporter, which results in increased uptake of iodide by thyroid tissue in Graves' disease

excess, e.g. amiodarone, may be important in precipitating hyperthyroidism in patients with subclinical Graves' disease.

The features of thyrotoxicosis are covered in Chapter 10. Graves' thyrotoxicosis has the potential to be associated with very high thyroid hormone levels. The TSH receptor is found in other tissues and TSHRAb binding (Table 11.2) may be responsible for the extra-thyroidal features of Graves' disease.

Management of Graves' disease

The thyrotoxicosis of Graves' disease is managed by rendering the patient euthyroid, while avoiding complications of treatment, and by reducing cardiac symptoms and risk. These topics are covered in Chapter 10.

Once rendered euthyroid, patients may be at risk of relapse of their disease, or hypothyroidism related to the autoimmune condition itself or its treatment, whether surgical or with radioactive iodine. Long-term follow-up should be offered to patients. A thyroid function test can be done annually and the organisation of this may be computerised so as to share the care with the family physician.

Management of Graves' Hyperthyroidism in Pregnancy

Pregnant patients with Graves' disease may require preconception counselling. Patients may also be seen who have been previously treated for Graves' hyperthyroidism, and a small group of hyperthyroid women may have inadvertently received radioiodine therapy. These aspects are not covered in this chapter. For women who are found to be hyperthyroid during pregnancy, medical therapy is preferred (Table 11.3), as radioiodine is contraindicated and surgery can usually be avoided. Maternal TSHrAb crosses the placenta and may cause fetal thyrotoxicosis or goitre.

Propylthiouracil (PTU) should be given in a dose of 100–150 mg twice daily until the patient becomes euthyroid, at which time the dose should be reduced to the lowest amount to maintain the euthyroid state with serum thyroxine (T_4) at the upper end of normal and continued up to and through labour. PTU is preferred to carbimazole; the latter can be used but it probably has increased transfer to breast milk. The so-called 'block and replace' regime in which thyroxine is given with antithyroid drug should not be used because the dose of antithyroid drug would inevitably be too high and cause fetal goitre and hypothyroidism. Infection or the development of pre-eclampsia may precipitate thyroid storm, requiring the use of thionamides, iodides, β-blockers, fluid replacement and possibly steroid therapy and plasmapheresis. PTU has a shorter half-life than carbimazole and is not present in as high a concentration in breast milk. Hence, women receiving PTU can breast-feed without significant risk to the neonate.

There is no significant effect of antithyroid drugs *in utero* on the long-term health of the neonate or child, assuming the dose during gestation has not caused iatrogenic fetal hypothyroidism. Propranolol may be used for a few weeks but prolonged use can result in retarded fetal growth, impaired response to anoxic stress,

---

Table 11.3   Management of Graves' hyperthyroidism in pregnancy

- Confirm diagnosis
- Start propylthiouracil
- Render patient euthyroid – continue with low-dose ATD up to and during labour
- Monitor thyroid function regularly throughout gestation (4–6 weekly) adjust ATD if necessary
- Check TSHR-Ab at 36 weeks' gestation, consider fetal ultrasound for goitre
- Discuss treatment with patient:
    effect on patient
    effect on fetus
    breast-feeding
- Inform obstetrician and paediatrician
- Review postpartum – check for exacerbation

together with postnatal bradycardia and hypoglycaemia. Surgery should be avoided if it is considered that medical therapy has a reasonable chance of success. However, subtotal thyroidectomy is indicated if control of the hyperthyroidism is poor on account of poor compliance or inability to take drugs or if the patient has a large compressive goitre. Surgery should be performed in the second trimester, as there is a higher risk of associated abortion at an earlier stage of gestation.

The euthyroid mother with Graves' disease and previous definitive treatment for thyrotoxicosis (surgery or radioactive iodine (iodine 131)) should be monitored. Although she has lost her 'bioassay' for TSHrAb and may even be taking thyroxine, her TSHrAb may cross the placenta and cause fetal thyrotoxicosis.

Thyroid Eye Disease

Patients with hyperthyroidism due to any cause may have upper lid retraction due to sympathetic stimulation of the levator muscle. Patients with Graves' disease may have a variety of ocular symptoms and signs, sometimes known as Graves' ophthalmopathy or thyroid-associated eye disease. The temporal progression of Graves' hyperthyroidism and ophthalmopathy (GO, or thyroid-associated ophthalmopathy – TAO) is independent. Graves' opthalmopathy appears before Graves' hyperthyroidism in 20%, at the same time in 40% and after Graves' hyperthyroidism in 40%. Symptoms include excessive watering, grittiness, pressure feelings and pain (Table 11.4).

The patient may notice protrusion of the eyes and diplopia. In severe cases loss of vision and extreme proptosis may occur. In nearly all cases evidence of autoimmune thyroid disease is obtained, but some patients have no thyroid abnormalities at all.

Table 11.4 Symptoms and signs of thyroid eye disease

Symptoms	Signs
Irritation/watering	Eyelid erythema
Pain at rest	Eyelid oedema
Pain on movement	Conjunctival infection
Diplopia	Caruncle swelling
Reduced visual acuity	Proptosis/exophthalmos
	Ophthalmoplegia

Graves' ophthalmopathy is usually mild but can cause extreme worry to both patient and physician. The clinical signs are usually seen in both eyes, but unilateral proptosis may occur, and differentiation from other causes of unilateral swelling (e.g. orbital tumour) must be made. Lid-lag on downward gaze with conjunctival congestion with swelling of the lateral rectus muscle are easily observed signs. Periorbital oedema and conjunctival infection also occur. Diplopia is due to fibrosis and tethering of extraocular muscles, most frequently the inferior rectus. This causes diplopia on upward gaze and may be associated with a rise in intraocular pressure. It is important to assess these signs as well as performing an examination of the optic fundus to look for signs of optic nerve compression. Referral to an ophthalmologist should be arranged early to distinguish active inflammatory ophthalmopathy from cold burnt out thyroid disease, which rarely progresses but may be severe.

The pathogenesis of Graves' ophthalmopathy is not fully understood but it occurs in association with autoimmune thyroid disorder, usually Graves' disease (Table 11.5).

In more than two-thirds of patients, both hyperthyroidism and ophthalmopathy develop within 2 years of each other. However, euthyroid patients who develop ophthalmopathy may never become hyperthyroid. It is probable that Graves' hyperthyroidism and ophthalmopathy have some pathogenic mechanisms, perhaps related to crossreactivity between autoantigens in the thyroid and orbital tissues. Recently it has been shown that there is an association between Graves' ophthalmopathy and cigarette smoking. Examination of orbital muscle and fibroblasts suggests that the condition is immunologically mediated, probably involving T-lymphocyte infiltration and activation, leading to inflammatory

Table 11.5   Pathogenesis of thyroid eye disease

- Autoimmune disorder
    T-cell infiltrate
    Presence of inflammatory cytokines
    Possible role of TSH receptor
    Possible role of orbital muscle antibodies
- Cigarette smoking
- Radioiodine (^{131}I) therapy
- High serum T_3 before hyperthyroid therapy

T_3 = triiodothyronine, TSH = thyroid-stimulating hormone.

damage to orbital contents. Unlike antithyroid drugs, radioiodine therapy (and probably subtotal thyroidectomy) carries a small risk of development or worsening of ophthalmopathy. Administration of prednisolone at the time of radioiodine therapy and for 3 months afterwards may ameliorate the condition. Routine steroid use after radioiodine is inappropriate as it will expose many patients to the side effects of high-dose steroids, only to prevent eye changes in a maximum of 15%. However, the risk factors for development of Graves' ophthalmopathy should be thoroughly assessed before consideration of steroid use. The most important factor is pre-existing *active* ophthalmopathy. Other predictors include smoking and high serum triiodothyronine (T_3) pretreatment.

Treatment of Graves' ophthalmopathy is difficult (Table 11.6) as there is no guarantee that the condition will resolve when the patient is euthyroid. Symptomatic treatment for mild cases with no optic nerve compression involves elevation of the head of the bed, wearing tinted spectacles and the use of artificial tears or other eye lotions to relieve irritation. The mainstay of medical therapy for compressive signs and symptoms is corticosteroids. High-dose prednisolone (120 mg/day) is required, with the dose being reduced gradually to 30 mg over the course of 6–8 weeks. If there is an imminent risk to vision, pulse prednisolone therapy (500–1000 mg methyl prednisolone intravenously on three successive days) is used.

Table 11.6 Management of thyroid eye disease

- *Symptomatic*
    Lubricant eye drops
    Elevation of the head of the bed
    Tinted glasses
    Mild diuretic

- *Anti-inflammatory*
    Steroid therapy
    Immunosuppressants (e.g. azathioprine, cyclosporin)
    Orbital radiotherapy

- *Surgical decompression*
    Coronal
    Ethmoidal
    Intranasal
    Lateral

Other immunosuppressive agents such as cyclosporin and azathioprine are also used and have a 'steroid' sparing effect. Steroid therapy is also used prophylactically in patients with Graves' ophthalmopathy who receive radioiodine therapy in view of the risk of exacerbation of ocular symptoms and signs.

Orbital radiotherapy has been found to be effective in causing a reduction in compressive symptoms in the condition. It is administered in conjunction with steroids to prevent acute oedema. Surgical decompression of the orbit has been used when vision is threatened seriously by optic nerve compression or the proptosis is so severe that corneal exposure is causing ulceration. However, the operation may be indicated at an earlier stage of the disease and should not necessarily be regarded as a last-ditch procedure.

Thyroid-Associated Dermopathy (Pretibial Myxoedema)

Thyroid-associated dermopathy, the least common of the three classic features of Graves' disease (the others are ophthalmopathy and hyperthyroidism), occurs in less than 5% of patients with ongoing or past history of hyperthyroidism. Rarely, it is associated with chronic autoimmune thyroiditis.

Its aetiology is not known. Despite the high levels of TSH receptor antibodies seen with the condition compared to those without dermopathy, there is no direct evidence to link TSH receptor recognising antibodies or T cells to the pathogenesis.

Pathology

There is increased glycosaminoglycan accumulation and disruption of collagen fibres within the dermis, resulting in non-pitting oedema.

Clinical features

Pretibial myxoedema has been seen in the toes, forehead and neck and other areas, in addition to the usual site. The condition may occur following radioiodine therapy in a similar fashion to ophthalmopathy. The condition features well-demarcated papules and nodules, non-pitting orange peel appearance of skin and a pigmented or violaceous appearance. Pruritus is common. Pretibial myxoedema may resolve spontaneously, stabilise or progress to elephantiasis.

Location

- pretibial skin
- dorsum of feet
- fingers
- hands
- elbows

Differential diagnosis

- chronic venous insufficiency
- chronic lymphatic obstruction
- chronic dermatitis

Investigations

- skin biopsy – required only when the clinical diagnosis is uncertain
- elevated TSH receptor antibodies usually encountered

Management

Most patients with thyroid-associated dermopathy are asymptomatic, but those complaining of pruritus or unpleasant cosmetic appearance require treatment.

Indications for treatment

- pruritus
- discomfort
- cosmetic reasons
- inability to wear footwear

Treatment

0.2% fluocinolone ointment is applied nightly under occlusive dressings, reducing the frequency of application as lesions regress. Somatostatin analogues may have a role in treatment of this condition, and this is being investigated.

Thyroid Acropachy

This condition is a rare manifestation of hyperthyroid Graves' disease and virtually all patients have thyroid-associated dermopathy. There is a symmetrical, painless soft-tissue swelling of hands and feet, with clubbing of fingers and toes. The differential diagnosis is with hypertrophic pulmonary osteoarthropathy (which is painful). No treatment is available.

Further Reading

Bahn RS, Heufelder AE. Mechanisms of disease: pathogenesis of Graves' ophthalmopathy. *New Engl J Med* 1993;**329**:1468–1475.

Davies TF. New thinking on the immunology of Graves' disease. *Thyroid Today* 1992;**15**:1.

DeGroot LJ, Gorman CA, Pinchera A *et al*. Therapeutic controversies. Radiation and Graves' ophthalmopathy. *J Clin Endocrinol Metab* 1995;**80**:339–49.

Fatourechi V. Localized myxedema. In: Braverman LE, Utiger RD (eds), *Werner & Ingbar's The Thyroid*, 7th edn. Philadelphia: Lippincott-Raven, 1996:553–8.

Harvey RD, Metcalfe RA, Morteo C *et al*. Acute pre-tibial myxoedema following radioiodine therapy for thyrotoxic Graves' disease. *Clin Endocrinol* 1995;**42**: 657.

Kendall-Taylor P. Thyrotoxicosis. In: Grossman A (ed.), *Clinical Endocrinology*. Oxford: Blackwell Scientific, 1998:328–58.

Lazarus JH. Hyperthyroidism. Seminar. *Lancet* 1997;**349**:339–43.

Lazarus JH, Kokandi A. Thyroid disease in relation to pregnancy – a decade of change. *Clin Endocrinol* 2000;**53**:265–78.

Leech NJ, Dayan CM. Controversies in the management of Graves' disease. *Clin Endocrinol* 1998;**49**:273–80.

Perros P, Crombie AL, Kendall-Taylor P. Natural history of thyroid associated opthalmopathy. *Clin Endocrinol* 1995;**42**:45–50.

Smith TJ, Bahn RS, Gorman CA. Connective tissue, glycosaminoglycans and diseases of the thyroid. *Endocrine Rev* 1989;**10**:366–91.

Sonino N, Grelli M, Boscaro M *et al*. Life events in the pathogenesis of Graves' disease. A controlled study. *Acta Endocrinologica* 1993;**128**:293.

Tunbridge WM, Evered DC, Hall R *et al*. The spectrum of thyroid disease in community: the Whickam survey. *Clin Endocrinol* 1977;**7**:481–93.

12

Hypothyroidism

Shahid T Wahid and Adam CJ Robinson

Introduction

The hypothalamic–pituitary–thyroid axis demonstrates a classical feedback loop system. Hypothyroidism is divided into two main categories: primary hypothyroidism, which is related to thyroid dysfunction, and secondary hypothyroidism, which is related to pituitary dysfunction. Tertiary hypothyroidism is very rare and related to thyroid hormone resistance (Figure 12.1). Each category has characteristic changes in the measured hormones of the thyroid axis (Table 12.1).

Most hormones are secreted in varying amounts to meet the exigencies of life, such as stress, nutrition and reproduction. Paradoxically, thyroid hormone is maintained at a constant level in nearly all circumstances. The main action of thyroid hormone is to increase tissue oxygen consumption. As a result there are a number of biochemico-cellular changes that achieve this (Box 12.1). Deficiency of thyroid hormone greatly reduces tissue oxygen consumption and has far-reaching consequences.

Table 12.1   Changes in thyroid-stimulating hormone (TSH) and free levels of thyroxine (fT_4) and triiodothyronine (fT_3) in the two main types of hypothyroidism

	Primary hypothyroidism	Secondary hypothyroidism
TSH	↑	↓
fT_4	↓	↓
fT_3	↔↓	↓↔

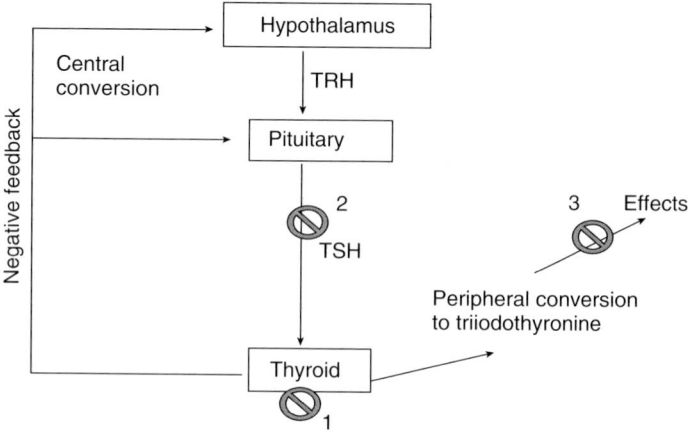

Figure 12.1 The hypothalamic–pituitary–thyroid axis and hypothyroidism. TRH (thyrotrophin-releasing hormone) acts on the pituitary to cause TSH (thyroid-stimulating hormone), which then acts on the thyroid. Primary hypothyroidism (**1**) represents damage to the thyroid itself with failure of thyroid hormone production. Secondary hypothyrodism (**2**) may follow hypothalamic or pituitary underfunction with consequent TSH deficiency. Most triiodothyronine (T3) is produced by peripheral conversion from thyroxine (T4). Failure of T3 action on its intranuclear receptor, thyroid hormone resistance, is sometimes termed tertiary hypothyroidism (**3**).

Box 12.1   Results of the action of thyroid hormones

- Increased cellular sodium pump activity
- Increased intracellular adenosine triphosphate levels
- Increased serum albumin production
- Increased haemoglobin production
- Increased number of mitochondrial cristae
- Increased mitochondrial adenosine diphosphate uptake
- Increased mitochondrial α-glycerophosphate dehydrogenase
- Increased cellular concentrations of glucose-6-phosphate dehydrogenase, pyruvate carboxylase and phosphoenolpyruvate carboxylase

Aetiology/Epidemiology

The incidence and prevalence of hypothyroidism is dependent upon the underlying cause (Box 12.2). Iodine deficiency is the commonest cause worldwide; this is especially so where populations do not have access to sea fish (Himalayas; Andes; parts of Africa, Asia; and Eastern Europe). In developed countries, the commonest causes of hypothyroidism are autoimmune hypothyroidism (Hashimoto's thyroiditis) and idiopathic atrophic hypothyroidism. The Whickham survey was conducted in the North East of England in 1977; the prevalence of newly diagnosed hypothyroidism in women was 3 per 1000 and that of treated hypothyroidism was 14 per 1000. When iatrogenic causes were removed, the overall prevalence was 10 per 1000. In men, the overall prevalence was just under 1 per 1000. In a study from the West Midlands the overall prevalence of hypothyroidism in 1210 subjects aged 60 and above was 4% for women and 1% for men. The incidence of hypothyroidism following radioiodine therapy is at least 10% in the first year and 3% per year thereafter, depending on the dosage of radioactivity used.

Box 12.2   Causes of hypothyroidism

Primary
- Autoimmune
    idiopathic atrophy
    Hashimoto's thyroiditis
- Iodine deficiency
- Iatrogenic
    radioiodine therapy
    thyroidectomy
    head and neck radiotherapy
- Thyroiditis
    subacute de Quervain's thyroiditis
    postpartum thyroiditis
    silent thyroiditis
    Riedel's thyroiditis
- Drugs
    antithyroid drugs, e.g. carbimazole
    lithium
    amiodarone
    alpha- and beta-interferon
    granulocyte colony-stimulating factor

(cont.)

Box 12.2   (cont.)

- Infiltrative disease
  - sarcoidosis
  - amyloidosis
  - lymphoma
- Congenital dyshormogenesis
  - thyroid enzyme defects
  - agenesis
  - fetal rubella infection

Secondary
- Hypothalamic disease
- Pituitary disease

Tertiary (very rare)
- Generalised thyroid hormone resistance

Diagnosis

Clinical features

A summary of recognised symptoms and signs is shown in Box 12.3: they can be very diverse due to the widespread tissue actions of thyroid hormones. Symptoms of hypothyroidism are usually non-specific and vague, and they can be insidious in onset, especially in the elderly. Often in mild disease symptoms and signs are absent. The skin changes are due to local infiltration with hyaluronic acid and mucopolysaccharides. The goitre in Hashimoto's thyroiditis, partially related to the high thyroid-stimulating hormone (TSH), can be variable in size but is characteristically firm to hard in consistency.

Investigations

Biochemical confirmation of hypothyroidism is essential. Many diseases such as depression or myalgic encephalomyelitis share symptoms with hypothyroidism; however, treatment of these conditions with thyroxine has no proven benefits and may cause harm. The development of high-precision TSH assays and the use of equilibrium dialysis and monoclonal antibody methods to measure free thyroxine (fT_4) and free triiodothyronine (fT_3) have largely overcome the problems of previous methods. The characteristic changes in TSH, fT_4 and fT_3 that occur in hypothyroidism have previously been detailed (see Table 12.1). In routine clinical

Box 12.3 Symptoms and signs of hypothyroidism

General
- Tiredness
- Weight gain
- Cold intolerance
- Goitre
- Dyslipidaemia

Cardiovascular
- Bradycardia
- Angina
- Cardiac failure
- Pericardial effusion
- Hypertension

Respiratory
- Pleural effusion
- Respiratory muscle myopathy
- Upper airways obstruction secondary to goitre
- Sleep apnoea

Neuromuscular
- Aches and pains
- Entrapment neuropathies
- Myalgia
- Hoarse voice
- Deafness
- Cerebellar ataxia
- Delayed relaxation of reflexes
- Depression
- Psychosis
- Painful neuropathies

Haematological
- Iron deficiency anaemia
- Macrocytosis
- Pernicious anaemia

Dermatological
- Dry skin
- Myxoedema
- Erythema ab igne
- Hypercarotenaemia
- Vitiligo
- Alopecia

Reproductive
- Infertility
- Menorrhagia
- Galactorrhoea
- Oligomenorrhoea

Gastrointestinal
- Constipation
- Ileus
- Ascites

Developmental
- Growth delay
- Mental retardation
- Delayed puberty

practice the majority of centres use TSH alone to diagnose hypothyroidism.

The endocrinologist should keep a degree of suspicion for secondary hypothyroidism. In pituitary failure, TSH is usually a late hormone deficiency: therefore, it should be clear TSH alone would be inadequate in diagnosis of hypothyroidism and fT_4 or total T_4 estimation would also be required. Some clinicians would advocate fT_4 measurement in addition to TSH in all cases of suspected hypothyroidism; this action would have major resource implications, as many hospitals screen over 10,000 patients a year.

Measuring antibodies to thyroglobulin or thyroid peroxidase (microsomal antibodies) is useful to confirm an autoimmune aetiology of primary hypothyroidism; values are typically strongly positive in Hashimoto's thyroiditis (titres > 1:2000). Other haematological and biochemical abnormalities that can occur in hypothyroidism are detailed in Box 12.4.

Box 12.4   Haematological and biochemical abnormalities in hypothyroidism

- Hypercholesterolaemia
- Raised serum creatine kinase
- Hypergammaglobulinaemia
- Anaemia
- Elevated erythrocyte sedimentation rate

In secondary hypothyroidism testing other hypothalomopituitary hormones and brain imaging is warranted (see Chapters 1 and 2). The thyrotrophin-releasing hormone (TRH) test was used in the past to diagnose hypothyroidism, when a blunt response would be expected. The TRH test is now obsolete in primary hypothyroidism, but still has a place in the diagnosis of rare tertiary hypothyroidism, when an excessive response would be expected. We recommend that serum calcium, plasma glucose, full blood count, liver enzymes and a standard autoantibody screen be conducted in young patients because of the association of autoimmune hypothyroidism with a number of autoimmune conditions (Box 12.5).

Box 12.5   Conditions associated with autoimmune hypothyroidism

- Addison's disease
- Type 1 diabetes mellitus
- Hypoparathyroidism
- Pernicious anaemia
- Vitiligo
- Alopecia areata

(cont.)

> **Box 12.5   (cont.)**
> - Thyroid-associated ophthalmopathy
> - Primary gonadal failure
> - Chronic active hepatitis
> - Coeliac disease
> - Dermatitis herpetiformis
> - Systemic lupus erythematosus
> - Rheumatoid arthritis
> - Sjögren's syndrome

Management

Treating primary hypothyroidism is often simple and can be managed in primary care. A temporary hypothyroidism related to thyroiditis should be borne in mind. A confirmed TSH greater than 10 would be a reasonable basis of a diagnosis of hypothyroidism. If there are no cardiovascular problems, 50–100 μg of T_4 can be given at the time of diagnosis and the dose titrated, using increments or decrements of 25 μg, by monitoring TSH and/or fT_4 every 6–8 weeks. Most patients will be stabilised on a dose of 75–200 μg daily. In subjects with ischaemic heart disease, an initial starting dose of 25 μg should be used, because an increase in the basal metabolic rate can provoke myocardial ischaemia. Some believe that the latter should also apply in the elderly or the very frail.

In a consensus statement published in the *British Medical Journal* in 1996 it is stated that the goal of therapy in hypothyroidism would be to use the dose of T_4 that restores the euthyroid state and relieves symptoms. It is stated that the dose of T_4 in most patients achieving symptom relief would result in a normal or slightly raised T_4 concentration and a normal or below normal TSH level. The American Thyroid Association stated 'the goal of therapy is to restore patients to the euthyroid state, which is done by normalising both T_4 and TSH concentrations'.

Excessive T_4 doses resulting in suppressed TSH concentrations have been associated with loss of bone mineral density (BMD), possibly resulting in increased fracture risk, increased risk of atrial fibrillation and increased cardiovascular and cerebrovascular mortality. It has been shown that a TSH-suppressive T_4 dose is not a risk factor on its own for reduced BMD, but that previous thyrotoxicosis and the postmenopausal state are more important. The link between a TSH-suppressive T_4 dose and increased cardiovascular and cerebrovascular mortality are not clearly delineated.

There is no consensus on the use of T_3 in the treatment of hypothyroidism. In a paper published in the *New England Journal of Medicine* in 1999 from Lithuania, a combination of treatment with T_4 and T_3 was reported to be of greater benefit in improving psychometric function and mood compared with patients on T_4 therapy alone. The trial was small and there was no difference in other 'hard' end-points. The trial included both autoimmune hypothyroidism and those given a suppressive dose of thyroxine for previous malignancy. It was therefore impossible to state some patients were overtreated, as the gold standard for replacement was the TSH. At the moment we believe there is insufficient evidence to recommend T_3 therapy, alone or in combination with T_4, and good physiological reasons for not doing so. However, T_3 therapy does have a role in the treatment of 'myxoedema coma' and in subjects who cannot tolerate T_4.

Although the therapy of hypothyroidism may seem simple on the surface, a lot of issues – from compliance to monitoring – still need to be borne in mind.

Special Situations

Subclinical hypothyroidism

Subclinical hypothyroidism describes the occurrence of a raised TSH concentration in the presence of a normal T_4 concentration. In the Whickham survey, 8% of women and 3% of men were reported as having subclinical hypothyroidism. After 20 years of follow-up in this group of subjects, the conversion rate to overt hypothyroidism was found to be 3% per year in thyroid-autoantibody-negative subjects and almost 6% per year in thyroid-autoantibody-positive subjects. Also, the higher the TSH concentration, the greater the conversion rate to overt hypothyroidism. Another interesting finding from the Whickham survey was that even those subjects with a TSH concentration in the upper half of the normal range (2–4 mU/L) were at increased risk of developing overt hypothyroidism, which was also further enhanced by the presence of thyroid autoantibodies. The latter data led to the *Drugs and Therapeutics Bulletin* circulating treatment guidelines for subclinical hypothyroidism in 1998 (Figure 12.2). Over the years a number of experts have suggested that if patients with subclinical hypothyroidism also have hypercholesterolaemia or underlying ischaemic heart disease they should automatically

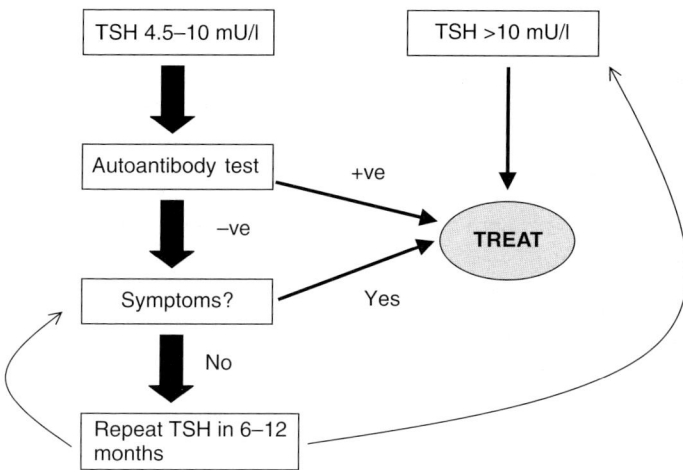

Figure 12.2 Treatment algorithm for subclinical hypothyroidism (based on *Drugs and Therapeutics Bulletin* guidelines). TSH = thyroid-stimulating hormone.

receive T_4 therapy. This stems from two studies: a coronary angiographic study found that subjects with subclinical hypothyroidism had a greater progression of atheroma lesions compared to euthyroid subjects; and, another study found that subclinical hypothyroidism is three times more common in subjects with hypercholesterolaemia compared to subjects with normal plasma cholesterol concentrations.

Pregnancy and oestrogen replacement therapy

In women on T_4 replacement therapy, pregnancy can increase T_4 requirements by 50–150% from the first trimester onwards; therefore, regular TSH monitoring is necessary. A case for screening all pregnant women for hypothyroidism was made by the recent work of James Haddow *et al.* (1999) This showed that the children of mothers who had a raised TSH (defined as a TSH level at or above the 99.7th percentile from a population sample of 25,216 pregnant women) during their pregnancy had abnormalities in certain neuropsychological tests compared with the children of mothers whose TSH was in the normal range during their pregnancy. The reason for increased T_4 requirements during pregnancy is thought to be in part due to the raised oestrogen levels. This is supported by recent work done by Baha Arafah (2001) when he compared women taking T_4 replacement therapy and women not taking T_4 therapy who began oestrogen replacement therapy for the menopause. There was an increase in TSH and a reduction in fT_4 serum levels in the women taking T_4 replacement therapy, whereas there was no change in the latter measures in the women not on T_4 therapy. This supports the need for TSH monitoring when initiating oestrogen replacement therapy in treated hypothyroid women. Hypothyroidism can occur up to 6 months after delivery as part of postpartum thyroiditis: in one-third it follows a period of hyperthyroidism, in one-third it is the sole manifestation and it remains permanent in one-third (the rule of thirds).

Myxoedema coma

Coma need not be present to make a diagnosis of myxoedema coma. The precipitating causes, altered mental state and defective thermoregulation, need to be considered and addressed.

Precipitating factors are outlined in Box 12.6. To minimise a mortality rate of 50%, prompt treatment is needed and awaiting biochemical confirmation is mistaken. Emergency investigations that provide nonspecific clues towards the diagnosis are outlined in Box 12.7. Management is outlined in Figure 12.3.

Box 12.6   Precipitating factors in myxoedema coma

- Infection
- Trauma
- Congestive heart failure
- Myocardial infarction
- Stroke
- Respiratory failure, leading to CO_2 retention
- Hypothermia
- Hypoglycaemia
- Drugs
   - diuretics
   - sedatives
   - anaesthetic
   - antidepressants

Box 12.7 Biochemical and cardiac investigation abnormalities in myxoedema coma

- Hyponatraemia
- Raised serum creatine kinase
- Hypoglycaemia
- Hypoxia
- CO_2 retention
- Low-voltage ECG
- Pericardial effusion on echocardiogram

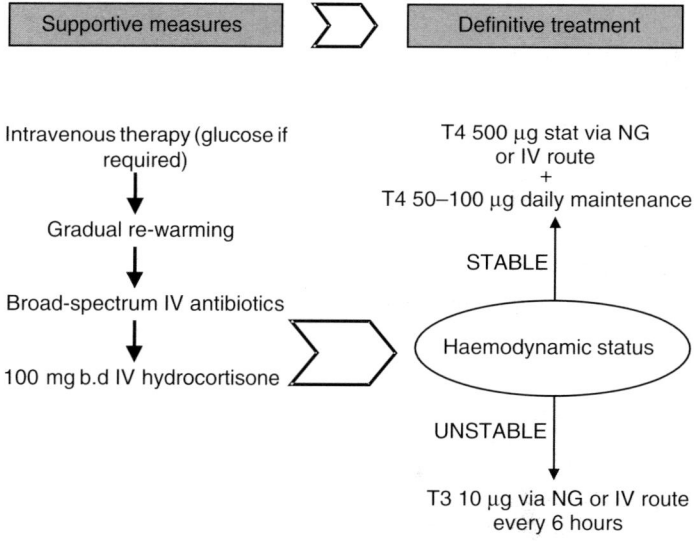

Figure 12.3 Management of myxoedema coma. T_3 = triiodothyronine; T_4 = thyroxine; b.d. = twice a day; IV = intravenous; NG = nasogastric tube; stat = immediately.

Autoimmune polyglandular endocrinopathies

Hypothyroidism can occur in up to 12% and 50% of patients with polyglandular endocrinopathy types 1 and 2, respectively. Regular TSH screening is therefore recommended, especially in those who are thyroid-autoantibody positive.

Amiodarone-induced hypothyroidism (AIH)

TSH is transiently raised in the first 3 months following the initiation of amiodarone. This is because of inhibition of T_4–T_3 deiodination in the pituitary. Treatment is not needed. AIH is more common in areas of high iodine intake, and incidence rates vary from 2 to 22%. The persistence of a raised TSH level with a low fT_4 level (normally raised by up to 40% by amiodarone) is evidence for the development of AIH. Low fT_3 levels do not indicate AIH, as this is an expected finding because amiodarone reduces the peripheral deiodination of T_4. The mechanisms of AIH include the Wolff–Chaikoff effect (whereby the large amount of iodide released by the metabolism of amiodarone inhibits thyroid hormone biosynthesis) and an underlying thyroid autoimmune predisposition makes the thyroid more susceptible to the inhibitory effects of iodide. It has been shown that patients with pre-existing thyroid microsomal antibodies have a relative risk of 13.5 for developing AIH compared to patients negative for thyroid microsomal antibodies. It is therefore recommended that patients have a TSH measurement and their thyroid autoantibody status confirmed before initiation of amiodarone so as to decide upon the need for TSH and fT_4 screening during treatment. Routine screening for AIH in thyroid autoantibody negative individuals is not recommended. If amiodarone can be discontinued (often it cannot), T_4 therapy need only be given for 3–12 months.

Thyroid-hormone resistance (tertiary hypothyroidism)

This condition is very rare. Resistance to thyroid hormone is due to mutations located in exon 9 and 10 which encode the T_3-binding domain of the TRβ thyroid hormone nuclear receptor. The variable tissue distribution of the TRβ receptor explains the variable phenotype of thyroid hormone resistance, which is traditionally defined as generalised resistance or selective pituitary resistance. The latter results in hyperthyroidism and is not discussed. In generalised resistance, pituitary and peripheral tissues are not always affected similarly, resulting in both hypothyroid and hyperthyroid manifestations. A similar degree of resistance in the pituitary and peripheral tissues can result in hypothyroidism (tertiary hypothyroidism). Treatment of tertiary hypothyroidism is still much debated. 3,5,3'-triiodothyroacetic acid (TRIAC) and highly purified dextrothyroxine have been used with some success in the past.

Further Reading

Arafah BM. Increased need for thyroxine in women with hypothyroidism during oestrogen therapy. *N Engl J Med* 2001;**344**:1743–9.

Bunevicius R, Kazanavicius G, Zalinkevicius R, Prange AJ. Effects of thyroxine as compared with thyroxine plus triiodothyronine in patients with hypothyroidism. *N Engl J Med* 1999;**340**:424–9.

Chu JW, Crapo LM. The treatment of subclinical hypothyroidism is seldom necessary. *J Clin Endocrinol Metab* 2001;**86**:4591–9.

Dayan CM. Interpretation of thyroid function tests. *Lancet* 2001;**357**:619–24.

Haddow JE, Palomaki GE, Allan WC, *et al.* Maternal thyroid deficiency during pregnancy and subsequent neuropsychological development of the child. *N Engl J Med* 1999;**341**:549–55.

Lazarus JH. Investigation and treatment of hypothyroidism. *Clin Endocrinol*, 1996;**44**:129–31.

McDermott MT, Ridgeway EC. Subclinical hypothyroidism is mild thyroid failure and should be treated. *J Clin Endocrinol Metab* 2001;**86**:4585–90.

Wass J, Ahlquist J (eds). *Hormone Replacement Therapy for Endocrine Deficiencies.* London: Royal College of Physicians of London, 1999.

13

Thyroid Enlargement/ Goitre

Helen C Cocks and Jayne A Franklyn

Introduction

This chapter will discuss thyroid enlargement in euthyroid subjects. Thyroid enlargement can be associated with hypothyroidism or hyperthyroidism, which should be investigated and treated as discussed in the previous chapters.

Goitre **is defined as any enlargement of the thyroid gland. It may be diffuse or nodular. Nodular disease may be multiple or solitary. A multinodular goitre is a structurally and functionally heterogeneous thyroid enlargement.**

Prevalence

Thyroid enlargement is common. Autopsy studies have shown that 50% of patients have one or more thyroid nodules. Ultrasound studies (using high-resolution scans) have confirmed this finding. Of these nodules, only 8% are palpable.

A survey of the population of northeast England revealed visible or palpable thyroid enlargement in 15% of the population. In the Framingham population (Massachusetts), 4.2% had a thyroid nodule. Lifetime risk for developing a thyroid nodule was estimated at between 5 and 10%. Both population studies showed females were affected 4 times more frequently than males. The incidence of multinodular goitre increases with age.

Thyroid cancer is rare, accounting for 0.5–1% of all new cancer diagnoses and deaths in England and Wales. The risk of malignancy in the patient with euthyroid nodular goitre is between 5 and 10%.

- **The management of thyroid disease requires a multidisciplinary approach involving the collaboration of endocrinologists, thyroid surgeons and radiotherapists/oncologists**
- **Early referral to a thyroid specialist from primary care and other specialities results in increased diagnostic accuracy, decreased cost due to elimination of unnecessary tests and savings also in patient time**
- **Early diagnosis of thyroid cancer is associated with improved outcome.**

Thyroid Enlargement

Aetiology

Endemic goitre (Box 13.1)

Worldwide iodine deficiency is the commonest cause of goitre. Iodine deficiency results in low levels of thyroid hormones and thus stimulation of thyroid-stimulating hormone (TSH). The severity of goitre increases with severity of iodine deficiency. It may appear in childhood but is most commonly seen around puberty. It affects females more than males.

> ### Box 13.1   Definition of an endemic goitre
>
> >10% prevalence of goitre in children aged 6–12 years in particular geographical region usually due to iodine deficiency.

Iodine deficiency is seen in the Himalayas, Andes, Africa and areas of Europe. It may be seen in the immigrant population.

Sudden introduction of high levels of iodine into such communities has led to thyrotoxicosis (jodbasedow phenomenon)

Sporadic nontoxic goitre

Much less common than endemic goitre, it affects women 8 times more than men and has a peak incidence at puberty.

The cause of sporadic goitre is not clear. TSH stimulation of growth is thought to be the mechanism, but elevated levels of TSH have not been detected: this may be because they are transitory. Similarly, a mild iodine deficiency at time of increased physiological demand such as puberty may account for the rise seen at this age. Dietary *goitrogen* intake may be superimposed on the above causal influences (Box 13.2).

Box 13.2 Goitrogens

Dietary
Brassica and Cruciferae plants (contain thiocyanates)
Cassava (cyanoglucosides metabolised to thiocyanates)
Seaweed (iodine excess)
Smoking (thiocyanates): thiocyanates compete with iodine for uptake into the thyroid gland

Environmental
Water pollution with nitrates
Calcium and fluoride in water supplies

Inherited defects. These are very rare causes of sporadic goitre:

- Hormone synthesis defects: (1) iodide transport, (2) organification, (3) dehalogenase and (4) iodotyrosine coupling defects
- Hormone transport defects
- Synthesis of excess thyroid-binding globulin (TBG).

Pathology

Nontoxic goitre results from compensatory hypertrophy and hyperplasia of follicular epithelium secondary to a defect in thyroid hormone output. In most cases the increased thyroid mass maintains a *euthyroid* state. Most start as a *diffuse goitre* or *colloid goitre*. Initially, there is hyperplasia, with the ongoing development of follicles that eventually become colloid filled. The follicles vary greatly in the amount of colloid that they contain. Most colloid goitres become *multinodular goitres*; hence, the latter can result from endemic or sporadic goitre. It is postulated that individual follicles have variable responsiveness to TSH, which affects their growth and function. Rupture of follicles can occur, with haemorrhage and scarring. Multinodular goitres can reach sizes of 2000 g. One lobe of the thyroid may be affected more than the other.

Clinical

The majority of thyroid disease is benign. It is important, however, to identify those patients who have malignant disease so that they may receive safe and effective treatment. The incidence of thyroid cancer in patients presenting with a euthyroid nodular goitre in a tertiary referral unit is estimated to be between 5 and 10%. However, it is likely that the risk of malignancy is considerably less in a nonselected group of patients. If the nodule is solitary, especially in men, the risks of malignancy are increased.

History

Time course. It is important to elicit the rate of growth, since a rapidly enlarging goitre or nodule may indicate cancer.

Pain. Discomfort in the neck is uncommon but may be a feature of benign inflammatory disease or haemorrhage into a cyst. In malignant disease, there may also be referred pain to the ear.

Pressure. Patients can complain of pressure symptoms in the neck. It is necessary to elucidate whether there is *dysphagia* or *dyspnoea*, indicating oesophageal or tracheal compression that may occur with large retrosternal goitre or can be associated with cancer.

Stridor. This results from either extreme tracheal compression or from a recurrent laryngeal nerve palsy: the latter is usually associated with malignancy but is not diagnostic of it.

Change in voice. This may also result from recurrent laryngeal nerve palsy.

Drug history. Prescription and over-the-counter medicine, e.g. carbimazole, propylthiouracil, lithium and iodine-containing drugs or foods such as kelp.

Risk factors

- History of radiation to the head and neck, particularly in childhood
- Place of emigration if relevant
- Family history of thyroid disease.

Examination

Inspection. Look for:

- Size and mobility on swallowing which may be lost in Riedel's thyroiditis or anaplastic carcinoma

- Facial congestion, which may be seen with a retrosternal goitre and superior vena caval obstruction.

Palpation. Nodules > 1 cm are usually palpable. Assess:

- size – if there is a retrosternal element, get the patient to extend his neck to see whether the lower limit is palpable
- consistency – nodular or diffuse goitre; dominant or solitary nodule; soft or hard
- sensation – tender or painless
- mobility – mobile or fixed
- lymphadenopathy – neck, supraclavicular and axillary
- vocal cord mobility – if cancer is suspected.

Anaplastic carcinoma is often hard and craggy.

A WHO classification exists for the classification of goitre by examination (Table 13.1).

Investigation of all thyroid enlargement

Fine needle aspiration cytology (FNAC)

This is the first line of investigation of any thyroid nodule, either a dominant nodule within a multinodular goitre or a solitary nodule (see later). It is a sensitive and specific (70–95%) means of diagnosing the uncommon thyroid cancer from the common benign goitre. There is controversy regarding FNAC from multinodular goitre. If a dominant nodule is changing, then it is likely the patient will need surgery, whatever the FNAC findings.

Sensitivity and specificity have been shown to be highest when aspiration is performed by an experienced person and when interpretation is made by a designated cytopathologist.

A major limitation in FNAC is the differential diagnosis of follicular and Hürthle cell adenoma from carcinoma since, in both,

Table 13.1 WHO classification of goitre by examination

Classification	Finding
0	No goitre palpable or visible
1a	Goitre detected by palpation only
1b	Goitre palpable and visible with neck extended
2	Goitre visible with neck in normal position
3	Large goitre visible from a distance

vascular and capsular invasion are diagnostic and this can only be determined by histological examination of an excised specimen.

USS-guided FNAC improves diagnostic accuracy, particularly in small nodules (< 1 cm), and decreases the number of inadequate aspirates. It has a role in repeat FNAC after previous inadequate specimens and in cysts that reaccumulate after aspiration.

Results of FNAC are reported as benign; indeterminate or insufficient; suspicious or malignant.

Blood tests

Free thyroxine (T$_4$) and TSH. Concentrations of these hormones should be measured in all patients with thyroid enlargement. Thyroid dysfunction is rarely associated with malignant disease and treatment for hypo- or hyperthyroidism often reduces goitre size. In euthyroid goitre, TSH concentrations may be suppressed without a rise in either free T$_4$ or triiodothyronine (T$_3$); this does not indicate a need for antithyroid treatment.

Thyroid autoantibodies. Thyroglobulin (TG), microsomal or thyroid peroxidase (TPO) antibodies are elevated in some patients with autoimmune goitre. The presence of these antibodies confers increased risk of hypothyroidism later.

Differentiated thyroid cancer in patients with Graves' disease may be more aggressive.

Serum thyroglobulin is a tumour marker for thyroid malignancy following definitive treatment (see later); however, it has no role in the routine investigation of goitre.

Serum calcitonin is a marker for medullary tumour of the thyroid (see later); however, there is no proven benefit in screening patients presenting with thyroid enlargement in the absence of clinical suspicion of familial syndromes, including medullary cancer.

Imaging

Historically, a variety of imaging techniques have been used in the diagnosis of thyroid pathology. These have largely been superseded by FNAC.

Scintigraphy. Some years ago scintigraphy was regarded as the 'gold standard' for investigation of the 'solitary thyroid nodule'. Radioactive isotopes of *iodine* or *technetium* are trapped by the thyroid and appear as areas of high uptake (hot nodules) or low uptake (cold nodules). Nodules >5 mm can be visualised.

Hot nodules are areas of thyroid overactivity; solitary hot nodules are uncommonly malignant. The incidence of malignancy in solitary cold nodules is up to 20%. Multinodular glands are likely to show heterogeneous uptake.

Radionuclide scans cannot distinguish benign and malignant nodules and have low sensitivity and specificity; hence, they have little role in the initial evaluation of goitre. A radionuclide scan may have a use when the FNAC result is suspicious. A 'hot' scan in this situation would argue against the diagnosis of malignancy.

Iodine scans are used postoperatively in patients with differentiated thyroid cancer to assess the presence of residual and recurrent disease (see later).

Plain X-rays. Plain X-rays of the chest and thoracic inlet can be useful to identify tracheal deviation in goitre and may show metastatic disease or concurrent pathology.

USS. This is more sensitive than palpation at detecting thyroid nodules and hence many clinically solitary nodules are shown to be part of a multinodular goitre. The risk of malignancy has been defined for solitary nodules detected clinically, and therefore whether the identification of a multinodular gland on USS changes that risk is unknown. USS is able to effectively distinguish between a solid and cystic nodule but is poorly specific and sensitive in the diagnosis of malignancy and hence has no role in routine investigation.

CT and MRI. Computed tomography and magnetic resonance imaging provide more detailed and accurate information on tracheal compression or deviation if necessary, but are not routinely used in the investigation of patients with thyroid enlargement.

Flow-volume loop studies

Such studies provide a sensitive and specific measure of upper airways obstruction and thus provide functional information superior to that obtained from routine radiography.

Management of (Multinodular) Goitre

Worldwide the prevalence of goitre can be decreased by the *iodination* of foods. In developed countries supplementing food, salt and bread has achieved this. In developing countries an intramuscular or oral dose of iodised oil acts as a depot for sustained release. Further supplementation of pregnant women, neonates and infants mini-mises the risk of hypothyroidism and the neurological effects of this.

The recommended daily amount of iodide is 100 μg (150 μg in pregnancy).

Indications for treatment of goitre are given in Box 13.3. Treatment options are displayed in Figure 13.1.

Box 13.3   Indications for treatment of goitre

- Tracheal or oesophageal compression
- Neck discomfort
- Cosmesis
- Anxiety
- Growth, especially retrosternal
- Venous congestion

Thyroxine (T$_4$)

T$_4$ use in the treatment of nontoxic goitre and solitary nodules is controversial due to the modest effect and potential side effects.

Thyroxine in doses causing TSH suppression is largely ineffective in reducing goitre size, especially in those with multinodular goitre or solitary nodules. There is no evidence that long-term T$_4$ therapy alters the natural history of multinodular goitre.

The potential side effects of TSH-suppressive doses of T$_4$ are the risk of subclinical thyrotoxicosis. Cardiac arrhythmias, particularly atrial fibrillation, can result in the older age group, who are also those likely to have large goitres.

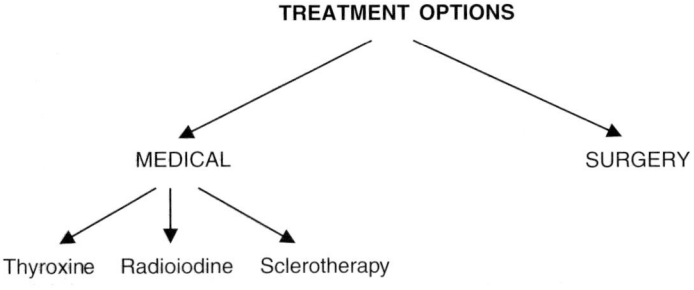

Figure 13.1   Treatment options for goitre.

Bone demineralisation in postmenopausal women may occur as a consequence of T_4 therapy in patients, especially when given in doses sufficient to suppress serum TSH.

Radioiodine

Radioiodine (RAI or iodine-131) is effective in decreasing thyroid volume in most patients with nontoxic goitre. A mean reduction of 40% of initial volume is seen at 1 year and 50–60% at 3–5 years. The decrease in size is directly related to the dose of iodine-131 used and indirectly related to goitre size. Although iodine-131 can be used to treat very large goitres, a reduction in size of only approximately 30% is seen at 1 year. A dose of 600 MBq or greater is used.

Compressive symptoms are improved and this can be measured with flow-loop studies.

Another advantage of RAI is that it can be used to treat recurrence of goitre after surgery.

Side effects

A total of 20–30% of patients with euthyroid goitre treated by RAI will become hypothyroid; the risk is higher in those with smaller goitre and in patients with antibodies to TPO or a family history of thyroid disease; paradoxically, 5% of patients develop autoimmune hyperthyroidism (Graves' disease). This is thought to be due to the irradiation-induced release of thyroid antigen.

Radiation thyroiditis is seen in about 3% of patients. Even in patients with large goitre, thyroid swelling and airway compromise is very uncommon.

Concern exists about the risk of teratogenesis and malignancy associated with RAI use for treatment of benign thyroid disease. Various studies have shown that the risk of birth defect following treatment with RAI is similar to that of the general population.

Current evidence shows that the overall relative risk of mortality from cancer has been shown to be decreased in patients treated for thyrotoxicosis; however, there is a small increase in relative risk of thyroid and small bowel cancer, although the absolute risks remain low. It is important to bear this in mind in follow-up of these patients.

Surgery

The indications for surgery in goitre are the same as for medical treatment. Subtotal thyroidectomy is the standard operation for patients with nontoxic goitre. This negates the need for thyroxine replacement in the short term in the majority of patients; however, if followed up, most patients will require thyroxine replacement eventually. If only one lobe is affected, a patients lobectomy may be performed. After lobectomy, disease may develop in the other lobe. Recurrence rates vary according to the surgery performed; they should be <10% in 10 years. For complications, see under thyroid cancer.

The Solitary Thyroid Nodule

The majority of 'solitary' nodules on palpation are in fact dominant nodules within a multinodular goitre. A classification of nodules is given in Box 13.4.

If a nodule is truly solitary there is a 20% risk of malignancy.

Box 13.4   Classification of nodules

Non-neoplastic nodules
Hyperplastic: spontaneous or compensatory (after surgery)
Inflammatory: acute, subacute, chronic

Benign
Solid, cystic or mixed
Adenoma (follicular/Hürthle)
Teratoma

Malignant
Papillary carcinoma
Follicular
Medullary
Anaplastic
Lymphoma
Metastatic from other primaries

An adenoma is completely encapsulated and is thought to be a monoclonal tumour. A cyst is not encapsulated: 15–25% of all nodules are cystic.

History and examination of patients with a solitary thyroid nodule is as previously mentioned, with particular attention to possible risk factors (see later) for thyroid cancer.

The Investigation of Choice is FNAC

First, FNAC allows differentiation of nodules that require surgery from those that do not. Secondly, with demonstration of a malignant nodule, the extent of surgery (subtotal thyroidectomy rather than lobectomy) can be defined. The FNAC result determines the management of a solitary (or dominant) nodule, as illustrated in Figure 13.2.

Benign solitary or dominant thyroid nodule

Patients with a benign FNAC result should be re-examined at 6 months. If there are no changes on examination and there has been negligible growth of the nodule, the patient should undergo a repeat FNAC at 1 year. The patient can be discharged if the result remains benign.

Suspicious FNAC

Patients with a suspicious FNAC result may undergo scintigraphy as a further diagnostic step. Hot nodules may be followed up by observation since they are unlikely to contain cancer. Warm or cold nodules should undergo surgical removal.

Optimal surgery in those with suspicious FNAC is *diagnostic lobectomy*. Histology will provide a definitive diagnosis (this is particularly important in distinguishing follicular and Hürthle cell adenomas from carcinomas). Subsequently, patients with a diagnosis of carcinoma should undergo definitive treatment, as discussed later.

Surgery should also be considered in:

1. patients with cysts > 4 cm diameter or that recur after three attempts at aspiration, since these are more likely to contain malignancy
2. patients with clinical symptoms of pressure, hoarseness, vocal cord paralysis, cervical lymphadenopathy and rapid enlargement of a thyroid nodule.

Treatment of Benign Solitary Nodules

Sclerotherapy

Cysts

FNAC alone may be enough to treat a thyroid cyst; however, approximately 50% of these recur after simple aspiration. Further aspiration can be followed by the injection of a sclerosant.

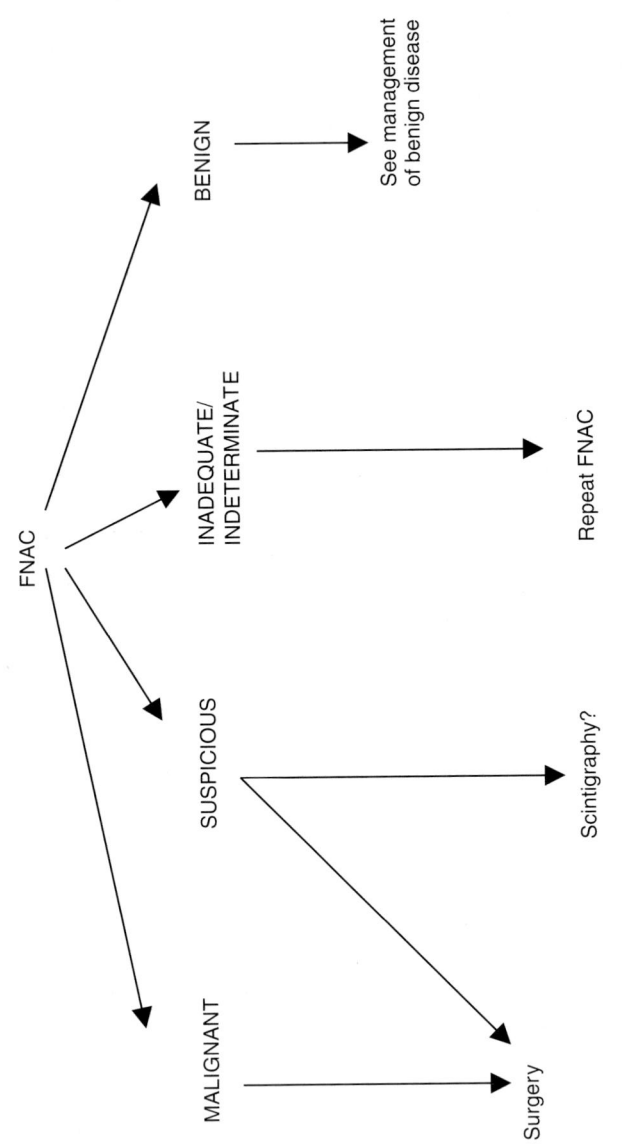

Figure 13.2 Management of a solitary (or dominant) nodule.

Tetracycline has been used most frequently. Larger cysts have a better response to sclerosant therapy.

Problems may result from extravasation, causing local irritation and inflammation. Recurrent laryngeal nerve palsy has also been documented after tetracycline use.

Ethanol may also be used as a sclerosant in thyroid cysts. A 95% solution is injected under ultrasound guidance and reaspirated 5 min later. Although some larger cysts need further injection 1 month later, there is a significant decrease in size at 12 months.

Nodules

Ethanol may also be used in the treatment of benign solid nodules. It is important that such patients have had two benign FNAC reports to exclude malignancies. Patients should be carefully selected for nodule sclerotherapy since there is a small risk of malignancy in patients with a benign aspirate at FNAC (< 2%).

Indications for treatment are as previously described, but the volume of the nodule must have remained stable: 1 ml of ethanol is injected per ml of nodule, which can be as given once only or repeated at intervals. A decrease in size is seen on average at 6 months, and is usually associated with a reduction in symptoms.

Ethanol sclerotherapy may be particularly attractive in patients who either do not want to undergo surgery or who are high risk for surgery.

Thyroxine

Modest short-term results have been seen with TSH-suppressive doses in patients with benign solitary nodules; however, randomised controlled trials have shown that there is no benefit of T_4 over placebo.

Surgery

Surgery for a solitary nodule takes the form of a lobectomy. In some instances this will be a diagnostic aid as described. Further surgery would be indicated only in the case of a malignancy (see later).

Thyroid Cancer

Clinically, thyroid cancer represents < 1% of all cancer deaths. At autopsy, microcarcinomas (< 1 cm) may be found in 5–36% of patients.

Differentiated thyroid cancer (DTC) is an indolent disease that has a high cure rate and low mortality rate when detected early and treated appropriately.

Incidence increases with age; the median age is 45–50 years. Thyroid cancer is rare below the age of 16. In children and adolescents, however, thyroid nodules are more likely to harbour malignancy. DTC is more common in females than in males, with a ratio of 2–3:1.

Classification of thyroid cancer

Malignant transformation can occur in any of the components of the thyroid gland. The majority of tumours arise from the follicular cells and other types are rare.

Differentiated thyroid cancer (DTC) refers to *papillary* and *follicular* adenocarcinomas that account for 85% of all thyroid cancers (Table 13.2). Papillary tumours can contain follicular elements but if there is any papillary architecture the tumour is termed a papillary tumour. The differential diagnosis of either a follicular cancer or adenoma is made on the histological finding of capsular and vascular invasion.

Medullary cancer

See later.

Anaplastic carcinoma

- Undifferentiated

Table 13.2   Differentiated thyroid cancers

Papillary	Follicular
80% thyroid cancer	10–15% thyroid cancer
80% multicentric	Usually focal
Associated with previous irradiation	Associated with iodine deficiency
Seen in children	Older age group (6th decade)
Lymph node spread common (60%)	Lymph node spread (10%)
20% pulmonary metastases at presentation	Haematogenous spread to lung and bone (20–30%)
Bone metastases rare	

- 5% of all thyroid cancer
- Typically seen in the elderly and females, often on a background of pre-existing thyroid enlargement which rapidly increases in size
- Often associated with local pain and referred pain to the ear
- Highly aggressive and invasive
- Treatment is usually ineffective, and the majority of patients are dead within 1 year of diagnosis.

Lymphoma

- Lymphoma of the thyroid gland is uncommon. It accounts for < 5% of all lymphomas and thyroid malignancies.
- Similar to anaplastic cancer, it is typically seen in elderly women and there is rapid enlargement of the gland.
- Histological and immunocytochemical diagnosis is important since treatment of lymphoma is different and carries a much better prognosis.
- It may be seen in patients with a previous diagnosis of Hashimoto's thyroiditis, although this association is uncommon.

Hürthle cell tumours

- This is a tumour of the eosinophilic, oncocyte or oxyphilic cell. This cell is derived from follicular epithelium but is much less able to produce thyroglobulin or concentrate iodine.
- Hürthle cell tumours can be benign or malignant; capsular or vascular invasion is diagnostic of malignancy, as in follicular cancer.
- Lymph node metastases are common.

Metastases

Primary tumours from other organs can metastasise to the thyroid gland: these are extremely rare.

Oncogenes

Several genetic transformations have been seen in thyroid cancers:

- *ras* oncogene mutations are seen in adenomas and cancers. They are more common in follicular carcinomas than in papillary carcinomas.

- *RET* oncogene transformation is seen in 3–33% of all papillary thyroid cancers unassociated with radiation exposure and in 60–80% of papillary cancers after radiation exposure.
- *TRK* mutations are seen exclusively in papillary cancer, but occur with less frequency than *ret* mutations.
- *p*53 inactivating point mutations are common in anaplastic carcinoma.

Risk factors

Radiation exposure

From 1920, ionising radiation was used to treat acne and to cause involution of enlarged lymphoid tissue such as the tonsils, adenoids and thymus in children.

Exposure to low-dose ionising radiation in childhood confers a risk of 1–7% of developing thyroid cancer in the 30 years following exposure. Exposure after the age of 15 does not confer this increased risk.

Environmental releases of radiation such as seen with the atomic bombing of Hiroshima and Nagasaki have shown similar trends.

In 1986 the Chernobyl nuclear disaster released vast amounts of radioactivity, including iodine-131,132 and 133 into the atmosphere. Since 1990 there has been an increase in the incidence of thyroid cancer in those who were below the age of 15 at the time of exposure. Men and women have been equally affected.

There is a 40% risk of cancer in a thyroid nodule in a patient exposed to radiation.

Radiation exposure may also cause nodular goitre.

Family history

Three per cent of patients have a first-degree relative with the same condition. There are inherited syndromes that are associated with high prevalence of thyroid cancer (Table 13.3).

Underlying thyroid disease

There is an increased risk of developing thyroid cancer on the background of Graves' disease. A nodule developing in a patient with Graves' disease has a high risk of malignancy. These tumours may have an aggressive nature. Similarly, Hashimoto's thyroiditis is weakly associated with an increased risk of lymphoma of the thyroid.

Table 13.3 Inherited syndromes of thyroid cancer

Condition	Findings
Familial polyposis coli	Large intestinal polyps and papillary thyroid cancer[a]
Gardner's syndrome	Polyps in large and small intestine, fibromas, osteomas, lipomas and papillary cancer[a]
Cowden's disease	Multiple hamartomas, breast tumours and follicular tumours
Multiple endocrine neoplasia type 2	Medullary cancer (see later)

[a]100-fold risk compared with the general population.

Solitary nodule

Patients with clinically solitary thyroid nodules have a higher incidence of thyroid cancer.

Gender

Men presenting with all types of goitre have a significantly increased risk of thyroid malignancy compared with women.

Iodine intake

In iodine-deficient areas there is a preponderance of follicular thyroid cancer, whereas where there is iodine excess, as in Iceland, papillary cancer is more commonly seen (Box 13.5).

Box 13.5 Risk factors for thyroid cancer

- Ionising radiation exposure
- Family history
- Pre-existing thyroid disease
- Solitary thyroid nodule
- Iodine intake
- Gender

Management of Differentiated Thyroid Cancer (DTC)

Patients should be assessed as previously discussed. Free T_4 and TSH should be routinely measured. The cornerstone for diagnosis of DTC is FNAC. Following this investigation, patients will fall into one of the categories shown. Those with suspicious or frankly malignant results should undergo surgery.

Further Investigations

CT and MRI

These imaging techniques both have a role in the assessment of the extent of larger tumours and their anatomical relations. A CT scan provides good visualisation of cartilage and bone. The disadvantage of CT scanning is that the patient is exposed to radiation and an iodide-containing contrast agent is used. This can block iodine uptake in the thyroid gland for up to 6 months and thus prevent any iodine treatment in this period and precipitate the development of hyperthyroidism. MRI scanning allows for the reconstruction of a three-dimensional image and excellent soft tissue imaging. There is no irradiation of the patient and no need for contrast medium. However, MRI is less widely available and more expensive than CT scanning.

Treatment

Surgery

Surgery is the first-line treatment for DTC. A definitive diagnosis should be made on the basis of FNAC and imaging. The extent of surgery and the need for adjuvant therapy can be predicted from a number of prognostic factors identified pre- and perioperatively.

Prognostic factors

Many staging systems have been described in the literature; they have variable accuracy and are too complex to use on a day-to-day basis. In the UK at present the *TNM* classification is used. This describes the extent of the tumour (T), the involvement of local nodal metastases (N) and the presence of distant metastases (M). It also includes age and histology as markers of risk. Overall, the prognostic factors shown in Table 13.4 are important.

Table 13.4 Prognostic factors

Patient factors	Tumour factors	Management factors
Age (< 20 or > 45 = high risk)	Size (< 1.5 cm papillary < 1.0 cm follicular = low risk)	Delay in treatment
Gender (male = high risk)	Histological grade	Operation performed
	Local invasion	Local expertise
	Metastatic spread	Postoperative adjuvant therapy

Controversy exists over the extent of surgery. A selective surgical approach has been suggested for patients who are low risk with low-risk tumour. All thyroid surgery requires a collar incision. Complications of surgery are given in Box 13.6.

Box 13.6 Complications of surgery

- Haemorrhage
- Hypocalcaemia
- Recurrent laryngeal nerve damage
- Hypothyroidism
- Tracheomalacia

Lobectomy

In general, papillary tumours < 1.5 cm or follicular tumours < 1 cm (in the absence of any other risk factors) can be safely managed by lobectomy with postoperative TSH suppression and annual thyroglobulin measurement (see later). Female low-risk patients who have larger papillary tumours (1–4 cm) may also be suitable for lobectomy. The more aggressive nature of follicular tumours means that conservative treatment is less favourable in tumours > 1 cm.

Thyroidectomy

All other patients should undergo a total or near total thyroidectomy (2–3 g of tissue are left). These have the advantage of lower recurrence rates. A near total thyroidectomy is advocated because it reduces the risk to the recurrent laryngeal nerves; however, in experienced hands, this risk should be < 1%. Even with a total thyroidectomy, there is some residual tissue in the thyroid bed, which can be ablated with radioiodine (see later). There should be preservation of at least one parathyroid gland. This can be re-implanted under the sternomastoid muscle or in the forearm if needed.

Retrosternal thyroid extensions may require a midline sternotomy for access.

Neck dissection

The extent of nodal dissection in the neck depends upon the extent of lymphatic involvement. Nodes from the midline should be routinely dissected. Further nodal levels should be removed if there is involvement, including those in the mediastinum. Other structures such as the sternomastoid muscle, internal jugular vein and accessory nerve should only be resected if they are involved in the cancer.

TSH suppression

TSH can stimulate tumour growth, and suppressive therapy has been shown to improve recurrence and survival rates when used as an adjunct to surgery. Thyroxine is given at a dose sufficient to suppress TSH in all patients who have surgery for thyroid cancer.

TSH serum levels should be < 0.1 mU/l, with T_3 levels within the normal range.

Thyroxine is also necessary as replacement in all patients who have no functioning residual tissue.

Liothyronine (replacement T_3) has a shorter half-life than T_4 and can be used instead.

Radioiodine

Pregnancy is an absolute contraindication to RAI.

Adjuvant therapy

Adjuvant radioiodine therapy is well established. Recurrence rates post-surgery have been shown to drop from 34 to 3% in patients with papillary cancer subsequently treated with RAI and from 45 to 6% in follicular cancer.

High TSH levels promote the uptake of iodine in the tissues and therefore high levels (TSH > 30 mU/l) are needed prior to radioiodine. Patients are required to stop their thyroid replacement to allow for a rise in their TSH levels; this will take 4 weeks after withdrawal of thyroxine and 10 days for liothyronine.

Patients should also adhere to a *low iodine diet* and have not had any recent radiological investigations using contrast agents (hence the need to avoid CT with contrast preoperatively).

Protocol
(See Figure 13.3 for Birmingham protocol.)

For RAI treatment, the patient is admitted to hospital in a single room that has radiation protection.

Radioiodine is given orally, and a scan is performed 3–4 days later with a gamma camera. The thyroid remnant or cancer takes up the iodine and the half-life here is at least 3 days. The biological half-life of the RAI is, however, about 1 day, so when the scan is performed the whole body radiation has become negligible.

RAI collects in the urine, and hence the patient should drink plenty of fluid to induce a diuresis and reduce the exposure to the pelvic organs. Similarly, the salivary glands take up iodine and, to avoid side effects (Box 13.7) of sialadenitis and xerostomia, salivation should be promoted by the sucking of citrus sweets.

Box 13.7   Side effects of RAI

- Local inflammation
- Gastritis
- Sialadenitis
- Pneumonitis

The patient is discharged when the measured whole body radioactivity has fallen to 30 MBq, or 15 MBq if using public transport.

Radioiodine is initially used for the *ablation* of thyroid remnants following total or near-total thyroidectomy. Its use has contributed to a decline in morbidity associated with surgery.

An ablative dose of 3 GBq (50–100 mCi) is given 4 weeks post-surgery. No scan is performed on this occasion.

Six weeks later the patient receives a *scanning dose* of 200 MBq (2–5 mCi) of radioiodine. A whole body scan is performed at 3 days to confirm ablation of the thyroid remnant and to look for any functioning residual disease or metastases.

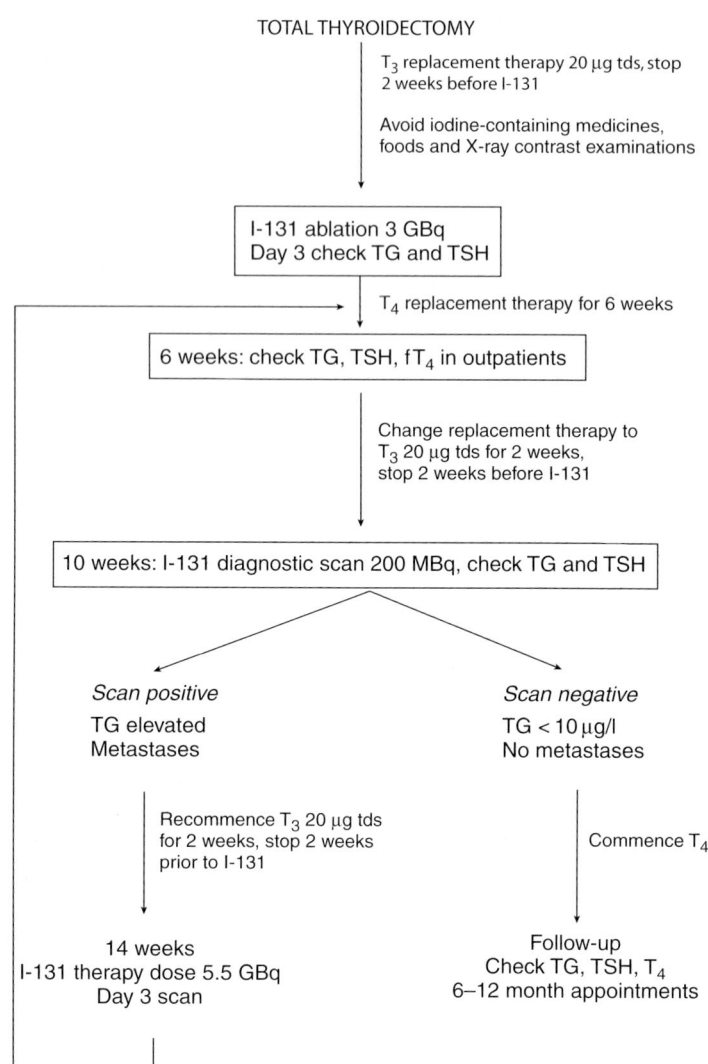

Figure 13.3 Birmingham protocol for the administration of radioactive iodine following total thyroidectomy. (TG = thyroglobulin)

If any uptake is demonstrated, a further *therapeutic dose* of 5.5 GBq is given. This is repeated every 3–6 months until there is no evidence of disease. A scanning dose is then given every year for 3 years and then every 2 years.

Palliative

Radioiodine for the treatment of metastases is generally considered palliative. A dose can be given every 4–6 weeks. There is no limit to the cumulative doses if iodine-131 is given to patients with distant metastases; however, the risk of leukaemia increases slightly when the cumulative dose is > 500 mCi.

Complete remission is seen in 45% of patients with metastases that take up iodine. The overall 10-year survival is 40%.

Studies have shown that there is no increased risk of infertility or fetal abnormalities after high-dose radioiodine.

Serum thyroglobulin (TG)

Thyroglobulin is only produced by thyroid follicular cells. It can therefore be used as a tumour marker following the removal of the thyroid gland and subsequent radioablation of any residual tissue. Elevated levels (> 10 μg/l) in patients on suppressive therapy or > 40 μg/l after the withdrawal of thyroxine indicate the presence of residual disease.

It is used alongside RAI scanning in the detection of residual or metastatic disease.

The TG concentration may not be elevated in a patient on thyroxine therapy and therefore should be repeated once thyroxine has been withdrawn prior to the administration of RAI. Thyroglobulin antibodies can alter results of TG determination and are found in 15–30% of patients with DTC. All patients should ideally be assessed for the presence of these antibodies.

The thyroglobulin-positive diagnostic RAI-scan-negative patient

Causes:

1. Falsely elevated thyroglobulin concentrations due to thyroglobulin antibodies
2. Low TSH levels at the time of the RAI scan or recent iodine intake, resulting in a false-negative scan

3. Micro metastases too small to visualise
4. Dedifferentiated tumour that has lost its ability to take up iodine.

Once the various reasons for points 1 and 2 above have been eliminated, there is a dilemma as to what to do. Further management should be based on risk factors and evidence of aggressive disease. Some clinicians advocate the administration of a *therapeutic dose* of RAI and a subsequent scan; the higher dose of iodine may show previously unseen lesions. This does, however, expose the patient to a further dose of RAI. Others clinicians are employing further scanning techniques to aid in diagnosis, including USS, MRI, Tc-99-labelled methoxyisobutyl isonitrile (sestamibi) and 18-fluorodeoxyglucose PET (positron emission tomography) scanning. Further surgery, external beam or chemotherapy (see later), can then treat residual or recurrent disease.

Human recombinant TSH (rhTSH)

High TSH levels are needed prior to RAI administration. This is usually achieved by discontinuation of thyroid hormone up to 4 weeks before the scan to allow for elevation of endogenous TSH levels. The hypothyroid state that develops can be debilitating for some patients.

A relatively new approach to avoid this is the use of human recombinant TSH to elevate the serum TSH levels needed for scanning to be effective. Patients receiving rhTSH may continue their thyroid hormone treatment.

It is not currently used routinely but is advocated in:

1. patients unable to generate sufficient endogenous levels of TSH after withdrawal of thyroid hormones (secondary hypothyroidism, high endogenous production of thyroid hormones from metastases or slow responders)
2. patients unable to tolerate thyroid hormone withdrawal.

Note that rhTSH is not indicated in patients who have tumours that do not concentrate iodide.

External beam radiation (radiotherapy)

- Used in treatment of DTC that does not take up iodine
- In conjunction with RAI in patients who have had incomplete resection
- To treat inoperable metastatic lesions.

Chemotherapy

Results have been poor, and chemotherapy should only be considered in patients with refractory, advanced DTC.

The overall survival of patients diagnosed with DTC is dependent on histological type and the presence of distal metastases (see Box 13.8).

Box 13.8   Overall survival

- Papillary   95%
- Follicular   80%
- From diagnosis of metastatic disease   25–40%

Anaplastic Thyroid Cancer

Any patient suspected of having anaplastic thyroid cancer from the history and examination should undergo an open biopsy to exclude lymphoma. Treatment is with radical radiotherapy with a tracheostomy if there is upper airway obstruction. The prognosis is poor, and death is almost inevitable within 6–12 months.

Lymphoma

Once a diagnosis of lymphoma has been made, the disease should be fully staged by total body CT. Radiotherapy and chemotherapy are the treatments for lymphoma.

Medullary Thyroid Cancer (MTC)

MTC is rare, accounting for < 10% of all thyroid cancer. It has an incidence of 1 in a million per year (60–80 cases in the UK).

It is a malignancy of the parafollicular C cells, which are embryologically derived from neural crest cells. These cells secrete *calcitonin*, which binds osteoclast receptors and inhibits bone resorption. Calcitonin secretion can be stimulated by pentagastrin; this forms the basis of a clinical investigation (see later).

MTC can be sporadic or familial (Box 13.9): it metastasises early to liver, lung and bone.

Multiple endocrine neoplasia 2

The features of multiple endocrine neoplasia (MEN 2) are given in Table 13.5.

Box 13.9   Medullary thyroid cancer

Sporadic
80%
No history or family history of hyperparathyroidism (HPT)
Phaeochromocytoma
Multiple endocrine neoplasia 2 (MEN 2)
Presentation at 30–50 years

Familial
20%
Positive family history of medullary cancer
HPT
Phaeochromocytoma
MEN II
Presentation earlier in life

Table 13.5   Clinical features of MEN 2

MEN 2A	MEN 2B
Medullary thyroid cancer	Medullary thyroid cancer
Hyperparathyroidism	Hyperparathyroidism
Phaeochromocytoma	Phaeochromocytoma
	Marfanoid habitus
	Ganglioneuromatosis

It is important to differentiate truly sporadic cases from the first presentation of familial disease. A family history of any of the tumours associated with MEN should be asked about and raise suspicion. C cell hyperplasia and multifocal disease seen at histology are usually indicative of familial disease. If clinical information is insufficient to make a diagnosis, then mutations of the *ret* proto-oncogene should be looked for. Transformation of the *ret* proto-oncogene is seen in > 90% of patients with familial MTC. These mutations are usually very specific. *Genetic screening* can be used as a means of diagnosing affected individuals with a family history and should be undertaken in close association with a clinical genetics department so that the implications of the tests are appreciated.

Clinical

Presents with:

- lump in thyroid
- metastatic neck node
- distant metastases
- paraneoplastic syndrome.

Diagnosis:

- FNAC is less sensitive for MTC
- serum calcitonin levels
- genetic screening.

Serum calcitonin. There is debate as to whether this should be measured on all patients with a thyroid nodule. This would give low yield and be expensive. However, studies show that early diagnosis of MTC improves survival. It is therefore important to keep a high index of suspicion for MTC in patients presenting with thyroid nodules.

Imaging techniques such as CT and MRI should be employed to determine the extent of the disease.

Treatment

Radical surgery. This treatment is the first-line treatment for all patients with MTC involving a total thyroidectomy with removal of any involved lymph nodes. A patient with a diagnosis of MTC from a diagnostic lobectomy should undergo completion thyroidectomy and nodal removal as required.

Radiotherapy. This treatment is not usually indicated.

Chemotherapy. This treatment has had some success in the treatment of MTC, but no routine regime exists.

Follow-up

Serum calcitonin levels are measured 30–40 days postoperatively. If both baseline and pentagastrin-stimulated levels are undetectable, then a cure is likely.

Outcome

Screening families can offer a survival rate of 100% at 10 years, but screening at a young age is essential. Outcome is directly related to age at diagnosis.

Early detection and treatment of stages 1 and 2 MTC (TNM classification) improves survival 85% for familial and 70% for sporadic MTC, a difference that reflects the younger age at diagnosis in familial MTC.

Overall survival rates for sporadic MTC are 60% at 10 years.

Thyroid Nodules in Children

A thyroid nodule in a person < 20 years old has a higher risk of being malignant. DTC in children is, however, unusual in accounting for 10% of all cases.

The incidence in this country has fallen since the use of ionising radiation to treat common childhood disorders has stopped. However, following the Chernobyl disaster, the incidence in areas affected by fallout has increased dramatically.

Tumours in children are often of a higher grade than those in adults and disease is often more advanced at the time of diagnosis, with pulmonary metastases in 20%. Despite this, above the age of 10, prognosis is excellent, especially with aggressive management. Below the age of 10, death from metastatic disease is more of a risk.

Further Reading

Franklyn JA. Lack of consensus in Europe in the management of nontoxic multinodular goitre. *Clin Endocrinol* 2000;**53**:3–4.

Franklyn JA, Maisonneuve P, Sheppard M *et al.* Cancer incidence and mortality after radioiodine treatment for hyperthyroidism: a population-based cohort study. *Lancet* 1999;**353**:2111–15.

Guidelines for the Management of Thyroid Cancer in Adults. London: Royal College of Physicians, 2002.

Hegedus L, Hansen BM, Knudsen N *et al.* Reduction of size of thyroid with radioactive iodine in multi-nodular non-toxic goitre. *Br Med J* 1988;**297**:661–2.

Kumar H, Daykin J, Holder R *et al.* Gender, clinical findings and serum thyrotropin measurements in the prediction of thyroid neoplasia in 1005 patients presenting with thyroid enlargement and investigated by fine-needle aspiration cytology. *Thyroid* 1999;**9**(11):1105–9.

Mazzaferri EL, Kloos RT. Current approaches to primary therapy for papillary and follicular thyroid cancer. *J Clin Endocrinol Metab* 2001;**86**:1447–63.

Mortensen JD, Woolner LB, Bemnnett WA. Gross and microscopic findings in clinically normal thyroid gland. *J Clini Endocrinol Metab* 1955;**15**:1270–80.

Pacini F, Vorontsova T, Demidchik E *et al*. Post Chernobyl thyroid carcinoma in Belarus children and adolescents: comparison with naturally occurring thyroid carcinoma in Italy and France. *J Endocrinol Metab* 1997;**82**(11):3563–9

Silverman SH, Nussbaum N, Rausen AR. Thyroid nodules in children: a ten-year experience at one institution. *Mount Sinai J Med* 1979;**46**:460–5.

Tunbridge WMG, Evered DC, Hall R *et al*. The spectrum of thyroid disease in a community: the Whickham survey. *Clin Endocrinol* 1977;**7**:481–93.

Wheeler MH. Investigation of the solitary thyroid nodule. *Clin Endocrinol* 1996;**44**:245–7.

14

Thyroiditis

Stephen Robinson and Dimitrous Goulis

Introduction

Thyroiditis is an end result of several processes that cause inflammation (Table 14.1), many causing temporary thyroid dysfunction. Although it is less common than Graves' disease or hypothyroidism, thyroiditis is important in the differential diagnosis of thyrotoxicosis and hypothyroidism. Possibly 10% of thyrotoxicosis is 'low uptake', and this proportion may be reduced over the last 30 years. Mostly, the thyroiditides are self-limiting, and patients return to a euthyroid state without long-term sequelae.

Typically, with any thyroiditis aetiology, there is a thyrotoxic phase followed by a hypothyroid phase and then recovery (illustrated in Figure 14.1 for subacute granulomatous thyroiditis). During the thyrotoxic phase, damaged follicular cells release stored thyroglobulin, thus increasing plasma thyroxine (T4) and

Table 14.1   The thyroidites

Condition	Notes	Pain
Subacute granulomatous	De Quervain's	+
Bacterial	Gram-positive or negative	++
Radiation		+/−
Palpation or trauma		+
Lymphocytic		−
Postpartum		−
Drug-induced	Amiodarone, interferon	−
	Interleukin-2	−
Fibrous	Rare	−

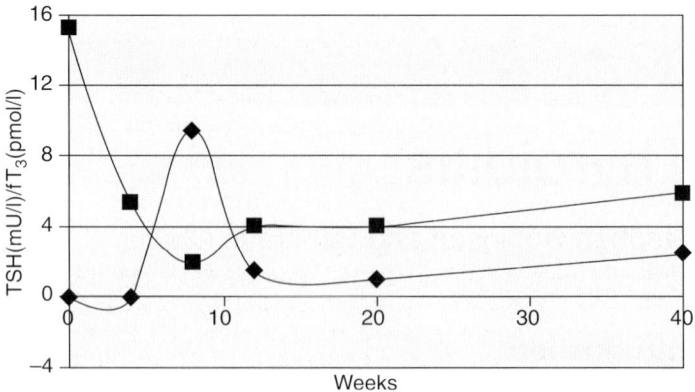

Figure 14.1   Course of postviral thyroiditis. ◆, TSH = thyroid-stimulating hormone; ■, fT3 = free triiodothyronine.

triiodothyronine (T3). This may be a one-off process, e.g. in a postviral thyroiditis, or an ongoing process, e.g. where amiodarone released slowly into the circulation over months may cause a more persistent thyrotoxicosis. During the thyrotoxic phase of thyroiditis, the thyroid is not trapping more iodine or producing more thyroid hormones, but the inflammation is associated with follicular cell damage or death and therefore thyroid hormone release. This is not under thyroid-stimulating hormone (TSH) regulation (nor stimulated by TSH receptor antibodies) and the thyroid hormone release is therefore unphysiological. Typically, damaged follicular cells take time to recover and there is a variable hypothyroid phase before normal thyroid function returns.

Subacute Granulomatous Thyroiditis

Subacute granulomatous thyroiditis is also known as de Quervain's or postviral thyroiditis. It is a granulomatous condition of the thyroid, typically lasting 3–6 months before full recovery. It is less common than Graves' disease and presents especially during the summer months, with 3–6 females for every male, presenting most commonly in the second to the fifth decade. The thyrotoxic phase is often proceeded by an upper respiratory tract infection. Viruses associated with the condition in decreasing order of likelihood include enteroviruses, coxsackievirus and mumps, measles and

Epstein–Barr viruses. Subacute thyroiditis is HDLB35-associated. Pathologically, the thyroid is enlarged with some oedema and there is follicular cell destruction. Fine-needle aspiration will demonstrate a mixed inflammatory infiltrate with neutrophils, lymphocytes, histiocytes and multinucleate giant cells without caseation.

Clinically, features include pain for 90% of patients. The pain may occur almost anywhere in the neck and radiate to the ears and may be unilateral in up to 30% of patients. The neck pain is typically a central dull ache and the patient may have a sore throat with pain on swallowing. General symptoms include malaise, fever, weight loss and anorexia. Obviusly, the latter feature is atypical in Graves' thyrotoxicosis. More typical features of thyrotoxicosis may be evident with sweating and tachycardia. The thyrotoxic phase typically lasts 4–10 weeks. The release of preformed thyroid hormones then stops before a hypothyroid phase lasting approximately 3 months, before full recovery.

The results of thyroid function will depend on when the disease is diagnosed. Early on, there will be a suppressed TSH with elevated free T_4 (fT_4) and free T_3 (fT_3); later, an elevated TSH with low fT_4. Early on in the disease the erythrocyte sedimentation rate (ESR) is often very elevated, possibly above 100 mm/h. The thyroid technetium uptake is low, even if only part of the thyroid is involved, as there is a suppressed TSH. Possibly, 40% of patients will have changes in viral antibodies.

Nonsteroidal anti-inflammatory drugs (NSAIDs) can be used to ease the pain. Steroids are thought to be more effective, starting at 40–60 mg/day and rapidly reducing the dose; however, there is no evidence that they shorten the thyrotoxic and hypothyroid phases. Carbimazole is ineffective as damaged thyrocytes are releasing more thyroid hormones rather than increased iodine trapping seen in the high-uptake thyrotoxicosis. In terms of treatment of thyroid function, the patient may benefit from a β-blocker in the thyrotoxic phase and thyroxine during the hypothyroid phase. Usually the patient will return to a euthyroid, pain-free state; but, occasionally, the condition can be ongoing.

Subacute Lymphocytic Thyroiditis

Subacute lymphocyte thyroiditis is also known as painless or lymphocytic thyroiditis. It is part of a spectrum of autoimmune thyroid disease similar to Hashimoto's hypothyroidism. The incidence may be altering: there was a peak in the 1970s when 20% of thyrotoxicosis was associated with silent thyroiditis, which is now approximately 10%. A proportion progressed to goitre and/or hypothyroidism indistinguishable from Hashimoto's thyroiditis. While lymphocytic thyroiditis is HLADR3-associated, excess iodine intake seems to precipitate the disorder and TSH is needed for it to progress.

The main differential diagnoses are with Graves' thyrotoxicosis and iodine-induced thyroid disorder. Patients may present with weight loss, nervousness, fatigue and heat intolerance. On examination, the patient may be thyrotoxic with tachycardia, hyperreflexia and tremor. An enlarged, firm thyroid is found in 50–60% of patients; this is usually painless.

Thyroid function findings will depend upon when the disease is diagnosed. Typically, it is 3–4 months before a patient moves from a thyrotoxic to a hypothyroid phase. The hypothyroidism will last 2 or 3 months before the patient returns to normal. The majority of patients will have positive thyroid peroxidase antibodies; technetium uptake is reduced. Fine-needle aspiration demonstrates a diffuse lymphocytic infiltrate.

The thyrotoxic phase can be treated with β-blockers; thionamides are of no value. Prednisolone has been used without clear benefit. Thyroxine would be required for the hypothyroid phase but treatment may not need to be permanent. Patients are likely to develop hypothyroidism in the long run; this contrasts with postviral thyroiditis. It would be recommended that patients had a yearly TSH estimation in order to diagnose hypothyroidism.

Trauma-induced Thyroiditis

Trauma – e.g. from a car seat belt, manipulation of the thyroid during fine-needle aspiration or neck surgery or even from vigorous palpation – may precipitate a transient thyroiditis. There may be a thyrotoxic and hypothyroid phase.

Radiation Thyroiditis

Radioactive iodine may precipitate a painful thyroiditis. This is unusual in the patients receiving iodine for thyroid malignancy as they should have had a subtotal or total thyroidectomy. These patients often have parotitis.

Occasionally, patients with thyrotoxicosis treated with radioactive iodine will develop a painful thyroiditis which typically resolves within 1 week of treatment.

Infective Thyroiditis

This may be acute, subacute or chronic. Microorganisms, including Gram-positive and Gram-negative bacteria which maybe anaerobic, may reach the thyroid from haematogenous spread or from a local source in the larynx. Tuberculous thyroiditis is becoming less common, whereas cytomegalovirus (CMV) infection is reported in immunocompromised patients.

Amiodarone-induced Thyrotoxicosis (AIT)

Amiodarone is indicated for the treatment and prevention of ventricular and superventricular dysrhythmias. Amiodarine is an iodinated benzofuran derivative which contains 75 mg of iodine per 200 mg tablet. Amiodarone given at a dose of 200–600 mg releases 75–225 mg of organic iodine/day; the normal daily intake is between 0.2 and 0.8 mg/day. Practically all patients treated with amiodarone will have changes to intrathyroidal physiology, thyroid hormone conversion and the hypothalamic–pituitary–thyroid axis. Amiodarone results in inhibition of thyroid hormone synthesis and release (the Wolff–Chaikoff effect describes chronic, rather than acute, iodine excess transiently decreasing thyroxine production), with decreased thyroid iodide trapping and enhanced T_4 rather than T_3 production. Amiodarone inhibits both type I (liver and peripheral) and type II (brain) 5'-deiodinase. The combination of this and the thyroidal effects results in increased serum T_4 and fT_4, whereas T_3 decreases by one-fifth. Reverse T_3 concentrations nearly double with amiodarone administration. The inhibition of central type II 5'-deiodinase results in a slight increase in TSH concentrations, even in the majority of patients who remain euthyroid. Amiodarone is concentrated in adipose issue as it is highly lipophilic. For the patient who has taken amiodarone for any length of time, these stores are slowly released into the circulation, which can result in reduced thyroid iodine uptake up to 1 year following discontinuation of amiodarone therapy.

If a population is iodine replete, pharmacological iodine administration may precipitate Hashimoto's hypothyroidism. Approximately 6% of patients taking amiodarone will become hypothyroid; this condition may occur 2–40 weeks after commencement of therapy.

Amiodarone may precipitate thyrotoxicosis in roughly 3% of patients; the actual incidence will depend on iodine intake (2% in the

United States, 10% in Italy). The prevalence seems high in young adults receiving amiodarone, e.g. in adults with congenital heart disease (19 of 92 became thyrotoxic in one study). On average thyrotoxicosis occurs 3 years after initiation of amiodarone. The jod-basedow phenomenon describes iodine supplementation in iodine-deficient populations, precipitating thyrotoxicosis. Most of these conditions are on the basis of a nodular goitre, but the prevalence will depend on iodine uptake in the population: it is more common in the relatively iodine-deficient populations, especially in Europe. Type I AIT precipitation of an underlying thyroid disorder may be a nodular or autoimmune thyrotoxicosis. The nodular goitre is more common in continental Europe; autoimmune thyrotoxicosis is probably more common in the United Kingdom. Therefore, on examination, the patient may have a nodular goitre, whereas with autoimmune disease the thyroid may be of a normal size or increased. A bruit may be present. Thyroid peroxidase antibodies are more likely to be present in the autoimmune type. Fine-needle aspiration of the autoimmune type may show typically hyperplastic features.

Type II AIT is destructive. The thyrotoxic phase is similar to that of postviral thyroiditis, although more prolonged, and pain is less commonly present. The ESR is not elevated and thyroid antibodies are typically negative. Damaged thyrocytes release thyroid hormones into the circulation. The patient is likely to suffer subsequent hypothyroidism.

It is important to try and differentiate these causes of AIT, as the treatments differ; however, this can be difficult. Typically, technetium uptake is low with either type I or type II AIT. Radioactive iodine (RAI) uptake in type I AIT is low but detectable (but has been described as normal or high). Colour flow Doppler has been used to try and differentiate the two causes, with decreased blood flow in type II AIT.

The treatment should be aimed at protecting from particularly cardiovascular effects of the thyrotoxicosis, rendering the patient euthyroid and then maintaining the patient euthyroid. Therefore β-blockade is useful, if not contraindicated. Carbimazole can be used for type I and type II AIT, but is more likely to be successful in type I AIT. Perchlorate, with its particular blockade of iodide uptake by the thyroid has been used especially in toxic nodular goitre type I AIT. If perchlorate is used, it should not be more than 1 g/day, with the danger of aplastic anaemia. Thyroidectomy may have to be performed in otherwise untreatable cases. Type II AIT can be treated with steroids, where response to treatment can be relatively rapid. When a patient has been rendered euthyroid, attention can be turned to maintaining this condition, especially if amiodarone is still required. Iodine may be slowly released from adipose stores for some time, maintaining a low RAI uptake, and this can delay the use of an ablative dose of RAI for up to 1 year. A technetium scan can be useful to demonstrate the suitability of RAI at this time: if there is little or no thyroidal uptake, then RAI will be unsuccessful in rendering the patient hypothyroid.

Sick Euthyroid Syndrome

Systemic non-thyroidal illness (NTI) is associated with a 'low T3 syndrome' or 'sick euthyroid syndrome'. This condition may occur in severely ill patients with almost any aetiology – after stress or surgery, liver disease, chronic renal failure, in the sick elderly patient – and is associated with a number of drugs.

In the sick euthyroid syndrome, production of T_3 is decreased, whereas clearance of T_3 is unchanged. Production of rT_3 (reverse T_3) is unchanged, whereas clearance of rT_3 is diminished. This may be related to reduced 5'-deiodinase activity causing decreased T_3 production with reduced breakdown of rT_3. The patient will have typically a low fT_3 and, early on, a decreased serum TSH. Thyroxine concentrations may be low or normal, whereas fT_4 concentrations may be increased. The drugs that cause a decreased peripheral metabolism of T_4 include amiodarone, corticosteroids, propranolol, propylthiouracil and some X-ray contrast agents. There is no evidence of any benefit of treatment of sick euthyroid syndrome with T_4 or T_3.

Postpartum Thyroid Dysfunction

Several autoimmune conditions are exacerbated in the postpartum state, possibly related to the lifting of the partial immune suppression of pregnancy. Between 2 and 16% of women postpartum will have some thyroid dysfunction. A variety of thyroid dysfunction may be seen postpartum and all their mechanisms are not clear. Possibly 5% are nonspecific, such as toxic nodular goitre or subacute thyroiditis. Ten per cent of postpartum thyrotoxicosis is related to Graves' disease. Differences have been attributed to the ethnic group under study and the methodology employed.

The thyrotoxic phase of autoimmune postpartum thyroiditis usually starts 2–4 months postpartum, although there may be no clinical thyrotoxic phase. The TSH is suppressed and the fT4 with fT3 are elevated. The thyroid uptake scan is very useful in differentiating

Graves' from postpartum thyroiditis at this stage. Typically, the breast-feeding mother would have to discard only the first milk after the scan. The TSH receptor antibodies are negative, although they need not be measured routinely. The thyrotoxic phase should not be treated with thionamides, but the low-uptake thyrotoxicosis is self-limiting. β-blockers may be required if the patient is particularly symptomatic.

Then, commencing 4–8 months postpartum, the mother develops a hypothyroid phase which is likely to be symptomatic. Many mothers will complain of tiredness, and the condition may be dismissed without biochemical investigation. Psychological or psychiatric disturbance occurs; plainly, a TSH should be measured in the assessment of postpartum depression. The mother may develop a goitre: fine-needle aspiration would demonstrate a lymphocytic infiltration. However, this investigation is not required unless there is uncertainty regarding the diagnosis with other tests. The TPO antibodies are usually positive. Treatment with T_4 may be required temporarily or, indeed, permanently in 25% of patients. Typically, thyroxine is used for 6–12 months before an attempt on no replacement. The disease will usually reoccur in subsequent pregnancies.

Further Reading

Berger SA. Zonszein J, Villamena P, Mittman N. Infectious diseases of the thyroid gland. *Rev Infect Dis* 1983;**5**:108–22.

Daniels GH. Amiodarone induced thyrotoxicosis. *J Clin Endocrinol Metab* 2001;**86**:3–8.

Dayan CM, Daniels GH. Chronic autoimmune thyroiditis. *N Eng J Med* 1996;**335**:99–107.

Guttler RB, Singer PA, Axline SG, Greaves TS, McGill JJ. *Pneumocystis carinii* thyroiditis: report of three cases and a review of the literature. *Arch Intern Med* 1993;**153**:393–6.

Martino E, Bartalena L, Bogazzi F, Braverman LE. The effects of amiodarone on the thyroid. *Endocrine Rev* 2001;**22**:240–54.

Muller AF, Drexhage HA, Berghout A. Postpartum thyroiditis and auto-immune thyroiditis in women of childbearing age: recent insights and consequences for antenatal and post natal care. *Endocrine Rev* 2001;**22**:605–30.

Roti E, Emerson CH. Postpartum thyroiditis *J Clin Endocrinol Metab* 1992;**74**:3–5.

Volpe R. Subacute thyroiditis. *Prog Clin Biol Res* 1981;**74**:115–34.

15

Gut Hormones and Gut Hormone Tumours

Shahrad Taheri and Karim Meeran

Introduction

The gastrointestinal tract can be considered an endocrine organ. It contains a large number of peptides that regulate the complex mechanisms of digestion, gastrointestinal motility and the maintenance of mucosal epithelial integrity. These peptides may act in an autocrine, paracrine or endocrine fashion, or as neurotransmitters and neuromodulators. Gut peptides and their receptors belong to various families determined by amino acid sequence and gene homology. Some peptides are expressed outside the gastrointestinal tract, e.g. the central nervous system (CNS), where they have other functions.

The secretin–glucagon superfamily of peptides includes secretin, glucagon, the proglucagon-derived peptides (glucagon-like peptide-1, GLP-1; glucagon-like peptide-2, GLP-2), glucose-dependent insulinotropic polypeptide (GIP; also known as gastric inhibitory peptide), vasoactive intestinal peptide (VIP) and related peptides, and growth hormone releasing factor (GRF). Secretin is the principal hormonal stimulant of pancreatic and biliary water and bicarbonate secretion. Glucagon, having opposite actions to insulin, is the first line of defence against hypoglycaemia. It acts on hepatocytes to inhibit glycogen synthesis, and to stimulate glycogenolysis, gluconeogenesis and ketogenesis. GLP-1 is a gluco-incretin (a factor released by the gut that stimulates insulin secretion). Both GIP (also a gluco-incretin) and GLP-1 are also enterogastrones (factors released from the intestine that inhibit gastric motility). GLP-2 has major effects on gastrointestinal epithelial growth.

VIP acts as an inhibitory neurotransmitter in the gut, where it relaxes the lower oesophageal sphincter, sphincter of Oddi and the anal sphincter. It is also a potent stimulator of intestinal secretion by inhibiting sodium reabsorption and stimulating chloride secretion. VIP also inhibits gastric acid secretion. Gastrin and cholecystokinin (CCK) belong to the gastrin–CCK family of peptides. The major action of gastrin is stimulation of gastric acid secretion through direct action on gastric acid secretion and also through the release of histamine from gastric enterochromaffin-like cells. CCK is the major hormonal stimulator of gall bladder contraction. The tachykinins are peptides commonly found in gut carcinoids and may contribute to some of the symptoms of patients with the carcinoid syndrome, such as flushing. Somatostatin, originally isolated from the hypothalamus, does not share any similarity to any other gut peptide. It has major inhibitory effects throughout the gastrointestinal tract, with somatostatin analogues being commonly used in the treatment of peptide-secreting gastroenteropancreatic neuroendocrine tumours (GEP tumours).

Despite the large number of peptides in the gut, only a few of these peptides, when secreted in excess by GEP tumours, result in defined clinical syndromes. GEP tumours are rare tumours that can be classified as functioning and non-functioning tumours. Functioning tumours include carcinoid tumours, insulinomas, gastrinomas, glucagonomas, VIPomas and somatostatinomas. Table 15.1 lists the sites of these tumours, their annual incidence and their major clinical features. These tumours are often slow growing and, usually, their clinical manifestations are due to excess peptide hormone secretion. Palliation for malignant disease can be achieved by suppression of peptide release or blocking of the action of the peptide hormone. Non-functioning tumours have a worse prognosis and present with local pressure symptoms or symptoms such as anorexia and weight loss.

Box 15.1 lists the treatment modalities used for GEP tumours. Although functioning tumours produce and secrete a single major peptide, these tumours frequently produce other gastrointestinal peptides. The clinical picture may therefore change with time and with treatment. For example, the elevated VIP levels may be reduced by surgical debulking of a VIPoma, only to be superseded by elevated gastrin levels, resulting in symptoms and complications of gastric hyperacidity. GEP tumours may also secrete parathyroid

Table 15.1. Major functioning gastroenteropancreatic (GEP) neuroendocrine tumours: their location, annual incidence and major clinical features. Pancreatic tumours may also secrete ACTH/CRH, resulting in Cushing's syndrome; GHRH, resulting in acromegaly; and PTHrP, resulting in hypercalcaemia

Site	Tumour type	Annual incidence	Major clinical features
Pancreatic	Insulinoma	1:1,000,000	Hypoglycaemia – neuroglycopenia and catecholaminergic response
	Gastrinoma (Zollinger–Ellison syndrome)	1:1,000,000	Unusual or complicated peptic ulcer disease, oesophagitis, diarrhoea
	VIPoma (Verner–Morrison syndrome)	1:10,000,000	Diarrhoea, electrolyte and acid–base disturbances, glucose intolerance, hypochlorhydria, hypercalcaemia, flushing, erythematous rash
	Glucagonoma	1:20,000,000	Necrolytic migratory rash, glucose intolerance, cachexia, anaemia, venous thrombosis, neuropsychiatric disturbances, bowel disturbance
	Somatostatinoma	1:40,000,000	Cholelithiasis, diabetes, steatorrhoea
Small bowel	Carcinoid	1:150,000	Flushing, diarrhoea, cachexia, cardiac complications, bronchospasm, pellagra, arthropathy, myopathy
	Gastrinoma		Features as above, multiple microgastrinomas in MEN1
	Somatostatinoma		Duodenal, usually present with bowel obstruction

ACTH = adrenocorticotrophic hormone; CRH = corticotrophin-releasing hormone; GHRH = growth hormone releasing hormone; PTHrP = parathyroid hormone-related protein.

Box 15.1. Therapeutic measures for gastroentero-pancreatic neuroendocrine (GEP) tumours

1. Surgery
A. Tumour resection
B. Tumour debulking surgery
C. Acid-reducing surgery for gastrinoma (now rarely used)
D. Liver transplantation
E. Valve replacement for carcinoid heart disease

2. Medical

Symptom control:
Carcinoid syndrome: Avoid alcohol; somatostatin analogues are useful for most symptoms (diarrhoea, flushing, bronchoconstriction); niacin supplements for pellagra-like skin symptoms. Second-line agents: histamine H_1 and H_2 antagonists, α-blockers, phenothiazines, α-interferon and glucocorticoids for flushing; serotonin antagonists (e.g. ondansetron), loperamide and α-interferon for diarrhoea
Insulinoma: Frequent meals, diazoxide, guar gum, verapamil, glucocorticoids
Gastrinoma: Proton pump inhibitors, H_2-blockers, somatostatin analogues
Glucagonoma: Oral and topical zinc, somatostatin analogues, insulin for diabetes, warfarin for thrombosis
VIPoma: Rehydration with saline, potassium and sodium bicarbonate is the mainstay of treatment. Somatostatin analogues are second-line agents. Third-line agents: glucocorticoids, indomethacin, lithium carbonate, clonidine, metoclopramide, loperamide and phenothiazines

Treatment of tumour:
Cytotoxic chemotherapy: multiple combinations (commonly streptozotocin and 5-fluorouracil), VIPomas most sensitive
Interferon therapy: Effective in tumour reduction in several tumours, but not well tolerated
Somatostatin analogues: Some cases of tumour regression with these analogues have been reported, radiolabelled analogues may prove to be useful in the future
Tumour embolization: Embolization with microspheres or chemoembolization
Immunotherapy: Experimental

hormone-related peptide (PTHrP), resulting in hypercalcaemia; growth hormone releasing hormone (GHRH), resulting in acromegaly; and CRH/ACTH (corticotrophin-releasing hormone/

adrenocorticotrophic hormone), resulting in Cushing's syndrome. GEP tumours may be associated with the autosomal dominant syndrome of multiple endocrine neoplasia type 1 (MEN1) with features of parathyroid disease, pituitary and pancreatic tumours. Since GEP tumours are rare, their diagnosis requires a high degree of clinical alertness in combination with appropriate biochemical (Box 15.2) and imaging investigations. Also, these tumours are best managed by a multidisciplinary team at a specialist centre.

Box 15.2. Biochemical diagnostic tests used for gastroenteropancreatic (GEP) neuroendocrine tumours

Insulinoma

Plasma and urine
Glucose, insulin, C-peptide, plasma and urine sulphonylurea screen; these are only valuable if patient is hypoglycaemic

The 72-hour fast
- Patient is admitted to hospital for close supervision
- Intravenous cannula is positioned and patency confirmed
- Only non-caloric drinks and water are permitted; activity is encouraged
- Plasma glucose is measured at regular intervals dictated by glucose values
- If the patient becomes symptomatic, blood is taken for plasma glucose, insulin and C-peptide, and blood and urine for sulphonylurea screening
- If plasma glucose is <2.2 mmol/l, the test is terminated and the above additional blood samples sent to the laboratory
- If patient not hypoglycaemic at 72 hours, the patient is exercised for 15–30 min and blood taken for blood is taken for plasma glucose, insulin and C-peptide; if plasma glucose is <2.2 mmol/l, blood is sent for insulin and C-peptide, and blood and urine for sulphonylurea screening
- The patient can then be fed
- Interpretation: 30% of patients develop symptoms at 12 hours into the fast, 80% within 24 hours and 100% at 72 hours. If insulin and C-peptide are elevated, proinsulin is measured (raised in insulinoma) as well as plasma ketones (low in insulinoma)

continued

Box 15.2. contd

C-peptide suppression test
- Intravenous cannula is positioned
- Exogenous insulin (0.1 U/kg) is infused over 60 min
- In insulinoma, insulin infusion fails to suppress C-peptide levels

Provocation tests
Tolbutamide, glucagon, intravenous or oral glucose tolerance test – these are generally unnecessary

Carcinoid syndrome

Urine
24-hour urinary 5-HIAA (5-hydroxyindoleacetic acid)

Gastrinoma

Plasma
Fasting plasma gastrin, proton pump inhibitors should be stopped for at least 2 weeks and H_2-blockers for at least 3 days before test

Basal acid output
Usually >15 mmol/h in gastrinoma; >5 mmol/h in patients with previous acid-reducing surgery

Secretin test
For borderline cases and patients who cannot be weaned off medication:
- Fast patient overnight and position intravenous cannula
- Secretin is given intravenously at a dose of 2 U/kg at time $T = 0$
- Blood samples (10 ml in lithium heparin tubes to which 200 ml of Trasylol [aprotinin] is added) are taken at $T= -15, 0, 2, 10, 15, 20, 30$ min
- Blood is immediately stored on ice and spun within 15 min; plasma is assayed for gastrin
- Interpretation: a rise in gastrin from baseline by 200 pg/ml (100 pmol/l) gives a sensitivity of 85% when performed in patients with fasting gastrin levels of < 400 pmol/l; a rise of 50% over basal values gives a sensitivity of 78%. Gastrin levels FALL in normals after administration of secretin

Glucagonoma, VIPoma, somatostatinoma, chromogranin A (pancreastatin) and chromogranin B (GAWK)

Plasma
10 ml collected (from overnight fasted patient) in lithium heparin tubes with 200 µl of Trasylol added and sent immediately to laboratory for plasma to be separated

Carcinoid Tumours

Carcinoid tumours are classically subdivided into foregut (from lung, stomach, proximal duodenum), midgut (from rest of small intestine to mid-transverse colon) and hindgut (from distal colon and rectum) tumours. Midgut carcinoids release serotonin, whereas foregut carcinoids may release serotonin, ACTH, gastrin, histamine and calcitonin. Hindgut carcinoids never produce serotonin, but may produce somatostatin and peptide YY. This classification has been questioned, with the term 'carcinoid' being the preferred name for midgut tumours located outside the appendix that result in the carcinoid syndrome – which consists of flushing, diarrhoea, carcinoid heart disease (associated with fibrosis of valves on the right side of the heart) and bronchial constriction. With long-standing disease, niacin deficiency results in pellagra-like skin symptoms. Occasionally, a carcinoid crisis occurs, with severe hypotension and haemodynamic instability requiring fluid and inotropic support. Rarely, the syndrome is associated with arthropathy and myopathy. Carcinoid tumours arising from the appendix constitute 80% of midgut carcinoids and are rarely associated with the carcinoid syndrome. With midgut tumours, the syndrome only occurs in the presence of liver metastases. The diarrhoea is probably secondary to serotonin secretion, whereas flushing is likely to be due to excess tachykinin and/or histamine secretion. Growth factors released from the tumour may contribute to the cardiac fibrosis. Apart from the well-defined carcinoid syndrome, gastrointestinal carcinoid tumours may present with bowel obstruction, bleeding and intussusception.

The biochemical diagnosis of the carcinoid syndrome requires demonstration of elevated urinary 5-hydroxyindoleacetic acid (5-HIAA; a serotonin metabolite). At least three 24-hour urine collections must be made to exclude the diagnosis, since secretion from the tumour may be intermittent. The levels of chromogranin A, neuropeptide K (a tachykinin) and human chorionic gonadotrophin (hCG) may also elevated, but are not routinely measured. Elevated plasma chromogranin A has been suggested as an early nonspecific tumour marker for carcinoid tumours and other GEP tumours and this is now measured in fasting gut hormone samples sent to the Hammersmith Hospital. A circulating peptide known as GAWK (defined by the single amino acid code for glycine–alanine–tryptophan–lysine), which is itself a fragment of a larger peptide, can be easily measured, and in fact is measured on all samples sent to the Hammersmith Hospital supraregional assay service when a gut hormone sample is requested (see Box 15.2). This is in fact a marker of chromogranin B. Flushing, which may be provoked by foods containing tyramine and alcohol, can also be clinically provoked by pentagastrin, but this is rarely necessary.

The tumour and metastases can usually be localised using radiolabelled somatostatin receptor scintigraphy. Computed tomography (CT), magnetic resonance imaging (MRI) and ultrasound scanning may be used to further localise and stage carcinoid tumours. The treatment of choice for isolated carcinoid tumours (such as bronchial tumours) is surgery. With midgut tumours resulting in the carcinoid syndrome, somatostatin analogues can control symptoms well in over 80% of patients and stabilise the disease, but rarely result in tumour regression. Octreotide is a long-acting somatostatin analogue that requires subcutaneous injections three times a day. After subcutaneous injection, it has a half-life of 6 hours, whereas native somatostatin has a half-life of only 3.5 min. Longer-acting somatostatin analogues (lanreotide; Somatuline LA) and longer-lasting preparations of octreotide (Sandostatin LAR), given intramuscularly every 14 and 28 days, respectively, are likely to be increasingly used. There are also a few case reports of tumour regression with somatostatin analogue therapy.

Interferon-α therapy can be useful in symptom control, but less than a one-third of tumours show regression with this treatment. Since interferon-α is associated with severe adverse effects, it is only used if an antiproliferative action is required. Cytotoxic chemotherapy is used for highly malignant anaplastic tumours, but the tumour response is poor. Embolisation of hepatic metastases is useful in symptom control and tumour regression. Tumour embolisation, which should be carried out in carefully selected patients by an experienced operator, relies on the fact that the hepatic parenchyma receives most of its blood supply from the portal vein, whereas metastases receive their blood supply from the hepatic artery. Therefore, branches of the hepatic artery supplying the metastases can be embolised, resulting in regression of metastases. The therapies described are tailored to the patient and the extent of the disease. For the carcinoid heart, valve replacement may be necessary to avoid right-sided heart failure.

Insulinoma

The majority of insulinomas are benign solitary adenomas, often less than 1 cm in diameter. Approximately 8% are associated with

MEN1. Insulinomas can occur at any age, but the majority occur in middle age with a female preponderance. When associated with MEN1, insulinomas occur at an earlier age, are often multiple, and can be malignant in up to 25% of cases. Excessive and inappropriate secretion of insulin results in symptoms of hypoglycaemia, which are of two types: symptoms of neuroglycopenia and symptoms due to the catecholaminergic response. Patients with neuroglycopenia may complain of headache, lethargy, dizziness, diplopia, blurred vision and amnesia. Hypoglycaemia rarely results in seizures, coma or permanent neurological deficit. The catecholaminergic response is associated with tremor, anxiety, palpitations, nausea, hunger and sweating. Hypoglycaemic episodes occur early in the morning and may be triggered by exercise. To prevent hypoglycaemic episodes, patients often increase their carbohydrate intake, usually resulting in excessive weight gain. There are many other causes of hypoglycaemia that have to be taken into account (Box 15.3).

Box 15.3. Causes of hypoglycaemia

Insulin or insulin-like mediated
Insulinoma
Non-β-cell islet tumours
Exogenous insulin
Insulin autoantibodies
Retroperitoneal sarcomas
Nesidioblastosis (β-cell hyperplasia)

Hormone deficiencies
Cortisol (Addison's disease)
Growth hormone (pituitary failure)
Glucagon
Catecholamine, e.g. postoperative resection of phaeochromocytoma

Drugs
Sulphonylureas (particularly in elderly), ethanol, quinine, haloperidol, salicylates

Enzyme deficiencies
Glycogen storage disease

Organ failure
Liver disease, renal failure, heart failure, starvation, sepsis, shock

Other
Intense exercise
Ackee fruit – Jamaican vomiting sickness syndrome

The diagnosis of hypoglycaemia depends on the demonstration of Whipple's triad: symptoms of hypoglycaemia, low plasma glucose (<2.2 mmol/l) and relief of symptoms with sugar intake. In insulinoma, hypoglycaemia is associated with inappropriately elevated plasma insulin (>30 pmol/l) and plasma C-peptide (>300 pmol/l), in the absence of sulphonylureas in the plasma and urine. Exogenously administered insulin is associated with raised plasma insulin and relatively low plasma C-peptide levels. Multiple tests have been proposed for the diagnosis of insulinoma, but the 72-hour fast is the gold standard test (see Box 15.2). The C-peptide suppression test is used for diagnosis of recurrent insulinoma and in patients who have a borderline positive 72-hour fast (see Table 15.2). Such provocative tests are rarely necessary.

Preoperative localisation of the tumour is carried out to aid curative surgical resection. CT scanning and transabdominal ultrasound can detect 20–40% of insulinomas. CT is most useful for staging and management of malignant insulinoma. We have used selective arterial stimulation with calcium in conjunction with hepatic venous sampling for tumour localisation, and now always perform this procedure before exposing a patient to surgery. In insulinoma, medical therapy is for patients awaiting surgery, for failed surgery, for inoperable metastatic disease or for poor operative risk patients. Frequent meals or snacks are often effective in symptom control. Guar gum can reduce insulin secretion in insulinoma and also allows increased interval between meals. The most commonly used drug is diazoxide (200–600 mg/day orally), which suppresses insulin secretion. Side effects such as fluid retention, hirsutism and weight gain occur in 10–50% of patients, whereas in some patients serious adverse effects including cardiomyopathy, bone marrow suppression and cardiac arrhythmias have been reported. Cytotoxic chemotherapy for malignant insulinoma includes the combination of streptozotocin and 5-fluorouracil, or streptozotocin with doxorubicin. The latter combination has been reported to result in a 69% tumour regression rate, with a median duration for remission of 18 months. The embolisation of hepatic metastases may also provide relief.

Gastrinoma (Zollinger–Ellison Syndrome)

In gastrinoma, the mean age at the onset of symptoms is 50 years with a male preponderance. Up to one-third of gastrinomas are associated with MEN1, whereas up to a half of MEN1 patients develop gastrinomas. The majority of gastrinomas arise in the gastrinoma triangle, an area containing the duodenum, pancreatic head and the hepatoduodenal ligament. At presentation, up to 50% of patients with gastrinoma have metastases, mainly to the liver. The diagnosis of gastrinoma should be considered in patients with unusual or complicated peptic ulcer disease that is refractory to treatment. Oesophagitis and diarrhoea are common, but hardly distinguish gastrinoma from other more common conditions. The diarrhoea is caused by increased acid secretion, secondary to elevated gastrin levels, neutralising digestive enzymes and damaging the intestinal mucosa. Diarrhoea that persists in spite of fasting and that is relieved by acid antisecretory drugs is suggestive of a gastrinoma. Since the increasing availability of potent acid antisecretory drugs, such as proton pump inhibitors (PPIs), the presentation of gastrinoma with complicated peptic ulcer disease in no longer common. Patients may present with a solitary ulcer, oesophageal reflux and/or diarrhoea.

Biochemically, gastrinoma is diagnosed by the demonstration of high levels of fasting serum gastrin in the face of high basal gastric acid secretion (>15 mmol/h). Several conditions can result in raised gastrin levels (Box 15.4). H_2-blockers and PPIs should be discontinued for at least 72 hours and at least 14 days, respectively, before fasting gastrin is measured. Since hypercalcaemia raises gastrin levels, hyperparathyroidism should be excluded in patients with MEN1. The secretin provocation test is carried out when gastrin levels are borderline and acid secretion results equivocal (see Box 15.2).

Tumour localisation is carried out to identify the small proportion of patients with solitary tumours who may benefit from curative surgery. Radiolabelled octreotide scanning usefully detects the primary tumour and any metastases. MRI provides information regarding hepatic metastases. Small tumours may be detected with endoscopic ultrasound and/or selective arterial angiography in combination with CT scanning. Intra-arterial secretin or calcium injection at the time of angiography aids localisation and is the only test that confirms that any visible lesion is functional. We now perform calcium-stimulated angiography on any patients before surgery is contemplated. Surgical exploration, in conjunction with intraoperative ultrasound, duodenal transillumination and duodenotomy can be carried out to localise small tumours not detected by the above techniques.

Symptomatic control can be achieved, without many side effects, with PPIs at dosages titrated to the patient's response and

---

Box 15.4. Causes of hypergastrinaemia and hyperglucagonaemia

Hypergastrinaemia

Associated with low gastric acid/achlorhydria
Atrophic gastritis – pernicious anaemia
Acid antisecretory drugs – proton pump inhibitors (PPIs), histamine H_2-blockers
Chronic renal failure
Helicobacter pylori infection
Post acid-reducing surgery

Associated with high gastric acid
H. pylori infection
Gastric outlet obstruction
Antral G cell hyperplasia
Retained gastric antrum post-surgery
Intestinal resection and short bowel syndrome
Gastrinoma (Zollinger–Ellison syndrome)

Hyperglucagonaemia

Prolonged fasting
Organ failure – liver, kidney
Drugs – oral contraceptive pill, danazol
Injury – trauma, burns, sepsis
Endocine – diabetic ketoacidosis, Cushing's syndrome
Familial

---

aimed at reducing gastric acid secretion to <10 mmol/h for the hour prior to the next dose of the drug. When high doses are required, patients benefit from the PPI dose being given twice a day rather than once a day. Somatostatin analogues and gastric surgery are rarely necessary. Solitary tumours are surgically excised in an aim to cure the patient. With metastatic disease, symptoms are controlled well with PPIs for many years, but when symptoms become difficult to control or the tumour behaves more malignantly, then somatostatin analogues, debulking surgery, chemotherapy, interferon-α therapy, hepatic tumour embolisation and treatment with radiolabelled somatostatin analogues are used, depending on local expertise.

In malignant gastrinoma, combination chemotherapy with streptozotocin and chlorozoticin or doxorubicin results in tumour regression with a median duration of up to 18 months. The majority of patients benefit from hepatic tumour embolisation through reduction of local pressure symptoms. Interferon-α therapy results in tumour regression in some patients but is not well tolerated. Liver transplantation in association with removal of the primary tumour has been attempted, but at present is not used routinely. The 5-year survival of patients with liver metastases is 20% compared with 81% in those without metastases. The management of nonmetastatic gastrinoma in MEN1 patients has been difficult, due to lack of information regarding the natural history of gastrinoma in these patients.

VIPoma (Verner–Morrison Syndrome)

VIPomas are usually solitary (1–7 cm diameter) with 37–68% having metastasised at the time of diagnosis, usually to the liver and regional lymph nodes. Extrapancreatic VIPomas occur along the autonomic nervous system, in the retroperitoneum, lungs, jejunum and liver, and in the adrenal. The mean age at presentation is 49 years, with a slight female preponderance. Ninety per cent of VIPomas are pancreatic. Elevated circulating VIP results in secretory diarrhoea (initially intermittent, but later continuous) with fluid, chloride, bicarbonate, potassium and magnesium loss from the small intestine. VIP is renally cleared and, as severe dehydration ensues, VIP concentrations in the plasma rise exponentially, fuelling the diarrhoea and dehydration. Hypochlorhydria occurs in 73% of cases. Stool volumes can reach up to 20 l/day, despite fasting, and potassium losses to greater than 400 mmol/day. The stool is otherwise normal. The severe hypokalaemia is frequently accompanied by a metabolic acidosis due to bicarbonate loss in the stool. The average duration of symptoms before diagnosis is about 3 years. Other features of the syndrome are hypercalcaemia, glucose intolerance and mild diabetes mellitus. In up to 20% of patients, flushing of the head and trunk may occur in association with a patchy erythematous rash.

The diagnosis of VIPoma requires the demonstration of secretory diarrhoea associated with elevated fasting plasma VIP levels. The plasma levels of peptide–histidine–methionine, pancreatic polypeptide and neurotensin may also be elevated. VIPomas, being large, can be localised by ultrasound, CT and radiolabelled somatostatin receptor scintigraphy. Up to 87% of VIPomas express somatostatin receptors. Rare small tumours may require more invasive localisation techniques.

The first-line treatment of VIPoma requires measures to restore fluid, electrolyte and acid–base balance and thus to break the vicious circle of dehydration and renal failure. Specific treatment involves somatostatin analogues, which inhibit VIP secretion. Third-line agents (see Box 15.1) are rarely necessary. Surgical tumour debulking can be beneficial in symptom control. Unlike other neuroendocrine tumours, VIPomas are sensitive to chemotherapy, showing good response to combination therapy with streptozotocin and 5-fluorouracil.

Glucagonoma

Glucagonomas secrete glucagon and other preproglucagon-derived peptides. The median age at presentation is 62 years, with a slight female preponderance. Twenty per cent of glucagonomas occur in association with MEN1. The nonspecific nature of the symptoms can delay the diagnosis for up to 10 years and may account for the fact that over 70% of the patients have metastatic disease at presentation. The most characteristic feature of glucagonoma is the presence of a *necrolytic migratory erythematous rash* that usually starts in the groin and perineum and migrates to the distal extremities. The lesions are highly pruritic and painful erythematous patches, which become raised and may be associated with bullae. These lesions break down and gradually heal, often leaving areas of hyperpigmentation, only to recur at another site. Secondary infections are common.

The underlying cause of the rash is unknown, but several factors such as direct action of glucagon on the skin, amino acid and fatty acid deficiency and zinc deficiency have been implicated in its aetiology. Associated mucosal involvement results in stomatitis, cheilitis and glossitis. Cachexia is also a common feature of glucagonoma and is difficult to treat. Other manifestations include impaired glucose tolerance, normocytic anaemia, nail dystrophy, diarrhoea, tendency to venous thrombosis and pulmonary embolism and neuropsychiatric symptoms.

Glucagonoma is biochemically diagnosed by highly elevated fasting plasma glucagon levels. Plasma glucagon may be elevated in other conditions, but these are easily distinguishable from glucagonoma (see Box 15.4). Elevated plasma gastrin, insulin, pancreatic polypeptide, VIP and urinary 5-HIAA levels have all been observed with glucagonoma. The majority of glucagonomas, being large and metastatic at presentation, can be localised with ultrasonography, CT or visceral angiography. Somatostatin receptor scintigraphy is most useful for determining the extent of metastatic disease. Endoscopic ultrasound is sensitive for the detection of pancreatic primaries. Localised solitary tumours may require multiple techniques for localisation.

Localised, solitary glucagonomas are surgically excised. The glucagonoma rash responds to oral and topical zinc and to somatostatin analogues. With time, the tumour may become less responsive to somatostatin analogues, requiring increasing doses and/or measures such as surgery and tumour embolisation to reduce tumour bulk. Warfarin anticoagulation is used for thrombotic episodes. Psychiatric symptoms such as psychosis or depression require psychiatric assessment and appropriate treatment. Palliative measures for metastatic glucagonoma include surgical debulking, hepatic tumour embolisation and cytotoxic chemotherapy.

Somatostatinoma

Somatostatinomas mostly occur in the pancreas but can also arise in the duodenum. Duodenal tumours present early with symptoms of obstruction. These tumours may be associated with neurofibromatosis type 1 and phaeochromocytomas. Pancreatic tumours present late with hepatic metastases and a syndrome characterised by the triad of cholelithiasis, diabetes and steatorrhoea. Other features include anaemia, hypochlorhydria, postprandial fullness, hypoglycaemia (occasionally) and weight loss. Highly elevated plasma somatostatin levels confirm the diagnosis. Tumour localisation uses the same techniques as described for the other tumours. Treatment is mainly surgical and the palliative measures are similar to those used for other tumours.

Further Reading

Anderson AS, Krauss D, Lang R. Cardiovascular complications of malignant carcinoid disease. *Am Heart J* 1997;**134**(4):693–702.

Bloom SR, Polak JM. Glucagonoma syndrome. *Am J Med* 1987;**82**(5B):25–36.

Bloom SR, Yiangou Y, Polak JM. Vasoactive intestinal peptide secreting tumors. Pathophysiological and clinical correlations. *Ann NY Acad Sci* 1988;**527**:518–27.

Hammond PJ, Jackson JA, Bloom SR. Localization of pancreatic endocrine tumours. *Clin Endocrinol (Oxf)* 1994;**40**(1):3–14.

Jensen RT. Overview of chronic diarrhea caused by functional neuroendocrine neoplasms. *Semin Gastrointest Dis* 1999;**10**(4):156–72.

Jensen RT. Management of the Zollinger-Ellison syndrome in patients with multiple endocrine neoplasia type 1. *J Intern Med* 1998;**243**(6):477–88.

Jensen RT. Gastrointestinal endocrine tumours. Gastrinoma. *Baillières Clin Gastroenterol* 1996;**10**(4):603–43.

Kulke MH, Mayer RJ. Carcinoid tumors. *N Engl J Med* 1999;**340**(11):858–68.

Marks V, Teale JD. Investigation of hypoglycaemia. *Clin Endocrinol (Oxf)* 1996;**44**:133–6.

O'Shea D, Rohrer-Theurs AW, Lynn JA, Jackson JE, Bloom SR. Localization of insulinomas by selective intraarterial calcium injection. *J Clin Endocrinol Metab* 1996;**81**(4):1623–7.

Service FJ. Classification of hypoglycemic disorders. *Endocrinol Metab Clin North Am* 1999;**28**(3):501–17, vi.

Todd JF, Meeran K. The tumour vanishes. *Clin Endocrinol (Oxf)* 2000;**53**(6):663–4.

Venook AP. Embolization and chemoembolization therapy for neuroendocrine tumors. *Curr Opin Oncol* 1999;**11**(1):38–41.

16

Osteoporosis

Juliet E Compston

Introduction

Osteoporosis is characterised by reduced bone mass and disruption of bone architecture, resulting in increased bone fragility and increased fracture risk. These fractures constitute a major health problem in the elderly population, causing significant morbidity and mortality and resulting in an estimated annual cost to the health services of £1.5 billion. One in three women and one in five men surviving to the age of 80 years will suffer a hip fracture due to osteoporosis. Demographic changes over the next few decades are predicted to lead to at least a doubling in the number of these fractures, largely as a result of increased longevity.

Epidemiology

Fragility fractures (defined as occurring after a fall from standing height or less) are the hallmark of osteoporosis. They may occur at a number of skeletal sites, but the most characteristic are as follows:

- spine
- proximal femur (hip)
- distal radius (Colles' fracture).

The incidence of these fractures increases with age; in women, the median age for Colles' fractures is 65 years and for hip fracture, 80 years. In women, vertebral fracture incidence reaches a peak between 65 and 80 years. In men, no age-related increase in forearm fractures is seen but hip fracture incidence rises exponentially after the age of 75 years. The prevalence of vertebral fractures rises with age in men, although less steeply than in women.

The estimated remaining lifetime risk of osteoporotic fracture in 50-year-old British white women has been estimated at 14% for the hip, 11% for the spine and 13% for the radius; for any osteoporotic fracture, the risk approaches 40% in women and 13% in men. For women this risk is similar to that of cardiovascular disease and approximately six times higher than that of breast cancer. In the United Kingdom it is estimated that approximately 60,000 hip fractures and 50,000 Colles' fractures occur annually; for vertebral fractures, the figure of 40,000 reflects only those which are clinically diagnosed and underestimates the true figure by up to two-thirds.

Clinical Features

Colles' fractures affect the distal radius and typically occur after a fall forwards on the outstretched hand. They can usually be treated on an outpatient basis, although approximately 20% of cases require hospitalisation. Long-term adverse sequelae are seen in up to one-third of patients. These include the following:

- pain
- sympathetic algodystrophy
- deformity
- functional impairment.

Spinal fractures may occur spontaneously or as a result of normal activities such as lifting, bending or coughing and are characterised by varying degrees of vertebral deformity (Box 16.1).

Types of vertebral deformity in osteoporosis are shown in Figure 16.1.

A minority of vertebral fractures (possibly around one-third) present with acute and severe pain at the site of the fracture, often radiating around the thorax or abdomen. The natural history of this pain is variable and, whereas in general there is a tendency for improvement with time, resolution is often incomplete. Multiple vertebral deformities have a number of permanent sequelae, as

---

Box 16.1   Vertebral deformity with osteoporosis

- Bioconcavity
- Wedging
- Compression or crush fractures

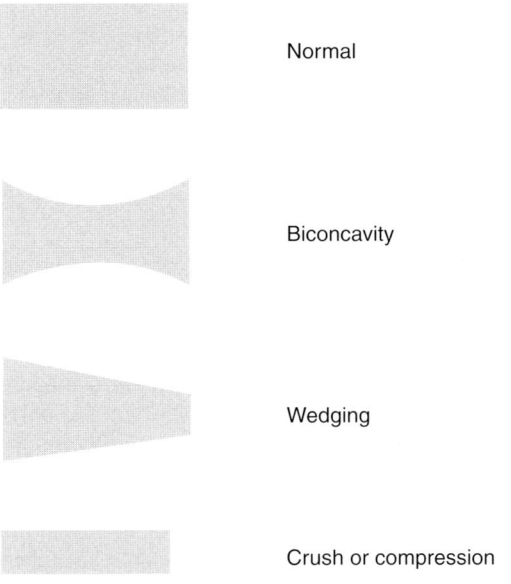

Figure 16.1 Types of vertebral deformity in osteoporosis.

shown in Box 16.2. The clinical impact of spinal fractures is thus substantial, although often underestimated.

Hip fractures cause the greatest morbidity and mortality. They may be intracapsular (femoral neck or subcapital) or extracapsular (intertrochanteric). They almost always follow a fall, either backwards or to the side, and require admission to hospital and

---

Box 16.2   Sequelae of vertebral fractures may include:

- Kyphosis
- Height loss
- Abdominal protuberance
- Loss of normal body contours
- Difficulty with normal daily activities
- Loss of self-confidence and self-esteem
- Social isolation

surgical treatment. Because hip fractures characteristically affect frail elderly people, postoperative morbidity and mortality is relatively high; at 6 months after fracture, mortality rates of 12–20% have been reported. Only a minority of patients regain their former level of independence following a hip fracture and up to one-third require institutionalised care.

Pathogenesis

Lifetime changes in bone mass are shown in Figure 16.2. Peak bone mass is attained in the third decade of life and age-related bone loss is believed to start in both men and women around the beginning of the fifth decade; thereafter, bone loss continues throughout life. In women, there is an increase in the rate of bone loss at the menopause, the duration of which is poorly characterised but may be 5–10 years.

The peak bone mass achieved in early adulthood is an important determinant of bone mass in later life and hence the risk of osteoporosis. Genetic factors strongly influence peak bone mass, accounting for up to 70–80% of its variance. Other determinants include the following:

- sex hormone status
- calcium and vitamin D intake
- nutrition
- physical activity.

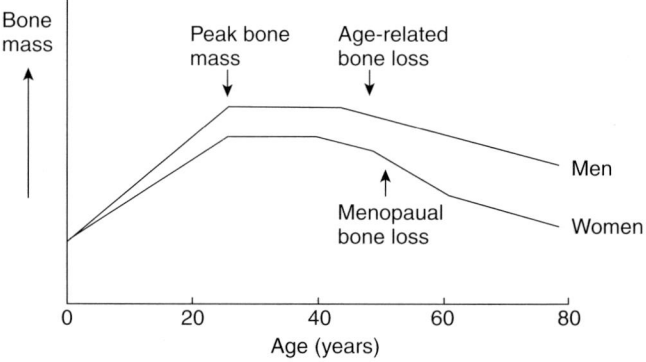

Figure 16.2 Lifetime changes in bone mass.

In women, oestrogen deficiency is a major pathogenetic factor in menopausal bone loss. In men, the relationship between age-related bone loss and declining testosterone levels is less well documented. In the elderly, vitamin D insufficiency and secondary hyperparathyroidism are common and contribute to age-related bone loss. Other factors which may contribute to age-related bone loss include declining levels of physical activity and intestinal calcium malabsorption.

Primary and secondary osteoporosis

Osteoporosis is traditionally classified as primary or secondary. Primary osteoporosis in women is due to a combination of oestrogen deficiency and ageing; in men, the pathogenesis is not well defined, but age-related reductions both in oestrogen and androgen production may be important. A number of secondary causes of osteoporosis have been identified, as shown in Box 16.3.

Box 16.3   Secondary causes of osteoporosis

Endocrine disorders
Primary and secondary
   hypogonadism
Thyrotoxicosis
Hyperparathyroidism
Cushing's syndrome
Hyperprolactinaemia

Malignant disease
Myelomatosis
Leukaemia
Lymphoma
Mastocytosis

Drugs
Alcohol abuse
Glucocorticoids
Heparin

Connective tissue disorders
Osteogenesis imperfecta
Marfan's syndrome
Ehlers–Danlos syndrome
Homocystinuria

Miscellaneous
Gastrointestinal disease
Chronic liver disease
Chronic renal disease
Post-transplantation
Immobilisation

Risk factors for osteoporosis

A number of endogenous and exogenous risk factors for osteoporosis have been identified (Box 16.4).

Risk factors for falling are major determinants of fracture risk, particularly for hip fracture in the elderly (Box 16.5). Their recognition is important, since many are modifiable.

Box 16.4   Risk factors for osteoporosis

Endogenous
Advancing age
Female gender
Caucasian or Asian race
Family history

Exogenous
Hypogonadism
Glucocorticoid therapy
Low body weight
Previous or prevalent fracture
Gastrointestinal disease
Chronic liver disease
Primary hyperparathyroidism
Hyperthyroidism
Hyperprolactinaemia
Prolonged immobilisation
Cigarette smoking
Excessive alcohol intake

Box 16.5   Risk factors for falling

- Reduced visual acuity
- Neuromuscular weakness
- Incoordination
- Reduced mobility
- Cognitive impairment
- Use of sedatives or tranquillisers
- Alcohol
- Environmental hazards, e.g. uneven paving stones, poor lighting and loose carpets and wires

Diagnosis

Bone densitometry

The diagnosis of osteoporosis has been revolutionised in the past two decades by the development of techniques which provide noninvasive measurements of bone mineral density at sites of clinical relevance such as the spine and proximal femur. Several techniques are available for the assessment of bone mass; these include the following:

- single photon absorptiometry
- single energy X-ray absorptiometry
- dual energy X-ray absorptiometry (DXA)
- quantitative computed tomography (CT)
- quantitative ultrasound.

Of these techniques, only DXA and quantitative CT have the ability to measure bone mineral density at both axial and appendicular sites; the remaining methods are restricted to the appendicular skeleton, most commonly the radius (single photon absorptiometry and single energy X-ray absorptiometry) and os calcis (quantitative ultrasound). At present, DXA is regarded as the optimal approach in clinical practice because of its ability to measure bone mineral density at axial and appendicular sites, its good reproducibility and the very low doses of radiation required. However, ultrasound is currently being evaluated and may become more widely adopted in the future.

The rationale for the use of bone densitometry in clinical practice is the continuous and inverse relationship between bone mineral density and fracture risk. For every standard deviation decrease in bone mineral density, there is a two- to three-fold increase in fracture risk; this is quantitatively similar to the relationship between blood pressure and stroke and superior to that observed for serum cholesterol and coronary heart disease. Bone mineral density at a range of sites, including spine, hip, radius and os calcis, is able to predict fracture risk, although the best predictive value, at least in the case of hip fracture, is provided by measurement at the potential fracture site.

Densitometric classification of osteoporosis

The relationship between bone mineral density and fracture risk forms the basis for the densitometric classification of osteoporosis, which is based on T scores – i.e. standard deviation scores above or below normal peak bone mass. The following definitions have been proposed by the WHO Study Group:

- osteoporosis: a bone mineral density T score at the hip and/or spine below -2.5
- osteopenia: a T score between -1 and -2.5
- established osteoporosis: a T score below -2.5 in the presence of one or more fragility fractures.

It should be recognised that the gradient of increasing fracture risk with decreasing bone mineral density is continuous and, therefore, there is no threshold below which fracture will always occur and above which it will not. Nevertheless, since a T score below -2.5 is associated with a high absolute risk of fragility fracture, it can be used as a starting point for making decisions about treatment. These criteria are based on data obtained in women and it remains uncertain whether they are applicable to men.

Indications for bone densitometry (Box 16.6)

Since population-based screening is not available at present, patients are selected for bone densitometry in clinical practice on the basis of risk factors and/or symptoms or signs suggestive of osteoporosis. Bone densitometry may be used in the following ways:

- to confirm or refute a diagnosis of osteoporosis in patients with radiological osteopenia, height loss or fracture

---

Box 16.6   Indications for bone densitometry

- Radiographic osteopenia and/or vertebral deformity
- Loss of height and/or thoracic kyphosis
- Hypogonadism
- Previous fragility fracture
- Glucocorticoid therapy
- Low body mass index (< 19 kg/m^2)
- Maternal history of hip fracture
- Diseases associated with an increased risk of osteoporosis, e.g. inflammatory bowel disease, chronic renal or liver dysfunction, hyperthyroidism, hyperparathyroidism

- to predict fracture risk in individuals with risk factor(s)
- to monitor the effects of treatment.

Bone densitometry should only be performed where the result will influence clinical management. It is not indicated in patients with clear evidence of established osteoporosis and in the very elderly, in whom low bone mass is almost universal, bone densitometry is rarely useful in directing clinical management. In addition, the presence of osteophytes, extraskeletal calcification and vertebral and/or spinal deformity in the elderly significantly reduces the accuracy of spinal measurements.

Radiography

Conventional radiography is an insensitive method for assessing bone loss, since radiological osteopenia can only be reliably detected after loss of 30–50% of bone mass. Nevertheless, when unequivocally present, radiological osteopenia is indicative of advanced bone loss. Diagnosis of peripheral fractures by X-rays is generally straightforward; however, the definition and diagnosis of vertebral fractures is more difficult because of inter- and intra-individual variations in vertebral shape and uncertainties as to the degree of change which constitutes a clinically significant fracture. In general, loss of 20% or more of anterior, middle and/or posterior height can be detected on visual assessment and indicates significant deformity. It should be noted that up to two-thirds of vertebral fractures are asymptomatic and lateral spinal radiographs therefore play an important role in the assessment of osteoporosis. Other conditions which are associated with vertebral deformity and may be confused radiologically with osteoporosis include osteoarthritis and Scheuermann's disease.

Biochemical markers of bone turnover

Biochemical markers of bone resorption and formation reflect whole body turnover and are indicators of the rate of bone loss at the time the measurement is performed. Increased bone turnover, as assessed by biochemical markers, is an independent risk factor for fracture, providing a rationale for the use of these markers in the prediction of fracture risk, particularly when combined with bone mineral density measurements. Biochemical markers of bone turnover are also useful, particularly in clinical trials, for assessing the short-term response to intervention; however, they exhibit considerable biovariability and there is also a large variance associated with their measurement so that application to the monitoring of response to treatment in individual patients is more problematic. It should be emphasised that biochemical markers of bone turnover are not useful in the diagnosis of low bone mineral density per se.

A number of products of collagen breakdown or of bone cells have been identified which may be used as markers of bone turnover. These are shown in Box 16.7.

Box 16.7   Biochemical markers of bone resorption and formation

Resorption
Urinary deoxypyridinoline
Urinary pyridinoline
Urinary type 1 collagen
     N- and C-telopeptides
Serum tartrate-resistant
     acid phosphatase

Formation
Serum osteocalcin
Serum bone alkaline phosphatase
Serum type 1 procollagen peptides

Exclusion of secondary causes of osteoporosis

Secondary causes of osteoporosis should be excluded where appropriate, using the following tests:

- full blood count
- liver function tests
- serum calcium, phosphate and alkaline phosphatase
- thyroid function tests.

If there are clinical reasons to suspect myeloma, plasma immunoelectrophoresis and Bence Jones protein should be performed in the first instance with a marrow trephine if indicated. If malignancy is suspected, an isotope bone scan should be considered. Secondary disorders are present in approximately 40% of osteoporotic men and investigation should also include serum testosterone and sex hormone-binding globulin, gonadotrophins, prolactin and 24-hour urinary cortisol.

Current Therapeutic Options for Osteoporosis

General considerations

A number of options are now available for the prevention of osteoporotic fractures in postmenopausal women (Box 16.8). For historical reasons the level of evidence on which the registration of these interventions is based varies widely; thus, adequately powered randomised, controlled trials with fracture as the primary endpoint exist only for alendronate, raloxifene, risedronate and combined calcium and vitamin D, whereas in the case of hormone replacement therapy (HRT), evidence for anti-fracture efficacy is based almost solely on observational data, which are subject to bias and are likely to overestimate beneficial effects because of the superior health status of women who choose to take HRT as opposed to those who do not.

Although for regulatory purposes a distinction is drawn between prevention and treatment of osteoporosis; this is not useful in clinical practice, nor is it logical, since all currently available agents act fundamentally in the same way, i.e. by inhibition of bone resorption. Furthermore, it is becoming increasingly clear that relatively short-term intervention with anti-resorptive agents produces significant reductions in fracture in women with established osteoporosis. It is therefore more useful to consider the indication for use as prevention of osteoporotic fracture, whether or not fracture has already occurred.

Box 16.8   Agents used in the prevention of osteoporatic fractures

- Hormone replacement therapy (HRT)
- Bisphosphonates (cyclical etidronate, alendronate, risedronate)
- Raloxifene
- Calcitonim
- Calcitriol
- Calcium and vitamin D

Hormone replacement therapy

Hormone replacement at the menopause, whether unopposed or combined with progestagens, prevents bone loss, and observational studies have shown that use of HRT is associated with reduction in fracture at the hip, spine and wrist. Formulations licensed for use in osteoporosis include oral and transdermal preparations of sequential combined, continuous combined and unopposed oestrogen. Tibolone, which has a combination of oestrogenic, androgenic and progestagenic effects is also available for use in osteoporosis.

At least in terms of its effects on bone mineral density, oestrogen replacement is effective both when given at the menopause and if started some years later; however, it is generally less well tolerated in more elderly women and compliance is correspondingly lower.

There is growing evidence for attenuation of the beneficial effects of HRT on the skeleton following cessation of therapy, both in terms of its effects on bone mineral density and protection against fracture. In a recent case control study of women with hip fracture, greater protection was observed in current as opposed to past hormone users and 5 years after cessation of HRT, the risk of hip fracture had reverted to that of a woman who had never had HRT. The implications of these findings are that lifelong treatment after the menopause is likely to be required to maintain optimal fracture protection and that the most cost-effective treatment strategies will be those which target high-risk women for treatment.

Short-term side effects of HRT include the following:

- vaginal bleeding
- breast tenderness
- nausea
- dyspepsia
- bloating
- headaches
- mood changes.

These short-term side effects are generally most severe during the first 3 months of treatment and are more common and more severe in elderly women who are some years past their menopause. Continuous combined 'no-bleed' preparations are now available for use in women who are at least 1 year postmenopausal. However, some vaginal bleeding is experienced by up to 30% of women during the first few months of such therapy.

Hormone replacement therapy may also have significant long-term risks and benefits, as shown in Box 16.9.

The major concern with long-term use is an increase in the risk of breast cancer; after 5–10 years' use, the relative risk increases by around 30%, which should be considered in the context of the

Box 16.9 Potential long-term risks and benefits of sex hormone replacement therapy

Risks
Breast cancer
Venous thromboembolism
Endometrial cancer

Benefits
Coronary heart disease
Cognitive function
Osteoporosis
Colon cancer

absolute risk for a disease which affects 1 in 12 postmenopausal women. Other adverse extraskeletal side effects include a two- to three-fold increase in risk of venous thromboembolism; in terms of absolute risk this is less significant, although HRT should be avoided in women with a past history of or risk factors for thromboembolic disease. Finally, there may be a small increase in the relative risk of endometrial cancer, even in those women taking combined regimens.

Potential long-term benefits of HRT include a reduction in morbidity and mortality attributable to coronary heart disease, although this remains to be confirmed in prospective studies. However, a recent study indicates that combined HRT in older women may not be effective in the secondary prevention of coronary heart disease; in that study, more deaths due to heart disease occurred during the first year in treated women than in controls and at no point during the 4-year follow-up period was any protection against heart disease observed in the treatment group. These results emphasise the need for prospective studies to establish the efficacy of HRT in the primary prevention of coronary heart disease and also indicate the need for caution in advising hormone use in women with a past history of heart disease.

Other potential but as yet unproven benefits of long-term HRT include improved cognitive function, protection against Alzheimer's disease and a reduction in risk of colon cancer.

Accurate evaluation of the risk/benefit ratio of HRT cannot at present be performed because of the lack of prospective data which are required to demonstrate the direction and magnitude of potential risks and benefits. Many women are reluctant to take indefinite HRT because of the increase in breast cancer risk, and treatment is thus often limited to a finite period of between 5 and

10 years. In addition, vaginal bleeding is an unwanted side effect for the majority of women and an important cause of the poor compliance which has been documented with long-term HRT.

Bisphosphonates

The bisphosphonates are synthetic analogues of the naturally occurring compound pyrophosphate. They inhibit bone resorption by complex and only partially understood mechanisms and may also inhibit mineralisation. The following bisphosphonates are currently licensed for use in osteoporosis:

- cyclic etidronate: taken in a 3-month cycle consisting of 400 mg daily of etidronate for 2 weeks followed by 500 mg daily of calcium for 76 days
- alendronate: given as a single daily dose of 10 mg, or a once-weekly dose of 70 mg
- risedronate: given as a single daily dose of 5 mg.

All three bisphosphonates have been shown to prevent bone loss in the spine and hip, both in healthy perimenopausal women and in more elderly women with osteoporosis. In large randomised controlled trials conducted in postmenopausal women with osteoporosis, both alendronate and risedronate have been shown to produce significant reductions in vertebral and nonvertebral fractures. For both agents, a significant reduction in vertebral fractures has been shown after only 1 years' treatment, the benefit being maintained for at least 3 years.

In the case of cyclic etidronate therapy, the clinical trials were not adequately powered to demonstrate fracture reduction but favourable trends for vertebral fracture were observed after 3 years' treatment and observational data from the General Practice Research Database also indicate protective effects against hip and other nonvertebral fractures.

Bisphosphonates are generally well tolerated. Hypocalcaemia may occur, but is rarely symptomatic, and hypophosphataemia has also been reported. Gastrointestinal side effects are most common; in the case of cyclic etidronate, these are usually related to the calcium supplement and can be averted by using an alternative calcium preparation. A small number of cases of erosive oesophagitis have been reported with alendronate. It is therefore important that patients take the drug according to the following instructions:

- take the tablet in morning on rising with a full glass of water

- do not take food, other drink or medications for at least 30 min after taking the tablet
- remain upright for 30 min after taking the tablet.

Alendronate is contraindicated in patients with oesophageal abnormalities or disease and should be withdrawn immediately if dyspepsia or dysphagia develop during therapy.

The optimum duration of bisphosphonate therapy is unknown. Despite the high skeletal retention of these compounds, preliminary indications are that bone loss resumes soon after treatment is discontinued although further studies are required in this area. There are theoretical concerns that prolonged suppression of bone turnover may have adverse effects on bone strength and, at present, treatment is usually given for a period of approximately 5 years.

Raloxifene

Raloxifene is a selective oestrogen receptor modulator (SERM) which has oestrogenic effects in the skeleton but without the unwanted effects of oestrogen in the breast and endometrium. In randomised controlled trials raloxifene has been shown to prevent menopausal bone loss in healthy early postmenopausal women; in addition, in a large randomised controlled trial of 7705 postmenopausal women with osteoporosis, a 30–50% reduction in vertebral fracture rate was demonstrated. Beneficial effects on bone mineral density are seen both in the spine and proximal femur; however, no reduction in non-vertebral fracture has been demonstrated.

Raloxifene is taken orally as a single daily dose. Adverse effects are rare but include the following:

- leg oedema
- leg cramps
- hot flushes
- venous thromboembolism.

Raloxifene does not alleviate, and may exacerbate, menopausal vasomotor symptoms and should therefore be avoided in perimenopausal women with active symptoms.

The extraskeletal effects of raloxifene are of considerable interest. In particular, a highly significant protective effect against oestrogen receptor positive breast cancer has emerged in the clinical trials. After 4 years' treatment there was a 75% reduction in new cases of breast cancer, this figure rising to 90% when only oestrogen receptor positive cases were considered. Consistent with its anti-oestrogenic effect on breast tissue, there is no increase in the frequency of breast and nipple tenderness in women taking raloxifene. Raloxifene use is not associated with vaginal bleeding or any increase in the incidence of endometrial hyperplasia or carcinoma. The effects of raloxifene on cognitive function and cardiovascular disease risk have not been established; the effects on serum lipid profile are similar but not identical to those observed with oestrogen.

The potential pros and cons of raloxifene versus HRT are shown in Box 16.10.

Box 16.10   Potential pros and cons of raloxifene versus hormone replacement therapy

Advantages
Lack of vaginal bleeding
Protection against breast cancer

Disadvantages
Does not alleviate (and may exacerbate) vasomotor menopausal
    symptoms
Possibly weaker effect on bone

Unknown
Effect on coronary heart disease
Effect on cognitive function and risk of Alzheimer's disease

Calcitonin

Calcitonin may be administered parenterally or intranasally; both forms of treatment have been shown to prevent spinal bone loss in postmenopausal women but treatment benefits at other sites such as the proximal femur and radius have not been clearly demonstrated. The effects of calcitonin on fracture rate are controversial, although some randomised controlled trial data indicate beneficial effects on vertebral fracture risk. Adverse effects with intranasal calcitonin are rare. Parenteral administration of calcitonin may be associated with the following side effects:

* nausea
* flushing
* diarrhoea
* vomiting
* tingling of hands.

These symptoms are usually transient but may persist for some hours after injection.

Vitamin D and calcium

There is increasing evidence that vitamin D and calcium supplementation protects against nonvertebral fractures in elderly subjects. Thus, in a randomised controlled trial of vitamin D and calcium in daily doses of 800 IU and 1.2 g, respectively, a significant reduction in hip and other nonvertebral fractures was seen after 12–18 months treatment in a cohort of very elderly women living in sheltered accommodation. Subsequently, a significant reduction in nonvertebral fractures was reported in community-dwelling men and women aged over 65 years in a randomised controlled trial of 700 IU vitamin D and 500 mg calcium daily. It is not possible from these studies to deduce the relative contributions of vitamin D and calcium to the observed benefit; vitamin D without calcium has been shown in some studies to reduce nonvertebral fracture rate in the elderly but this finding has not been universal. The important question of whether vitamin D alone reduces hip fracture thus remains unanswered at present.

Calcitriol

Calcitriol (1,25-dihydroxyvitamin D, the active metabolite of vitamin D) preserves bone mineral density in women with postmenopausal osteoporosis and some but not all studies indicate that it also reduces vertebral fracture rate. In one study a reduction in nonvertebral fracture rate was also observed. Calcitriol is given orally in a dose of 0.5–1.0 µg daily; hypercalciuria and hypercalcaemia may occur and serum calcium levels should be monitored at regular intervals.

Calcium

Beneficial effects of calcium on bone mineral density have been documented in children and adults, particularly at appendicular skeletal sites. In lumbar spine bone, these effects are generally less evident and may be transient; the benefits of calcium are also less marked in perimenopausal women, presumably because of the dominant effects of oestrogen deficiency. Although several small studies have reported a reduction in vertebral fracture rate in calcium-supplemented individuals, evidence from adequately powered studies is not available and calcium should be regarded as an adjunct to treatment rather than as definitive therapy.

Nonpharmacological interventions

Several nonpharmacological interventions may be beneficial in the management of patients with osteoporosis:

- hip protectors
- physiotherapy, including hydrotherapy and transcutaneous electrical nerve stimulation (TENS)
- occupational therapy
- fall assessment and advice
- weight-bearing exercise
- lifestyle advice.

Hip protectors have been shown to protect against hip fracture in randomised controlled trials in the elderly and should be considered in all those at high risk and in those who have already sustained a hip fracture. Physiotherapy has an important role to play in the management of pain and restricted mobility, and measures such as hydrotherapy and TENS are often effective. In elderly patients, occupational therapy is also often helpful, and assessment of the risk of falling should be performed with advice on reducing risk where appropriate.

Weight-bearing exercise can produce modest, site-specific increases in bone mineral density in younger adults but its skeletal effects in postmenopausal women are less certain and it should not be regarded as a definitive treatment. In the elderly, exercise may reduce the risk of falling and, if a fall should occur, improve the neuromuscular protective responses; however, the efficacy of this approach in reducing fracture risk has yet to be proven in randomised controlled trials.

Lifestyle advice is an important component of the management of all patients with or at risk from osteoporosis. Adequate nutrition and body weight should be advised, with particular attention to calcium intake and vitamin D status. Smoking and alcohol abuse should be discouraged and exercise advocated.

Other aspects of treatment

Pain associated with acute vertebral fracture is often underestimated and can be difficult to manage. Very strong analgesics should be avoided where possible, since these may increase the risk of falling, and bed rest should be restricted to a minimum to avoid further bone loss associated with immobilisation. Calcitonin is often effective in the treatment of pain associated with vertebral fractures; salcatonin is usually given subcutaneously in a dose of 100 IU daily or on alternate days for a period of 3–6 weeks.

Treatment of Glucocorticoid-Induced Osteoporosis

Cyclical etidronate, risedronate and alendronate therapy have all been shown to be effective in the prevention of glucocorticoid-induced osteoporosis. Management can be divided into general measures and primary and secondary prevention. General measures are as follows:

- keep the dose of glucocorticoids to a minimum and review frequently
- ensure adequate dietary calcium and vitamin D status
- correct hypogonadism if present (both in males and females)
- give lifestyle advice.

Primary prevention

There is evidence that the most rapid bone loss in patients receiving glucocorticoids occurs in the first 3–6 months of treatment, emphasising the need for early intervention in those at highest risk. The indications for primary prevention are as follows:

- high-dose glucocorticoid therapy (e.g. 15 mg oral prednisolone daily) for > 3 months
- strong risk factors, e.g. previous fragility fracture, age > 65 years.

In such cases, prophylaxis should be commenced concurrently with the glucocorticoids, and bone densitometry prior to starting treatment is not required.

Secondary prevention

In patients on oral prednisolone 7.5 mg daily (or equivalent) for 6 months or more who have not received primary prevention, bone densitometry should be performed to assess fracture risk. The relationship between bone mineral density and fracture risk has not been firmly established in the context of glucocorticoid-induced osteoporosis but there is some evidence that fractures occur at a higher bone mineral density than in postmenopausal osteoporosis. For this reason, the intervention threshold recommended is a T score of -1.5 at the spine or hip. In addition, secondary prevention should be advised to all patients who sustain a fragility fracture while taking glucocorticoids.

Treatment of Osteoporosis in Men

Alendronate, 10 mg daily, is the only treatment currently licensed for prevention of osteoporotic fractures in men. Beneficial effects on bone mineral density have also been reported in trials of testosterone and cyclical etidronate but effects on fracture risk have not been reported for either agent.

Further Reading

Compston JE. The role of vitamin D and calcium supplementation in the prevention of osteoporotic fractures in the elderly. *Clin Endocrinol* 1995;**43**,393–405.

Eastell R, Reid DM, Compston J *et al.* UK consensus group on management of glucocorticoid induced osteoporosis: an update. *J Internal Med* 1998;**244:**271–92.

Looker, Bauer DC, Chesnut CH *et al.* Clinical use of biochemical markers of bone remodelling: current status, future directions. *Osteoporosis International* 2000;**11**(6):467–80.

Wood AJJ. Treatment of postmenopausal osteoporosis. *New Engl J Med* 1998;**338:**736–46.

Writing group of the Royal College of Physicians and Bone and Tooth Society. *Osteoporosis; clinical guidelines for prevention and treatment.* Royal College of Physicians Update. London: RCP, 2000.

17

Calcium

David A Heath

Basic Physiology

Serum calcium is closely controlled and the total serum calcium normally ranges between 2.20 and 2.60 mmol/l.

Approximately 50% of the total calcium is bound to proteins, especially albumin, and the total calcium is affected by changes in the serum protein concentration. Although correction factors are available, they are not precise and are likely to be inaccurate if a large correction is made.

The hormonal control of calcium metabolism is predominantly regulated by parathyroid hormone and vitamin D. Calcitonin is of little or no importance in human calcium regulation.

Parathyroid hormone (PTH) is a polypeptide hormone acting on a receptor found in kidney and bone. It can be measured using a two-site immunometric assay.

Vitamin D, or calciferol, is produced predominantly in the skin with minor amounts ingested in our diet. Conversion to 25-hydroxy-vitamin D occurs in the liver, followed by the production in the kidney of the active metabolite 1,25-dihydroxyvitamin D.

Parathyroid hormone-related protein (PTHrP) is a protein produced in small amounts by many normal cells, especially of squamous origins. It has local autocrine or paracrine actions. It acts in an identical manner to PTH on the PTH receptor. It is not normally present in significant amounts in the circulation. However, a variety of malignant tumours can produce excessive amounts, which appear in the circulation and cause hypercalcaemia.

The parathyroid and renal tubular cells have a surface receptor which recognises circulating ionised calcium concentration – the calcium-sensing receptor (CaR). This receptor is responsible for regulating the release of PTH from the parathyroid cells and controlling calcium reabsorption in the tubule. Inherited modifications of CaR can alter the relationship between ionised calcium and PTH release and renal calcium reabsorption. This can lead to disorders causing either hyper- or hypocalcaemia.

DISORDERS OF CALCIUM METABOLISM

Hypercalcaemia

The vast majority of cases of hypercalcaemia encountered in medical practice have either primary hyperparathyroidism or malignancy. Although there are many other causes of hypercalcaemia, they are rare outside specialist clinics. The initial approach to a new case of hypercalcaemia should be to look for evidence of hyperparathyroidism, or malignancy.

Hypercalcaemia is due to either hyperparathyroidism or malignancy in 97% of cases.

Primary hyperparathyroidism

The fact that calcium is measured in the majority of patients who are investigated by biochemical tests has brought to light many previously unrecognised cases of hyperparathyroidism (Box 17.1). Many of the cases identified are either completely asymptomatic or have a series of nonspecific symptoms. Complications of the disease, such as renal stones, are unusual (less than 10% of cases) and overt bone disease is rare (less than 1% of cases). As a consequence, most cases of hyperparathyroidism are not clinically particularly ill and rarely get immediately referred as acute admissions.

Hyperparathyroidism is, therefore, by far the commonest cause of hypercalcaemia that is referred for outpatient investigation. The

---

Box 17.1   Primary hyperparathyroidism

- Patients are usually relatively well
- By far the commonest cause of hypercalcaemia referred for outpatient investigation
- Diagnosis usually only requires demonstrating an elevated serum PTH

coincidental occurrence of vitamin D deficiency may mask the hypercalcaemia.

Symptoms

Approximately 50% of patients are asymptomatic. Symptoms, when present, are nonspecific and often include tiredness, difficulty climbing stairs, vague aches and pains, increased thirst and polyuria and constipation.

Age of onset

Hyperparathyroidism is unusual in the young and much more common in older age. In the elderly, women are affected four times more commonly than men.

Diagnosis

In the face of hypercalcaemia, an elevated PTH level always means primary hyperparathyroidism. A normal PTH is compatible with hyperparathyroidism but particularly in the asymptomatic patients should suggest the possibility of familial benign hypercalcaemia. All other causes of hypercalcaemia have suppressed (but often detectable) PTH concentrations. Calcium, phosphate, renal function, PTH and vitamin D can be assessed.

Imaging

Radioisotope scanning with sestamibi is the most successful technique for pre-operative localisation of parathyroid tumours. Ultrasounds, CT and MRI are less successful. These techniques are particularly valuable in the management of cases where initial surgery has been successful.

Treatment

There is currently no effective medical treatment of hyperparathyroidism. Surgery is the only option other than conservative management. Conservative management is being increasingly considered in elderly patients with few or no symptoms. Surgery is definitely indicated in young patients and where complications of the disease have developed, e.g. renal stones or bone disease. Although there is no randomised control trial, surgery almost certainly reduces fracture rate in primary hyperparathyroidism.

Bisphosphonates have been used where surgery is contraindicated. However, there are no data on improvement in fracture risk in this group of patients. If the calcium is greater than 3.0 mmol/l, parathyroidectomy is recommended.

Surgical management. Surgery must be performed by an experienced parathyroid surgeon, most of whom do not require preoperative localisation to be performed.

Over 90% of patients have a single, benign parathyroid adenoma. The rest have four-gland hyperplasia or multiple adenomas. Parathyroid carcinomas are very rare.

Patients should be well hydrated before surgery. Surgery is successful in around 95% of cases and should result in a normal calcium within 24–36 hours of surgery.

Management of postoperative hypocalcaemia. Mild hypocalcaemia (serum calcium 1.90 mmol/l or higher) is not uncommon following surgery and usually does not require active treatment. Severe, symptomatic hypocalcaemia occurring 3–5 days postoperatively is uncommon but may occur in patients with parathyroid bone disease or in patients who have had multiple parathyroid glands removed. In the former case, the condition is due to large amounts of calcium returning to the bones (hungry bone syndrome) and it eventually resolves, and in the latter case permanent hypoparathyroidism is usually the cause. Both situations require large amounts of intravenous calcium (calcium gluconate 15 mg/kg intravenously in 1 litre 0.9% saline over 4 hours) to be given together with alphacalcidol (starting at 1–2 μg daily) or calcitriol until normocalcaemia occurs. Treatment can then be slowly withdrawn to see if permanent hypoparathyroidism is present.

Familial hyperparathyroidism

Familial hyperparathyroidism can occur in multiple endocrine neoplasia (MEN) type 1 or 2 (Chapter 19): it is common in MEN1 and uncommon in MEN2. Hyperparathyroidism usually develops in the 3rd to 4th decades.

Hypercalcaemia of malignancy

Hypercalcaemia complicates many forms of malignancy, especially those tumours arising from squamous epithelium. Hypercalcaemia is usually associated with a large tumour mass and is seen most typically in tumours that are advanced and often disseminated. Bone secondaries are not, however, an essential feature. As a consequence, hypercalcaemia typically develops in patients known to have active malignant disease, or where the malignancy is easily identified. Because of the advanced state of the malignancy, patients are usually unwell prior to the development of the hypercalcaemia and then deteriorate rapidly as the hypercalcaemia presents (Box 17.2). Hypercalcaemia associated with malignancy is the commonest cause of hypercalcaemia found in hospital.

Box 17.2   Hypercalcaemia of malignancy

- Patients are usually obviously unwell
- The malignancy is usually advanced
- PTH concentrations are low, PTHrP may be elevated
- Intravenous fluids with an intravenous bisphosphonate will control the hypercalcaemia

---

Symptoms

As already mentioned, patients are usually unwell from the malignancy and then symptoms of hypercalcaemia may develop, such as thirst, nausea and vomiting and constipation.

Diagnosis

In most cases, diagnosis is easy as the malignant process is known to be present. If not, there are usually features to suggest malignancy. Anaemia, abnormal liver function tests and a low albumin are common associated features. PTH should be suppressed.

Aetiology

Most cases are due to the release of hormonal agents from the malignancy – the commonest being PTHrP. Bony metastasis are not necessary for this to occur.

Treatment

Surgical cure of the malignancy is rarely possible. Appropriate chemotherapy should be given, if possible.

Symptomatic patients require admission to hospital for intravenous fluid therapy, usually with the addition of intravenous bisphosphonate therapy, e.g. disodium pamidronate 30–60 mg infused over 2–4 hours. Serum calcium falls slowly and may take 4–5 days to reach normal values.

Unless the malignant process can be controlled, the hypercalcaemia will recur and then bisphosphonate infusions can be given on an outpatient basis – every 3–4 weeks.

Steroids are typically ineffective, except where the tumour is known to be of haematological or lymphoid origin.

Familial benign or hypocalciuric hypercalcaemia

This is a condition which can easily be confused with asymptomatic primary hyperparathyroidism and was, in fact, identified originally by the fact that parathyroidectomy did not cure what had been thought to be cases of hyperparathyroidism (Boxes 17.3 & 17.4).

Box 17.3   Familial benign hypercalcaemia (FBH)

- Always suspect this disorder if PTH concentrations are normal in a hypercalcaemic patient
- Look for affected family members
- *Do not* consider parathyroidectomy

Box 17.4   To exclude familial benign hypercalcaemia (FHH) a high 24-hour urinary Ca^{2+} should be demonstrated

The calcium clearance to creatinine clearance ratio should be > 0.01. This ratio can be reduced to:

$$\frac{\text{Urine calcium (mmol/l)} \times [\text{Plasma creatinine (}\mu\text{mol/l) / 1000}]}{\text{Plasma calcium (mmol/l)} \times \text{Urine creatinine (mmol/l)}}$$

The hypercalcaemia is usually mild and the patient well. The PTH is usually normal but occasionally elevated; hence the confusion with primary hyperparathyroidism. The condition is inherited in an autosomal dominant manner, with affected individuals being hypercalcaemic from birth. The urine calcium excretion is often low, but rarely in a way that differentiates the condition from hyperparathyroidism. The most certain way of making the diagnosis is to identify other hypercalcaemic family members who are asymptomatic. The finding of hypercalcaemia with normal PTH concentration, and especially hypercalcaemic children, differentiates the condition from the MEN syndromes.

The condition is benign and requires no treatment, except in one situation. Very rarely, neonates can develop a severe hyperparathyroid state with marked hypercalcaemia, failure to thrive, parathyroid bone disease and very high PTH concentrations. Emergency total parathyroidectomy may be required. The vast majority of affected neonates are not affected in this way.

The explanation of the disorder is an inherited mutation of the *CaR* gene which shifts the set point for the regulation of PTH secretion in response to changes in ionised calcium. The renal tubule also has an altered calcium reabsorption, thus explaining the hypocalciuria often noted.

Other Causes of Hypercalcaemia

Renal failure

Hypercalcaemia is a common complication of chronic renal failure due to a variety of causes. The use of calcium carbonate as a phosphate binder and vitamin D metabolites to prevent renal bone disease can both cause hypercalcaemia. Prolonged parathyroid stimulation can give rise to tertiary hyperparathyroidism and the development of hypercalcaemia.

Hypercalcaemia occasionally complicates the polyuric recovery phase of acute renal failure.

Vitamin D therapy

The use of large doses of calciferol (e.g. 50,000 units or more per day) or 1–2 μg of alphacalcidol or calcitriol can lead to hypercalcaemia. The fact that the patient is on potent vitamin D metabolites is usually known about, so that the diagnosis is usually apparent.

Sarcoidosis

Although hypercalcaemia is commonly known to be associated with sarcoidosis, it is a rare complication. It occurs in less than 1–2% of cases of sarcoidosis. The sarcoid process is not always obvious. The hypercalcaemia is due to excess production of

1,25-dihydroxyvitamin D by the abnormal granulomatous tissue. PTH concentrations are low and the hypercalcaemia is completely corrected by oral steroid therapy, e.g. 20 mg prednisolone daily.

Thyrotoxicosis

Hypercalcaemia is a rare complication of severe thyrotoxicosis. PTH values are suppressed. The hypercalcaemia may take 4–6 weeks of antithyroid therapy to resolve.

Milk-alkali syndrome

Although the name persists, milk is now rarely involved. Milk-alkali syndrome is typically associated with the heavy ingestion of proprietary alkaline indigestion remedies, e.g. Rennies. PTH is low. Mild renal failure is common. Once ingestion is stopped, the hypercalcaemia usually resolves within 24 hours.

Immobilisation

This is uncommon and occurs in situations whereby increased turnover is associated with immobilisation of a major part of the body. It is seen most frequently when youths develop paraplegia or are immobilised in hip spicas.

Paget's disease

This is listed purely to say that despite being in many textbooks as a cause of hypercalcaemia, this is *not the case!* Hypercalcaemia in a patient with Paget's disease usually means coincidental hyperparathyroidism.

Hypocalcaemia

Hypocalcaemia is a less common biochemical abnormality than hypercalcaemia. The commonest cause is an apparent hypocalcaemia secondary to low serum proteins. Such changes are common in many acute or chronic disorders. If measured, the ionised calcium is normal. Even with very low serum proteins, the total calcium is unlikely to be below 1.8 mmol/l and it should never be confused with causes of severe symptomatic hypocalcaemia. The simultaneous measurement of calcium and albumin should always make this situation obvious.

Acute and chronic renal failure

Hypocalcaemia occurs in both acute and chronic renal failure. In acute renal failure, it is a consequence of the high serum phosphorus concentration, whereas in chronic renal failure there is the additional failure to produce 1,25-dihydroxyvitamin D in the kidneys. In both situations, secondary hyperparathyroidism develops. In chronic renal failure without effective treatment, the combination of a failure to produce 1,25-dihydroxyvitamin D and high PTH concentrations can lead to a severe bone disorder, with both osteomalacia and parathyroid bone disease – renal osteodystrophy.

Vitamin D deficiency

Vitamin D deficiency causes hypocalcaemia, which is usually fairly well compensated by the development of secondary hyperparathyroidism. As a consequence, the serum calcium is usually at the lower end of normal, or just below normal. Serum phosphorus is usually low and the alkaline phosphatase increased. Occasionally, the serum calcium is very low. Subclinical vitamin D deficiency is very common in Asians in Britain for reasons that are not entirely clear. Although most Asians are asymptomatic, clinical disease can develop at times of increased vitamin D requirements, e.g. neonates, growing children, during the teenage growth spurt and pregnancy. In adults, multiple, chronic bone pain is common, together with a difficulty walking or climbing stairs, or getting out a bath or a low chair.

Vitamin D deficiency can also occasionally complicate small intestinal disease or cholestatic liver disease.

Diagnosis

Clinical suspicion is essential as the condition is easily missed. Biochemical changes are often very mild. X-ray changes, if present, can be very helpful. In children, changes are present in the metaphysis – e.g. the knee or wrist – whereas in adults, Looser's zones around the femoral neck or in the pubic rami are most likely.

The finding of an elevated PTH is a useful confirmatory finding but measuring vitamin D concentrations are unhelpful. The PTH is useful in monitoring vitamin D replacement in osteomalacia.

Treatment

Treatment should be with low doses of calciferol, 500–1000 units/day for a period of at least 3 months (Box 17.5). In simple vitamin D deficiency, there is no need to use the active vitamin D metabolites.

Box 17.5   Vitamin D deficiency – rickets and osteomalacia

- Commonest in Asians; rare in white or black people
- Vague symptoms and often only slight biochemical changes
- Therapeutic trail of low-dose vitamin D therapy is worth considering

---

Vitamin D-dependent rickets

This is a rare inherited disorder due to an inherited defect of the renal 1α-hydroxylase enzyme. The biochemical and radiological changes are identical to those seen in simple vitamin D deficiency, but healing of the disease requires 10–50,000 units of vitamin D/day, or the use of an active metabolite.

Vitamin D-resistant or hypophosphataemic rickets

This is the commonest cause of rickets or osteomalacia in white subjects, but is uncommon. The hallmark is a very low serum phosphorus and a *normal* serum calcium, without evidence of secondary hyperparathyroidism. This is a disorder of phosphorus transport rather than vitamin D metabolism.

Treatment is with phosphate supplements and vitamin D (to correct the secondary hyperparathyroidism induced by the phosphate therapy).

An identical clinical picture can be associated with slow-growing tumours, often of the skin or subcutaneous tissues – oncogenic rickets. This should be suspected in all cases of apparent adult-onset hypophosphataemic rickets.

Hypoparathyroidism

Hypoparathyroidism most commonly occurs as a result of surgical operations on the neck – thyroidectomy, parathyroidectomy or laryngopharyngectomy. It may occasionally be transient for several weeks after surgery, but usually is permanent. Much more rarely, the condition will occur spontaneously, with one form being associated with other autoimmune conditions and moniliasis.

Biochemically, hypoparathyroidism is associated with hypocalcaemia, hyperphosphataemia, a normal serum alkaline phosphatase and a low serum PTH.

Treatment

Acute symptoms require intravenous calcium for initial control. Long-term treatment is with a potent vitamin D metabolite – 1 µg of One-Alpha or 1,25-dihydroxyvitamin D. Routine oral calcium supplements are rarely necessary. Regular checks of the serum calcium are required with the aim of keeping the serum calcium around the lower end of the normal range.

Pseudohypoparathyroidism

This is a very rare condition whereby there is a peripheral resistance to the actions of PTH due to a defective G-protein component of the adenylate cyclase unit in the kidney and bone. The biochemical changes are identical to hypoparathyroidism but serum PTH is elevated. Some forms of the condition are associated with typical phenotype features such as short stature, moon face and shortened metacarpals and metatarsals.

Autosomal dominant hypocalcaemia

This condition is due to an abnormality of the calcium-sensing receptor, whereby hypocalcaemia occurs typically with a normal serum PTH concentration. It is, therefore, the mirror opposite to FBH (see above). Some patients have, in fact, a low PTH, thus appearing identical to hypoparathyroidism. Many of the reported cases following long-term vitamin D therapy have developed renal failure and/or nephrocalcinosis, thought to be secondary to treatment. As most cases are asymptomatic, treatment should be aimed at producing serum calcium values that approach the lower end of normal and without increasing the urinary calcium excretion to abnormal values.

Hypocalcaemia due to hypomagnesaemia

Severe hypomagnesaemia causes profound hypocalcaemia which is resistant to treatment with vitamin D metabolites. Correction of the hypomagnesaemia completely rectifies the biochemical changes. Hypomagnesaemia, when severe, prevents PTH release and hence the hypocalcaemia.

Such severe degrees of hypomagnesaemia can occur frequently following prolonged treatment with certain drugs such as aminoglycosides and cisplatin. It may also complicate major small bowel resection or disease and chronic alcoholism.

Further Reading

Silverberg SJ, Bilezikain JP. Evaluation and management of primary hyperparathyoidism. *J Clin Endocrinol Metab* 1996;**81**(6):2036–40.

Silverberg SJ, Bilezikian JP, Bone HG, Talpos GB, Horwitz MJ, Stewart AF. Therapeutic controversies in primary hyperparathyroidism. *J Clin Endocrinol Metab* 1999;**84**(7):2275–85.

Vestergaard P, Mollerup CL, Frokjaer VG, Christiansen P, Blichert-Toft M, Mosekilde L. Cohort study of risk of fracture before and after surgery for primary hyperparathyroidism. *BMJ* 2000;**321**:598–602.

18

Sodium and Water

Stephen G Ball

Introduction

Sodium is the major circulating cation, and the maintenance of plasma sodium concentration within the range of 135–144 mmol/l is critical to the maintenance of electrolyte and body fluid homeostasis. This chapter describes the physiology and pathophysiology of this process, concentrating on the role of the hypothalamic peptide vasopressin: its molecular/cell biology; physiology; and the clinical problems associated with defects in its production and action.

The Cell Biology and Physiology of Sodium and Water Balance

Molecular cell biology of vasopressin

Vasopressin (VP) is a basic nonapeptide, with a disulphide bridge between the cysteine residues at positions 1 and 6 (Figure 18.1). Most mammals have the amino acid arginine at position 8. In the pig family, arginine is substituted by lysine. Nonmammalian species have a variety of peptides very similar to VP, probably reflecting derivation from a common ancestral gene.

The vasopressin–neurophysin gene

The *VP* gene lies in tandem array with that for oxytocin on chromosome 20, separated by 8 kb DNA in man. The *VP* gene is composed of 3 exons, and encodes a polypeptide precursor with a

Amino acid position

	1	2	3	4	5	6	7	8	9	Distribution
Arginine vasopressin:	Cys-Tyr-Phe-Glu(NH$_2$)-Asp(NH$_2$)-Cys-Pro-Arg-Gly(NH$_2$)									Most mammals
Lysine vasopressin:								Lys		Pig family

Figure 18.1　Amino acid sequence of vasopressin gene.

modular structure: an amino-terminal signal peptide; the VP peptide; a mid-molecule peptide termed a neurophysin (Np); and a carboxyl-terminal peptide (Figure 18.2).

Hypothalamic-specific expression of the *VP* gene is conferred through selective repressor elements within the structural gene and its 5' flanking sequence. Control of *VP* gene expression is mediated through positive and negative regulatory elements in the proximal promoter. Several transcription factors bind to these elements: AP1, AP2 and CREB stimulate expression, whereas the glucocorticoid receptor (GR) negatively regulates expression.

Synthesis, release and metabolism of vasopressin

Synthesis of the VP precursor occurs in the cell bodies of specific magnocellular neurosecretory neurones within the supraoptic (SON) and paraventricular (PVN) nuclei of the hypothalamus. Generation of the mature hormone entails post-translational modification of the large primary precursor. Following translation, the carboxyl-terminal domain of the precursor is glycosylated, and the product packaged in vesicles of the regulated secretory pathway. These migrate along the axons of the magnocellular neurones, during which the VP precursor is cleaved by basic endopeptidases. The final products of processing, the mature hormone and the associated Np, are stored as a complex in secretory granules in the terminals of the magnocellular neurones, within the posterior pituitary. Increased firing frequency of vasopressinergic neurones opens voltage-gated Ca^{2+} channels in these nerve terminals which, through transient Ca^{2+} influx, results in fusion of the neurosecretory granules with the nerve terminal membrane and release of VP and its Np into the systemic circulation in equimolar quantities. Apart from acting as carrier proteins for VP during axonal migration, Nps appears to serve no specific biological function.

The circulating half-life of VP is 5 to 15 min. It circulates unbound to plasma proteins. However, VP does bind to specific receptors on platelets; VP concentrations in platelet-rich plasma are five-fold higher than in platelet-depleted plasma. Several endothelial and circulating endo- and aminopeptidases degrade VP. A specific placental cysteine aminopeptidase degrades VP rapidly during pregnancy and the immediate postpartum period.

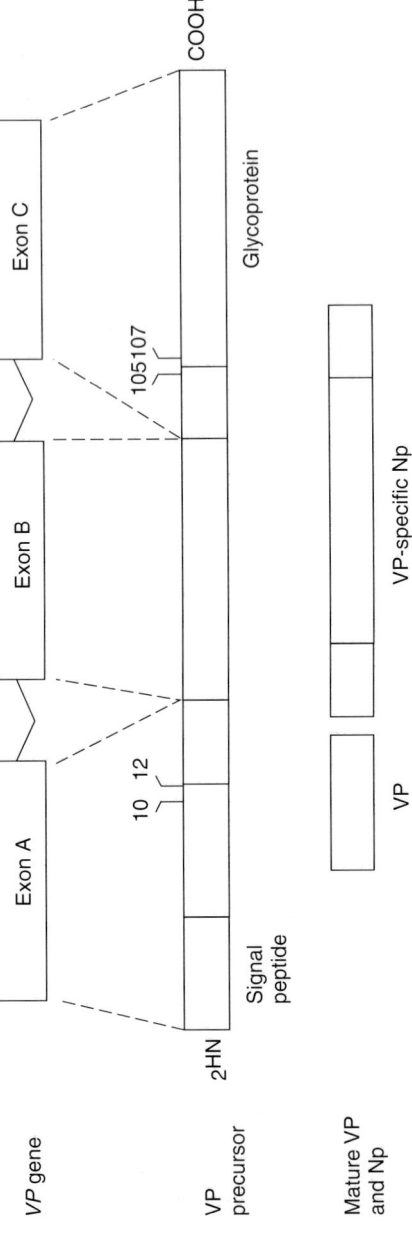

Figure 18.2 Structural organisation of the vasopressin (*VP*) gene, and processing of its product. Numbers annotating the VP precursor correspond to amino acid positions. Np: neurophysin.

The physiology of vasopressin

Actions of vasopressin in sodium and water balance

Vasopressin receptors.   There are three VP receptor (V-R) sub-types, encoded by different genes (Table 18.1). All have seven transmembrane spanning domains, and all are G-protein coupled. They differ in tissue distribution, signal transduction mechanisms and function. The V2 receptor is found in the distal nephron. The human *V2-R* gene has been mapped to Xq28. In contrast to many other hormone receptors, the V2-R is upregulated by its ligand.

Effects of VP on renal water excretion.   Although VP has multiple actions, its principal physiological effect is in the regulation of water resorption in the distal nephron.

The hairpin structure and electrolyte transport processes of the nephron allow the kidney to both concentrate and dilute urine in response to the prevailing circulating VP concentration. Active transport of solute out of the thick ascending loop of Henle generates an osmolar gradient in the renal interstitium, which increases from renal cortex to inner medulla, a gradient through which distal parts of the nephron pass en route to the collecting system. The presence of selective water channel proteins (aquaporins) in the wall of the distal nephron allows resorption of water from the duct lumen along an osmotic gradient, and excretion of concentrated urine.

Ten different human aquaporins (AQPs) have been identified to date. AQP1 is present in the apical and basolateral membranes of the proximal tubule and descending loop of Henle. Loss of function mutations in the *AQP1* gene result in no clinical disturbances in water conservation. However, AQP1 may serve a crucial role in situations in which the renal counter-current exchange system is impaired. AQP3 and AQP4 are constitutively expressed on the basolateral membrane of collecting duct cells. They facilitate the movement of water from collecting duct cells into the interstitium. VP modulates expression of AQP3, but not AQP4. The AQP3 and AQP4-null mice are clinically normal. AQP2 is expressed on the luminal surface of collecting duct cells, and is responsible for water transport from the lumen of the nephron into collecting duct cells. Expression of AQP2, which functions as a homotetramer, is VP-dependent; VP produces a biphasic increase in expression of the protein. Generation of intracellular cyclic adenosine monophosphate (cAMP) by ligand activation of the V2-R stimulates *AQP2*

Table 18.1 Vasopressin receptor subtypes

Parameter	Vasopressin receptor		
	V1	V2	V3
Expression	Vascular smooth muscle: liver platelets CNS	Basolateral membrane of distal nephron	Pituitary corticotroph
Molecular features	418 amino acids (human)	370 amino acids (human)	424 amino acids (human)
Second messenger system	Gq/11 mediated phospholipase C activation: Ca^{2+}, inositol triphosphate and diacyl glycerol mobilisation	Gαs mediated adenylate cyclase activation, cAMP production and protein kinase A stimulation	As V1
Physiological effects	Smooth muscle contraction Stimulation of glycogenolysis Enhanced platelet adhesion Neurotransmitter and neuromodulatory function	Increased production and action of aquaporin-2	Enhanced ACTH release

ACTH = adrenocorticotrophic hormone, cAMP = cyclic adenosine monophosphate.

gene expression through CRE and AP-1 elements in the *AQP2* promoter. In addition, VP accelerates trafficking of presynthesised protein from intracellular vesicles, and the assembly of functional water channels in luminal cell membranes.

VP has additional effects at other parts of the nephron; it decreases medullary blood flow and stimulates an active urea transporter in the distal collecting duct. VP can also stimulate active sodium transport into the renal interstitium. These effects contribute to the generation and maintenance of a hypertonic medullary interstitium and augment the action of VP on water channels of the distal nephron.

Regulation of vasopressin release

Neurophysiology of VP release. Vasopressin is produced and regulated by the neurohypophysis, a portion of the lower central nervous system (CNS) consisting of three parts:

- the SON and PVN of the hypothalamus, containing the cell bodies of the magnocellular neurosecretory neurones that synthesise and secrete VP and oxytocin
- the supraoptico-hypophyseal tract, which includes the axons of these neurones, projecting to the posterior pituitary
- the posterior pituitary, where the axons terminate on capillaries of the inferior hypophyseal artery.

In man, vasopressinergic neurones are found in the ventral SON, and centrally within the PVN. The PVN contains additional, smaller parvicellular vasopressinergic neurones which cosecrete corticotrophin-releasing hormone (CRH), and have a role in the regulation of adrenocorticotrophic hormone (ACTH) release.

VP release is modulated by sensory signals that chiefly reflect osmotic status and blood pressure/circulating volume. The relationships of the SON and PVN with the autonomic afferents and CNS nucleii responsible for osmo- and baroregulation are thus key to the physiological regulation of VP.

Functional osmoreceptors are situated in anterior circumventricular structures: the subfornicular organ (SFO) and the organum vasculosum of the lamina terminalis (OVLT). Local fenestrations in the blood–brain barrier allow this neural tissue direct contact with the circulation. VP neurones themselves may have additional, independent osmoreceptor properties. Interestingly, VP receptors are present on vasopressinergic neurones of both the PVN and SON, highlighting the potential for autocontrol of VP release through the action of magnocellular neurites. Thirst appreciation is dependent upon osmosensitive hypothalamic nuclei, possibly the AV3V region, anatomically distinct from those regulating VP release.

Baroregulatory influences on VP release derive from aortic arch, carotid sinus, cardiac atrial and great vein afferents via cranial nerves IX and X projecting to the nucleus tractus solitarius (NTS) in the brainstem, from where further afferents project to the SON and PVN. The SON and PVN receive additional adrenergic afferents from other brainstem nucleii, such as the locus caeruleus.

Osmoregulation of VP Plasma osmolality is the most important determinant of VP secretion. The osmoregulatory system for thirst and VP secretion maintains plasma osmolality within narrow limits: 284–295 mOsm/kg. The relationship between plasma osmolality and plasma VP concentration is described by three characteristics:

- the shape of the line describing changes in plasma VP concentration with changing plasma osmolality
- the osmotic threshold or 'set point' for VP release
- the sensitivity of the osmoregulatory mechanism.

Increases in plasma osmolality increase plasma VP concentrations in a linear manner (Figure 18.3). The abscissal intercept of this line indicates the mean 'osmotic threshold' for VP release (284 mOsm/kg): the mean plasma osmolality above which plasma VP starts to increase. Though there is no level of plasma osmolality below which VP release is completely suppressed, this concept remains a pragmatic means of characterising the physiology of osmoregulation. The slope of the line reflects the sensitivity of osmoregulated VP release: increasing from a basal rate through activation of stimulatory osmoreceptor afferents and decreasing to minimal values when this drive is removed and synergistic inhibitory afferents are activated. Although there are considerable inter-individual variations in both threshold and sensitivity of VP release, these parameters are remarkably reproducible within an individual over time.

There are several physiological situations where the relationship between plasma osmolality and VP concentration is lost:

- rate of change of plasma osmolality – rapid increases in plasma osmolality result in exaggerated VP release

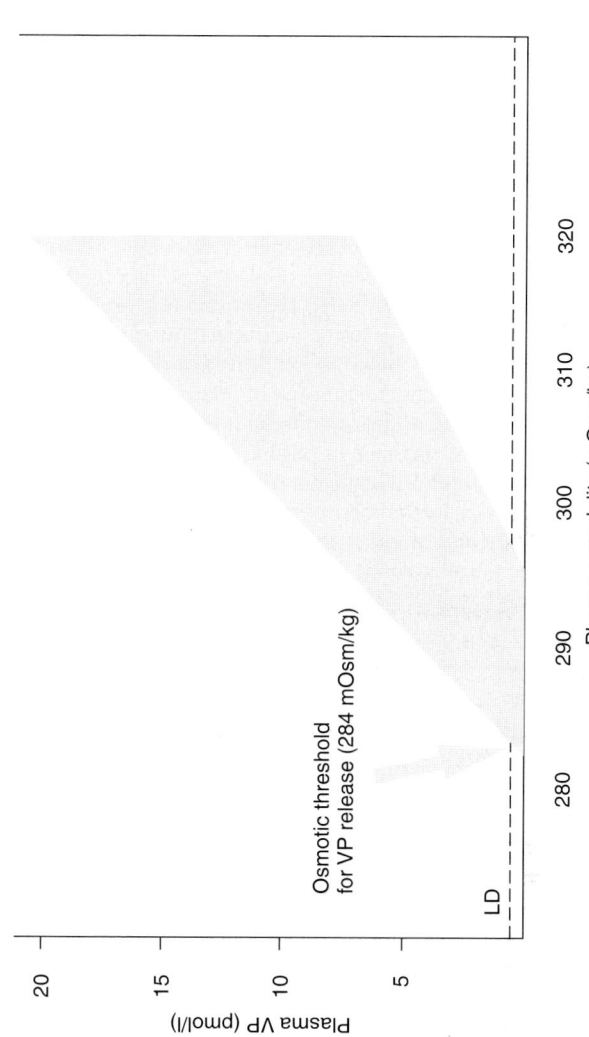

Figure 18.3 Relationship between plasma osmolality and plasma VP concentration. VP concentration determined during progressive hypertonicity induced by infusion of 855 mmol/l saline in a group of healthy adults. LD represents the limit of detection of the assay, 0.3 pmol/l. The relationship between thirst (measured on a visual analogue scale) and plasma osmolality is almost identical.

- drinking – rapid suppression of VP release through afferent pathways originating in the oropharynx
- pregnancy – the osmotic threshold for VP release is lowered.

In addition, plasma VP concentrations increase with age, together with enhanced VP responses to osmotic stimulation. At the same time, thirst appreciation is blunted and fluid intake reduced. These changes, together with age-related decreases in renal handling of water loads and generation of maximal urine concentration, predispose the elderly to both hyper- and hyponatraemia.

Baroregulation of VP. Significant reduction in circulating volume stimulates VP release through the activation of mechanoreceptors in the cardiac atria and central veins. Hypotension stimulates VP release through the activation of aortic arch and carotid sinus afferents. Falls in arterial blood pressure of 5–10% are necessary to increase circulating VP concentrations in man. In contrast to osmoregulated VP release, progressive reduction in blood pressure produces an exponential increase in plasma VP. Baroregulated VP responses can be modified by other neurohumoral influences triggered as part of the coordinated neurohumoral response to changes in circulating volume and blood pressure: ANP inhibits and norepinephrine augment baroregulated VP release.

Other regulatory mechanisms. Nausea and emesis are potent stimuli to VP release, independent of osmotic and haemodynamic status. Manipulation of abdominal contents is another powerful stimulus to VP release. Both may contribute to high plasma VP values observed after surgery and may contribute to apparent or real postoperative SIADH (syndrome of inappropriate antidiuretic hormone).

Thirst

Thirst, and the ensuing drinking response, are key to maintaining sodium and water balance. The basis of thirst and the regulation of water ingestion involve complex, integrated neural and neurohumoral pathways. Animal data place the osmoreceptors regulating thirst in the circumventricular AV3V region of the hypothalamus, anatomically distinct from those mediating VP release. Projections to higher centres remain largely unmapped.

There is a linear relationship between thirst and plasma osmolalities in the physiological range. The mean osmotic threshold for thirst perception is 281 mOsm/kg, similar to that for VP release.

Thirst occurs when plasma osmolality rises above this threshold. As with osmoregulated VP release, the characteristics of osmoregulated thirst remain consistent within an individual on repeated testing, despite wide inter-individual variation.

As with VP release, there are specific physiological situations in which the relationship between plasma osmolality and thirst breaks down. The act of drinking reduces osmotically stimulated thirst, just as it does VP release, whereas both thirst appreciation and fluid intake are blunted in the elderly. Thirst can also be stimulated by extracellular volume depletion, both through volume-sensitive cardiac afferents and the generation of circulating and intracerebral angiotensin II, a powerful dipsogen.

Integrated physiology of vasopressin and fluid homeostasis

The physiological regulation of water balance is intimately linked with that of circulating volume; common systems are involved in both processes. As sodium is the major cationic osmolyte, the inter-relationships of sodium and water excretion with circulating volume regulation are key to appreciating the position of VP in the physiology of fluid homeostasis.

At plasma osmolalities of 285–295 mOsm/kg, osmolar balance can be maintained by VP-dependent regulation of renal water loss: a rise in plasma osmolality within this range produces a progressive increase in plasma VP and antidiuresis. Although further increases in plasma osmolality stimulate further VP release, this does not result in further reduction of renal water excretion: correction of plasma osmolality back to the range over which VP can maintain osmolar balance requires thirst-stimulated drinking. As the osmolar threshold for thirst is similar to that for VP release, the maintenance of water balance through a combination of VP release and thirst is a seamless, coordinated process.

If excessive fluid volumes are consumed, greater than those demanded by thirst, plasma VP levels are suppressed to < 0.3 pmol/l, resulting in maximum diuresis. Ingestion of water in excess of this causes a reduction of plasma osmolality into the sub-normal range, and hyponatraemia.

VP release is also regulated by other, nonosmotic stimuli. This multicomponent regulation has a hierarchy, with significant physiological and pathophysiological sequelae. Moderate hypo-volaemia shifts the relationship of plasma osmolality and plasma VP concentration to the left, osmoregulation being maintained around a lower osmolar set point. As the degree of hypovolaemia progresses, baroregulated VP release overrides the osmolar set point, and antidiuresis is maintained despite potential hyponatraemia. Coincident activation of the systemic and intracerebral renin–angiotensin systems stimulates drinking and augments VP release, in addition to independent pressor and antinatriuretic effects. The homeostatic response to hypovolaemia thus involves an integrated neurohumoral cascade, of which VP is a key component.

Clinical Problems in Sodium and Water Balance

The pathophysiology of sodium and water balance reflects the importance of maintaining plasma sodium concentration and osmolality within the physiological range, and the key role of the VP and thirst axes in this process. Some clinical problems involve defects in either VP production or action. A further group of conditions reflects primary defects in thirst. In some cases, the two may coincide, reflecting the close anatomical and functional relationship of both processes. However, not all clinical problems in sodium and water balance reflect primary abnormalities in this axis.

Diabetes insipidus

Classification

Diabetes insipidus (DI) is characterised by production of dilute urine in excess of 3 l/24 hours (> 40 ml/kg/24 hours in adults, > 100 ml/kg/24 hours in infants). One of following three mechanisms is responsible (Table 18.2):

- deficiency of VP – hypothalamic diabetes insipidus (HDI)
- renal resistance to the antidiuretic action of VP – nephrogenic diabetes insipidus (NDI)
- inappropriate, excessive water drinking – dipsogenic diabetes insipidus (DDI) or primary polydipsia.

Hypothalamic diabetes insipidus

HDI (also known as neurogenic, central or cranial DI) is the result of deficient osmoregulated VP secretion. Plasma VP concentrations

Table 18.2   Classification of diabetes insipidus

Hypothalamic diabetes insipidus

Primary	Genetic	*DIDMOAD (Wolfram) syndrome*
		Autosomal dominant
		Autosomal recessive
	Developmental syndromes	*Septo-optic dysplasia*
		Laurence–Moon–Biedl syndrome
	Idiopathic	
Secondary/ acquired	Trauma	*Head injury*
		Post-surgery
		(transcranial, transsphenoidal)
	Tumour	*Craniopharyngioma, pinealoma, germinoma, metastases, pituitary macroadenoma*
	Inflammatory	*Granulomata*
		sarcoidosis, histiocytosis
		Infection
		meningitis, encephalitis
		Infundibulo-neurohypophysitis
		Guillain–Barré syndrome
		Autoimmune
		(anti-VP neurone antibodies)
	Vascular	*Aneurysm*
		Infarction
		Sheehan's syndrome
		sickle cell disease
	Pregnancy (associated with vasopressinase)	

Nephrogenic diabetes insipidus

Primary	Genetic	*X-linked recessive (V2-R defect)*
		Autosomal recessive (AQP2 defect)
		Autosomal dominant (AQP2 defect)
	Idiopathic	
Secondary	Chronic renal disease	*Polycystic kidneys*
		Obstructive uropathy
	Metabolic disease	*Hypercalcaemia*
		Hypokalaemia
	Drug induced	*Lithium*
		Demeclocycline
	Osmotic diuretics	*Glucose*
		Mannitol
	Systemic disorders	*Amyloidosis*
		Myelomatosis
	Pregnancy	

(cont.)

Table 18.2 (*cont.*)

Dipsogenic diabetes insipidus	
Compulsive water drinking	
Associated with affective disorders	
Drug induced?	
Structural/organic	*Sarcoid*
hypothalamic disease	*Tumours involving hypothalamus*
	Head injury
	Tuberculous meningitis

are inappropriately low with respect to prevailing plasma osmolalities. Presentation with H DI implies destruction or loss of function of more than 80% of vasopressinergic magnocellular neurones. It is rare, with an estimated prevalence of 1:25,000, and equal gender distribution. Although persistent polyuria can lead to dehydration, given free access to water, most patients can maintain water balance through appropriate polydipsia.

Aetiology. Most cases of HDI are acquired. Trauma from head injury, or surgery, can produce HDI through damage to the hypothalamus, pituitary stalk or posterior pituitary. Pituitary stalk trauma may lead to a triphasic disturbance in water balance, an immediate polyuria characteristic of HDI followed within days by a more prolonged period of antidiuresis suggestive of VP excess. This second phase may last several weeks, and can be followed by reversion to HDI or recovery. Such a 'triple response' reflects initial axonal damage, the subsequent unregulated release of large amounts of presynthesised VP, and ultimately, either recovery or development of permanent HDI (determined by the magnitude of initial damage to vasopressinergic neurones). The polyuric phase is associated with the presence of circulating inhibitors of VP action, which may be partly processed VP precursors. Not all phases of the response may be apparent in any one individual.

Although hypothalamic tumours or pituitary metastases (e.g. breast or bronchus) can present with HDI, primary pituitary tumours rarely cause HDI. In childhood, hypothalamic tumours, such as craniopharygioma and germinoma/teratoma, are a relatively common cause. Together with developmental defects, such as septo-optic dysplasia (SOD), they account for up to 50% of cases. HDI can present in pregnancy: high placental vasopressinase activity decompensates previously limited antidiuretic capacity through increased VP degradation. Polyuria and polydipsia can revert to normal after delivery, although permanent HDI may develop if the natural history of the defect is progressive.

Familial forms account for 5% of HDI. Wolfram, or DIDMOAD syndrome (Diabetes Insipidus, Diabetes Mellitus, Optic Atrophy, and Deafness) is a rare, recessive multicomponent disorder. It has several phenotypic features in common with mitochondrial (*mt*) cytopathies. However, no specific *mt* gene mutation has been confirmed in this disorder, and linkage has been shown with autosomal markers. It is proposed currently that both *mt* and autosomal genes contribute to the pathogenesis.

Autosomal dominant familial HDI is caused by loss of function mutations in exons 1 and 2 of the VP gene. It typically presents in childhood, although the age of presentation varies considerably, reflecting variation in the progressive loss of VP secretion. Mutant VP precursors accumulate in the endoplasmic reticulum of vasopressinergic neurones, to which they are neurotoxic, which is the basis of both the progressive loss of VP release and the dominant inheritance.

Investigation. The aim of investigation is as follows:

- to confirm the polyuric state
- to define the basis of the polyuria
- to explore primary aetiologies.

After establishing significant polyuria, and excluding hyperglycaemia, hypokalaemia, hypercalcaemia and significant renal insufficiency, attention should be focused on the VP axis.

Although direct measurement of plasma VP in response to osmotic stimulation differentiates HDI from other causes of polyuria, access to reliable VP assays has been limited. Thus, a test using a surrogate endpoint of VP release has been developed, assessing the capacity to concentrate urine during the osmotic stress of controlled water deprivation. Renal sensitivity to exogenous VP can be determined as part of the test (see Protocols, Appendix 1). Diagnostic results are as follows:

- HDI – urine osmolality less than 300 mOsm/kg accompanied by plasma osmolality greater than 290 mOsm/kg after dehydration; urine osmolality should rise above 750 mOsm/kg after desmopressin (DDAVP). DDAVP (des amino D-arginine vasopressin) is V2-receptor specific.

- NDI – failure to increase urine osmolality above 300 mOsm/kg after dehydration, with no response to DDAVP
- DDI – appropriate urine concentration during dehydration, without significant rise in plasma osmolality.

In practice, the test is often indeterminate for the following reasons:

- incomplete defects
- mild forms of DI
- partial NDI secondary to dissipation of the intrarenal medullary concentration gradient due to prolonged polyuria (independent of aetiology).

An accurate diagnosis of HDI can be made by direct measurement of plasma VP during the controlled osmotic stress of a hypertonic 5% saline infusion. Patients with HDI have either undetectable VP levels, or values falling to the right of the nomogram relating plasma VP to plasma osmolality. In NDI, plasma VP is inappropriately high for the prevailing osmolality, consistent with VP resistance. In DDI, the relationship of plasma VP to plasma osmolality is normal. The test is not interpretable if it produces significant nausea, a powerful nonosmotic stimulus of VP release.

A pragmatic alternative to VP measurements during hypertonic stress, in situations where a water deprivation test has proved nondiagnostic, is a controlled therapeutic trial of DDAVP: 10–20 µg of intranasal DDAVP/day for 2–4 weeks, with monitoring of plasma sodium every 2–3 days. Patients with DDI exhibit progressive dilutional hyponatraemia, whereas those with NDI remain unaffected. Patients with HDI experience improvement in polyuria and polydipsia, but remain normonatraemic.

Imaging of the hypothalamus, pituitary and surrounding structures with magnetic resonance imaging (MRI) is essential in HDI, to exclude mass lesions. HDI is associated with the loss of the normal hyperintense signal of the posterior pituitary on T1-weighted images. Signal intensity is correlated strongly with VP content of the gland.

Treatment. The treatment of choice for those with significant symptoms is the synthetic, long-acting VP analogue DDAVP, given as an intranasal spray (5–100 µg daily), parenterally (0.1–2.0 µg daily) or orally (100–1000 µg daily) in divided doses. There is wide individual variation in the dose required to control symptoms. Dilutional hyponatraemia is the most serious potential adverse effect. This can be avoided by omitting treatment on a regular basis (perhaps weekly), to allow a short period of breakthrough polyuria and thirst. Doses may need to be increased in pregnancy; this may be due to placental vasopressinase.

Nephrogenic diabetes insipidus

NDI is the result of renal resistance to the antidiuretic effects of VP. Primary familial forms are rare. X-linked recessive familial NDI is caused by inherited loss of function mutations of the V2-R. Over 70 different mutations have been described, affecting all aspects of receptor function: expression; ligand-binding; and G-protein coupling. Most lead to complete loss of function; a few are associated with a mild phenotype.

Of kindreds with familial NDI, 10% have an autosomal recessive form, with normal V2-R function. Affected individuals harbour loss of function mutations of the AQP2 gene. Most mutations occur in the region coding for the transmembrane domain of the protein. An additional kindred has been described in which there is a mutation of the carboxy-terminal intracellular tail of AQP2. The NDI of this kindred is inherited as an autosomal dominant trait, mutant protein sequestering the product of the wild type AQP2 allele as mixed tetramers, in a dominant-negative manner.

More commonly, NDI is due to a variety of acquired metabolic or drug effects. The final common pathway producing NDI in many of these is downregulation of AQP2 expression. NDI secondary to lithium toxicity can persist after drug withdrawal, and can be irreversible.

Secondary/acquired cases of NDI are managed by removing the underlying cause, and ensuring adequate hydration. Additional measures for persistent, severe symptoms rarely reduce urine volumes by more than 50%, although this may still be worthwhile. High-dose DDAVP (4 mg intramuscularly, twice a day) may produce a response in partial NDI, especially if the lesion is acquired. Additional treatment options, either alone or in combination, include the following:

- thiazide diuretics – hydrochlorothiazide (25 mg/24 hours)
- nonsteroidal anti-inflammatory drugs (NSAIDs) – ibuprofen (200 mg/24 hours)
- low salt diets.

All probably work through reducing glomerular filtration rate, and interfering with the diluting capacity of the distal nephron.

Dipsogenic diabetes insipidus

DDI is a polyuric syndrome secondary to excess fluid intake. Although structural abnormalities may be the cause, it is generally a manifestation of primary hyperdipsia, psychiatric disease or secondary to drug effects. It is associated with abnormalities of thirst perception:

- a low osmotic threshold for thirst
- exaggerated thirst responses to osmotic challenge
- inability to suppress thirst at low osmolalities.

The structural and/or functional bases for any of these abnormalities have not been identified. The association of DDI with affective disorders is well recognised. Up to 20% of patients with chronic schizophrenia have polydipsia. Although abnormal drinking may reflect the primary thought disorder, abnormalities in osmoregulated VP release and thirst have been described. Whether these reflect long-term effects of drug therapy, or primary defects in central processing, are unclear.

The treatment of DDI should address the underlying disorder. This can be difficult. Clozapine may reduce polydipsia in those patients with refractory schizophrenia and a history of hyponatraemia on dopamine antagonists. Whether this is an effect on central thirst mechanisms, or disordered thought, remains to be clarified. Individuals with persistent DDI are at risk of hyponatraemia if treated with DDAVP. Reduced fluid intake is the only rational treatment.

Hyponatraemia

Pathophysiology

Hyponatraemia, defined as a plasma sodium concentration less than 130 mmol/l, is a common source of morbidity in clinical practice, occurring in about 15% of hospitalised patients. Hyponatraemia is not invariably associated with a low serum osmolality; high concentrations of other circulating osmolytes (e.g. glucose), or a reduced plasma aqueous phase secondary to dyslipidaemia can result in hyponatraemia but normal plasma osmolality.

True hyponatraemia can occur through one of three mechanisms:

- reduction of renal free water clearance – increased total body water

- excessive water intake in excess of total body water loss – increased total body water
- sodium depletion – increased renal sodium loss in excess of free water loss.

An appreciation of the inter-relationships of sodium, water and volume regulation is key to understanding the basis of hyponatraemia.

The pathophysiological, pharmacological and clinical context is critical to understanding the often multiple mechanisms involved and, in turn, the development of a rational approach to intervention and prevention (Table 18.3).

Hypovolaemia

Even when hyponatraemia is a true indicator of hypo-osmolality, it may reflect an appropriate physiological response. To maintain circulating volume in hypovolaemia, baroregulated VP release proceeds despite plasma osmolalities well below the osmotic threshold for VP release. This can result in hyponatraemia, which can become chronic. Clinical assessment identifies the extracellular volume status of most patients. However, problems can arise in distinguishing mild forms of hypovolaemia. This is important for planning intervention. Hyponatraemia due to the uncommon central salt wasting is important to differentiate from that of VP excess. They can both occur following brain injury from trauma or neurosurgery, but central salt wasting is a hypovolaemic condition requiring fluid resuscitation rather than restriction. Careful clinical assessment, calculation of urine sodium excretion and adjunctive invasive monitoring may be required.

Syndrome of inappropriate antidiuretic hormone (SIADH)

Pathophysiology. An individual with hypo-osmolar plasma but a normal circulating volume, in whom the plasma VP concentration is high for the prevailing osmolality, has SIADH due to VP excess. A variety of conditions are associated with SIADH. Four patterns of abnormal VP secretion have been identified. Absolute plasma VP concentrations may not be strikingly high; the key finding is that that they are inappropriate for the prevailing plasma osmolality. When this obligate antidiuresis is not accompanied by decreased water intake, haemodilution is inevitable.

Table 18.3 Causes of hyponatraemia

Pseudohyponatraemia		
Hyperglycaemia		
Hyperlipidaemia		
Nonphysiological osmolyte		
Sodium depletion		
Renal loss	*Diuretics*	
	Salt wasting nephropathy	
	Hypoadrenalism	
Extra-renal loss	Gut loss	
	Central salt wasting	
Excess water intake		
Dipsogenic DI		
Sodium-free, hyposomolar irrigant solutions		
Dilute infant feeding formula		
Reduced renal free water clearance		
Hypovolaemia	*Drugs*	
	Renal failure	
	Portal hypertension and ascites	
	Hypoalbuminaemia	
		Sepsis and vascular leak syndromes
		Central salt wasting
		Fluid sequestration
Cardiac failure		
Nephrotic syndrome		
Hypothyroidism		
Hypoadrenalism		
SIADH		

Aetiology. Many conditions have been reported to cause SIADH (Table 18.4). SIADH is a nonmetastatic manifestation of small-cell lung cancer and other malignancies. Some tumours express VP ectopically. However, excessive posterior pituitary VP secretion also occurs in association with malignancy. The mechanism(s) of apparent inappropriate VP release in many cases of SIADH are not clear. The normal osmoregulated VP release found in the type D syndrome suggests an increase in renal sensitivity to VP, or the action of an additional antidiuretic factor.

Clinical features. The major features in the diagnosis of SIADH are given in Box 18.1. The most frequent difficulty in practice is in distinguishing SIADH from chronic, mild hypovolaemia. In both

Table 18.4   Causes of SIADH (syndrome of inappropriate diuretic hormone)

Neoplastic disease	Chest disorders
Carcinoma (bronchus, duodenum, pancreas, bladder, ureter, prostate)	*Pneumonia*
Thymoma	*Tuberculosis*
Mesothelioma	*Empyema*
Lymphoma, leukaemia	*Cystic fibrosis*
Ewing's sarcoma	*Pneumothorax*
Carcinoid	*Aspergillosis*
Bronchial adenoma	
	Drugs
	Sulphonylreas
Neurological disorders	*Opiates*
Head injury, neurosurgery	*Alkylating agents and Vinca*
Brain abscess or tumour	*alkaloids*
Meningitis, encephalitis	*Thiazides and loop diuretics*
Guillain–Barré syndrome	*Dopamine antagonists*
Cerebral haemorrhage	*Tricyclic antidepressants*
Cavernous sinus thrombosis	*MAOIs*
Hydrocephalus	*SSRIs*
Cerebellar and cerebral atrophy	*3,4-MDMA ('Ecstasy')*
Shy–Drager syndrome	*Anticonvulsants*
Peripheral neuropathy	*DDAVP, oxytocin*
Seizures	
Subdural haematoma	**Miscellaneous**
Alcohol withdrawal	*Idiopathic*
	Psychosis
	Porphyria
	Abdominal surgery

> **Box 18.1   Diagnosis of SIADH (syndrome of inappropriate diuretic hormone)**
>
> Hyponatraemia with appropriately low plasma osmolality
> Urine osmolality greater than plasma osmolality
> Renal sodium excretion > 20 mmol/l
> Absence of hypotension, hypovolaemia and oedema-forming states
> Normal renal and adrenal function

groups, urine osmolality tends to be higher than plasma osmolality, and plasma VP concentrations will be detectable or elevated. Neither is therefore diagnostic of SIADH. Measurement of urinary sodium concentration is helpful.

Drug-induced hyponatraemia

Drugs induce hyponatraemia through reducing free water clearance and/or through sodium/volume depletion. In addition, intravenous fluid therapy, a common source of iatrogenic hyponatraemia, can result in hyponatraemia when the administered water load exceeds renal and insensible water losses.

Drug-induced reduction in free water clearance. There are three mechanisms of drug-induced reduction in free water clearance:

- drug-induced SIADH
- drug-associated VP-like activity
- potentiation of endogenous VP action.

SIADH is a common mechanism of drug-induced hyponatraemia, and can reflect direct stimulation of VP release from the hypothalamus, indirect action on the hypothalamus or aberrant resetting of the hypothalamic osmostat. The prevalence of hyponatraemia in patients taking high-dose dopamine antagonists is greater than 25%. It is not restricted to one class of these agents, and has been reported with newer antipsychotic compounds such as risperidone. The role of abnormal thirst in this phenomenon remains to be defined. Hyponatraemia secondary to antidepressants is well recognised, occurring with most SSRIs (selective serotonin reuptake inhibitors), and the related drug venlafaxine. It can arise in the first few weeks of treatment, and those patients on concurrent diuretic therapy are particularly at risk.

Anticonvulsants are a common cause of hyponatraemia, the frequency in patients treated with carbamazepine (CBZ) ranging from 4.8 to 40%. CBZ-induced sensitisation of both central osmoreceptors and renal responses to VP has been described.

Treatment with VP analogues is a recognised cause of iatrogenic hyponatraemia. Hyponatraemia has been reported in patients treated with VP analogues for nocturnal enuresis. Excess fluid intake is a contributing factor in over 50% of cases. It has also been reported in patients treated with long-acting analogues for the management of gastrointestinal haemorrhage, where both hypovolaemia and intravenous fluid resuscitation are likely to be contributory. Oxytocin is structurally similar to VP and has antidiuretic effects at high doses. Oxytotic drugs are used to augment uterine contraction, often coupled with intravenous fluid replacement therapy. The combination of obligate antidiuresis and obligate fluid load can produce hyponatraemia in both mother and neonate.

Nonsteroidal anti-inflammatory drugs potentiate the action of VP indirectly, by inhibiting the synthesis of intrarenal prostaglandins that functionally antagonise the effects of VP. Hyponatraemia due to NSAIDs is rare without concurrent diuretic use or volume depletion. VP-independent aquaporin expression may constitute one of the mechanisms by which both CBZ and sulphonylureas induce hyponatraemia, although both also have central effects. As with other drugs, concurrent diuretic use is an additional risk factor.

Sodium depletion: increased renal sodium loss in excess of free water loss. Because of the intimate relationship between plasma volume and sodium concentration, pharmacological targeting of the processes regulating plasma volume can have profound effects on plasma sodium levels. As such processes are a key target in the treatment of congestive cardiac failure (CCF), a common condition, this problem is a predictable consequence of treatment with some of the most commonly prescribed agents in clinical use. Disruption of renal solute and water handling can also occur as a consequence of drug toxicity. Such responses are less predictable.

Diuretics block the resorption of filtered sodium by the nephron. They all increase renal sodium loss, and thus predispose to hyponatraemia. However, they differ in this predisposition, reflecting differences in their site of action.

Renal sodium loss sufficient to produce volume depletion is a stimulus for nonosmotic VP release. In the presence of an intact counter-current concentrating system, this leads to increased distal nephron water resorption, exacerbating hyponatraemia. Thiazide diuretics block the electro-neutral sodium–chloride transporter in the distal tubule, but do not interfere with the formation of the medullary counter-current osmolar gradient; thus, these agents produce sodium loss without impairing renal concentrating ability, and can produce profound hyponatraemia. Spironolactone inhibits aldosterone-dependent synthesis of the distal tubular sodium–potassium–hydrogen ion exchange transporter. Its effects on renal sodium and water loss are similar to thiazides, as are those of the other diuretics targeting transport processes in the distal nephron. In contrast, loop diuretics block the sodium–potassium–chloride transporter in the thick ascending limb of the loop of Henle, interfering with the generation of the medullary osmolar gradient. This limits the hyponatraemia associated with these agents, despite significant volume contraction and nonosmotic VP release, as it limits the concentrating ability of the distal nephron.

Some drugs cause renal salt wasting, volume depletion and hyponatraemia by direct nephrotoxicity. Increased fluid intake may have a role in the hyponatraemia associated with cytotoxic therapy; high fluid loads are often prescribed with these drugs, to avoid toxicity. Nausea is a powerful nonosmotic stimulus for VP release, and its role in the hyponatraemia associated with cytotoxics remains unclear.

Management of hyponatraemia

The morbidity and mortality of hyponatraemia are predominantly related to CNS dysfunction (Box 18.2). Values of serum sodium around 100 mmol/l are life-threatening. However, patients can remain asymptomatic, especially if hyponatraemia develops slowly. This is probably a reflection of CNS adaptation, brain oedema being limited by efflux of organic solutes. However, CNS adaptation can complicate the management of hyponatraemia. Changes in brain volume, in response to changes in osmolar gradient across the blood–brain barrier as serum sodium changes during the treatment of hyponatraemia, can trigger CNS demyelination (central pontine myelinolysis). This osmotic demyelination is a rare but serious complication of hyponatraemia and its treat-

---

Box 18.2   Clinical features of hyponatraemia

Headache	Seizure
Nausea	Coma
Vomiting	Osmotic demyelination
Muscle cramps	Brainstem herniation
Lethargy	Death
Disorientation	

---

ment. Neurological manifestations may include quadriplegia, ophthalmoplegia, pseudobulbar palsy and coma. Osmotic demyelination can develop within 1–4 days of rapid (>12 mmol/24 hours) correction of plasma sodium, irrespective of the method employed to achieve it. It can occur even when sodium levels are corrected slowly, and other factors (hepatic failure, potassium depletion, malnutrition) may play a role in susceptibility.

Chronic asymptomatic hyponatraemia, with plasma sodium concentrations greater than 125 mmol/l, may not require specific treatment. More severe degrees of hyponatraemia, particularly if symptomatic, require some form of intervention. However, there is no consensus on optimal treatment. Correction of the underlying causes, where identifiable, is appropriate. This may include withdrawal of drugs, appropriate hormone replacement, avoidance of excess fluid intake or correction of hypovolaemia. These measures should prevent worsening hyponatraemia but may not address the deficit in plasma sodium, which may require additional intervention. Any additional intervention should adhere to two key principles:

- correction should not risk morbidity and mortality (such as that from osmotic demyelination) in excess of that associated with the initial degree of hyponatraemia
- correction should be at sufficient pace to reverse life-threatening features of hyponatraemia as quickly as is feasible and safe.

Inherent in this approach are several considerations: the degree of symptoms attributable to hyponatraemia; the time over which hyponatraemia has developed; and the target plasma sodium to be achieved. Hyponatraemia developing over several days is associated with adaptive responses in organic osmolytes within the CNS. Rapid correction of plasma sodium in such circumstances risks changes in brain volume that can precipitate osmotic demyelination. Hyponatraemia developing over several hours is not associated with such adaptive responses. Rapid correction of sodium may be more appropriate in such circumstances, if hyponatraemia is associated with severe symptoms.

Patients with mild to moderate symptoms of hyponatraemia that cannot be attributed to rapid falls in plasma sodium should be managed conservatively. If the patient is not hypovolaemic, this can be with fluid restriction: 500–750 ml/24 hours, aiming to raise plasma sodium to 125–130 mmol/l at a rate not exceeding 8 mmol/l/24 hours. Plasma sodium should be measured every 12 hours; if levels rise too quickly, fluid restriction should be relaxed. Prolonged fluid restriction can be distressing, and additional measures may be required in patients with chronic hyponatraemia due to SIADH. Traditionally, these have attempted to either block the release of VP or to generate renal resistance to its antidiuretic actions. Drugs that suppress neurohypophyseal VP secretion (e.g. phenytoin) have met with limited success. SIADH can be treated by inducing NDI with demeclocycline (600–1200 mg/day). This may take several weeks to have a maximal effect. Synthetic, nonpeptide V2-R antagonists increase solute-free water excretion. This new class of aquaretics will greatly improve the management of this condition.

The use of hypertonic saline is controversial and not without risk of central pontine myelinolysis.

Hypernatraemia

Aetiology

Hypernatraemia is a consequence of one of two processes (Table 18.5):

- water loss in excess of concurrent sodium loss
- sodium gain in excess of concurrent gain in water.

Net water loss is the most common mechanism; net gains in sodium resulting in hypernatraemia are usually iatrogenic. Hypernatraemia can only be sustained if thirst is impaired or access to water restricted. It follows that certain groups of patients are at increased risk:

- patients with impaired consciousness
- infants

Table 18.5 Causes of hypernatraemia

Net loss of water	Net gain of sodium
Unreplaced insensible loss	Hypertonic sodium infusions
Hypodipsia	Hypertonic feeding
Hypothalamic DI	
Nephrogenic DI	
Diuretics	
Post-acute tubular necrosis polyuria	
Post-obstructive diuresis	
Intrinsic renal disease	
Gastrointestinal losses	
Burns	
Diabetic hyperosmolar nonketotic coma	

- the elderly
- patients with hypodipsia.

Clinical features

As with hyponatraemia, mortality and morbidity of hyperna-traemia are largely related to CNS dysfunction. However, as the problem arises most commonly in the very young or old, and in those with pre-existing neurological conditions, clinical features may be difficult to interpret (Box 18.3). Predominant water loss may lead to concurrent signs of hypovolaemia. Reduction in brain volume as neuronal contents equilibrate with increased cerebrospinal fluid (CSF) and plasma osmolality may lead to cere-bral bleeding with subarachnoid haemorrhage. Reductions in volume are countered by adaptive increases in organic solute production, although these do not correct detrimental increases in intracellular osmolality.

Box 18.3 Clinical features of hypernatraemia

Muscle weakness	Seizure
Restlessness	Coma
Lethargy	Cerebral bleeding
Disorientation	

Management

Management addresses two issues:

- removing or treating the underlying cause
- correcting the hypertonicity with fluid replacement.

Direct precipitating causes must be addressed where possible, and ongoing fluid losses and requirements covered. These measures should prevent worsening hypernatraemia. The aim of additional replacement therapy is to reduce plasma sodium concentration to 145 mmol/l. In long-standing hypernatraemia, or hypernatraemia of uncertain duration, this should be at a rate of 0.5 mmol/l/hour, to a maximum of 10 mmol/l/day. Hypernatraemia developing over a period of a few hours (generally only applicable to cases of iatrogenic sodium loading) can be corrected at a rate of 1 mmol/l/hour. Hypovolaemia sufficient to compromise circulatory function should be initially corrected with 0.9% sodium chloride or colloid. Although 0.9% sodium chloride may be hypotonic with respect to hypernatraemic plasma, the volume required to normalise plasma sodium in hypernatraemia is prohibitive. Hypotonic fluid therapy (5% dextrose or 0.45% sodium chloride) is thus the appropriate choice for correction of hypernatraemia: the more hypotonic the fluid chosen, the lower the volume or rate of administration required. The preferred route of administration is oral, or via a feeding tube, as this buffers rates of change of sodium. Intravenous therapy may prove the only feasible route.

Excessively rapid correction of hypernatraemia may precipitate cerebral oedema, and must be avoided. It is imperative that the fluid regimen is reassessed at regular intervals, guided by careful clinical assessment and laboratory monitoring.

Hypodipsia

Adipsic and hypodipsic disorders are characterised by inadequate spontaneous fluid intake due to a primary defect in osmoregulated thirst (Tables 18.6 and 18.7). Patients may present with hypovolaemia and dehydration: despite this, they deny thirst and do not drink. If the defect is mild, the resultant hypernatraemia is often well tolerated. More severe disorders can lead to somnolence, seizures, coma and renal impairment. Because of the close anatomical relationship of the osmoregulatory centres for thirst and VP release, adipsic syndromes are often associated with defects in

Table 18. 6   Classification of adipsic/hypodipsic syndromes

Adipsia/hypodipsia syndrome	Osmoregulated thirst	Osmoregulated VP release
Type A (essential hypernatraemia)	*Osmotic threshold increased* *Normal sensitivity*	*Osmotic threshold increased* *Normal sensitivity* *Normal nonosmotic stimulation*
Type B	*Normal osmotic threshold* *Reduced sensitivity*	*Normal osmotic threshold* *Reduced sensitivity* *Normal nonosmotic stimulation*
Type C	*No response to osmotic stimulation*	*Persistent low level VP release* *No response to osmotic stimulation* *Normal nonosmotic stimulation*
Type D (rare)	*No response to osmotic stimulation*	*Normal*

Table 18. 7   Causes of adipsic/hypodipsic syndromes

Neoplastic (50%)
Primary
Craniopharyngioma
Pinealoma
Meningioma

Secondary
Pituitary tumour
Bronchial carcinoma
Breast carcinoma

Vascular (15%)
Internal carotid ligation
Anterior communicating artery aneurysm
Intrahypothalamic haemorrhage

Granulomatous (20%)
Histiocytosis
Sarcoidosis

Miscellaneous (15%)
Hydrocephalus
Ventricular cyst
Trauma
Toluene poisoning

osmoregulated VP release and HDI, exacerbating electrolyte and water balance problems.

The principles of management are to maintain an obligate fluid intake of 2 l/24 hours and adjust this on the basis of other fluid loss. The principles of management are to achieve normal sodium levels through a combination of fixed dose DDAVP (to result in a urine output of 1–2 l/day) and a variable daily fluid intake calculated to balance renal and insensible losses. The effectiveness of the regimen should be monitored through daily weighing and regular checks on plasma sodium.

Further Reading

Adrogue HJ, Madias NE. Hypernatraemia. *New Engl J Med* 2000; **342**:1493–9.

Agre P, Brown D, Nielsen S. Aquaporin water channels: unanswered questions and unresolved controversies. *Curr Opin Cell Biol* 1995;**7**:472–83.

Ball SG, Baylis PH. Mechanisms of drug induced hyponatraemia. *Adv Drug Reaction Bull* 1998;**192**:734–7.

Ball SG, Vaidja B, Baylis PH. Hypothalamic adipsic syndrome: diagnosis and management. *Clin Endocrinol* 1997;**47**:405–9.

Baylis PH. Vasopressin and its neurophysin. In: Degroot LJ (ed), *Endocrinology*, 3rd edn. Philadelphia: WB Saunders, 1995.

Baylis PH, Cheetham T. Diabetes insipidus. *Archi Dis Childhood* 1998;**79**:84–9.

Bichet DG, Arthus M-F, Barjon JN *et al*. Human platelet fraction arginine-vasopressin: potential physiological role. *J Clin Invest* 1987;**79**:881–7.

Higgins J, Gleeson R, Holohan M, Cooney C, Darling M. Maternal and neonatal hyponatraemia: a comparison of Hartmanns solution with 5% dextrose for the delivery of oxytocin in labour. *Eur J Obstetr Gynaecol Reprod Biol* 1996;**68**:47–8.

Hofman S, Bezold R, Jaksch M, Kaufold P, Obermaier-Kusser B, Gerbitz K-D. Analysis of the mitochondrial DNA from patients with Wolfram (DIDMOAD) syndrome. *Molecul Cell Biochem* 1997;**174**:209–13.

Ito M, Jameson JL, Ito M. Molecular basis of autosomal dominant neurohypophyseal diabetes insipidus. Cellular toxicity caused by the accumulation of mutant vasopressin precursors within the endoplasmic reticulum. *J Clin Invest* 1997;**99**:2897–905.

Iwasaki Y, Oiso Y, Saito H, Majzoub JA. Positive and negative regulation of the rat vasopressin gene promoter. *Endocrinology* 1997;**138**:5266–74.

Laycock JF, Hanoune J. From vasopressin receptor to water channel: intracellular traffic, constraint and by-pass. *J Endocrinol* 1998;**159**:361–72.

McKenna K, Thompson C. Osmoregulation in clinical disorders of thirst and thirst appreciation. *Clin Endocrinol* 1998;**49**:139–52.

Marples D. Water channels: who needs them anyway? *Lancet* 2000;**355**:1571–2.

Polymeropoulos MH, Swift RF, Swift M. Linkage of the gene for Wolfram syndrome to markers on the short arm of chromosome 4. *Nature Genetics* 1994;**8**:95–7.

Robson VLM, Noorgard JP, Leung AKC. Hyponatremia in patients with nocturnal enuresis treated with DDAVP. *Eur J Pediatr* 1996;**155**:959–62.

Russell JT, Brownstein MJ, Gainer H. Biosynthesis of vasopressin, oxytocin and neurophysins: isolation and characterization of two common precursors (propressophysin and prooxyphysin). *Endocrinology* 1980;**107**:1880–91.

Seckl JR, Dunger DB, Bevan JS *et al.* Vasopressin antagonist in early postoperative diabetes insipidus. *Lancet* 1990;**355**:1353–6.

Waller SJ, Ratty A, Burbach JPH, Murphy D. Transgenic and transcriptional studies on neurosecretory cell gene expression. *Cell Molec Neurobiol* 1998;**18**:149–71.

Yasui M, Zelenin SM, Celsi G, Aperia A. Adenylate cyclase-coupled vasopressin receptor activates AQP2 promoter via a dual effect on CRE and AP1 elements. *Am J Physiol Renal Fluid & Electrolyte Physiol* 1997;**272**:F443–50.

Zimmerman EA, Ma L-Y, Nilaver G. Anatomical basis of thirst and vasopressin secretion. *Kidney Intern* 1987;**32**(suppl 21):514–19.

19

Multiple Endocrine Neoplasia

Rajesh V Thakker

Introduction

Multiple endocrine neoplasia is characterised by the occurrence of tumours involving two or more endocrine glands within a single patient. The disorder has previously been referred to as multiple endocrine adenopathy (MEA) or the pluriglandular syndrome. However, glandular hyperplasia and malignancy may also occur in some patients and the term multiple endocrine neoplasia (MEN) is now preferred. There are two major forms of multiple endocrine neoplasia, referred to as type 1 and type 2, and each form is characterised by the development of tumours within specific endocrine glands (Table 19.1).

Thus, the combined occurrence of tumours of the parathyroid glands, the pancreatic islet cells and the anterior pituitary is characteristic of multiple endocrine neoplasia type 1 (MEN1), which is also referred to as Wermer's syndrome. However, in multiple endocrine neoplasia type 2 (MEN2), which is also called Sipple's syndrome, medullary thyroid carcinoma (MTC) occurs in association with phaeochromocytoma, and three clinical variants, referred to as MEN2a, MEN2b and MTC-only, are recognised (Table 19.1). Although MEN1 and MEN2 usually occur as distinct and separate syndromes as outlined above, some patients occasionally develop tumours that are associated with both MEN1 and MEN2. All these forms of MEN may either be inherited as autosomal dominant syndromes, or they may occur sporadically, i.e. without a family history. However, this distinction between sporadic and familial

Table 19.1   The multiple endocrine neoplasia (MEN) syndromes, their characteristic tumours and associated biochemical abnormalities

Type	Tumours	Biochemical features
MEN1	Parathyroids	Hypercalcaemia and ↑ PTH
	Pancreatic islets	
	Gastrinoma	↑ Gastrin and ↑ basal gastric acid output
	Insulinoma	Hypoglycaemia and ↑ insulin
	Glucagonoma	Glucose intolerance and ↑ glucagon
	VIPoma	↑ VIP and WDHA
	PPoma	↑ PP
	Pituitary (anterior)	
	Prolactinoma	Hyperprolactinaemia
	GH-secreting	↑ GH
	ACTH-secreting	Hypercortisolaemia and ↑ ATCH
	Non-functioning	Nil or α subunit
	Associated tumours	
	Adrenal cortical	Hypercortisolaemia or primary hyperaldosteronism
	Carcinoid	↑ 5-HIAA
	Lipoma	Nil
MEN2a	Medullary thyroid carcinoma	Hypercalcitoninaemia[a]
	Phaeochromocytoma	↑ Catecholamines
	Parathyroid	Hypercalcaemia and ↑ PTH
MEN2b	Medullary thyroid carcinoma	Hypercalcitoninaemia
	Phaeochromocytoma	↑ Catecholamines
	Associated abnormalities:	
	Mucosal neuromas	
	Marfanoid habitus	
	Medullated corneal nerve fibres	
	Megacolon	

Autosomal dominant inheritance of the MEN syndromes has been established. Key: ↑, increased; PTH, parathyroid hormone; VIP, vasoactive intestinal peptide; WDHA, watery diarrhoea, hypokalaemia and achlorhydria; PP, pancreatic polypeptide; GH, growth hormone; ACTH, adrenocorticotrophin hormone 5-HIAA, 5-hydroxyindoleacetic acid.

[a] In some patients, basal serum calcitonin concentrations may be normal, but may show an abnormal rise at 1 min and 5 min after stimulation with pentagastrin, 0.5 µg/kg.

cases may sometimes be difficult, as in some sporadic cases the family history may be absent because the parent with the disease may have died before developing symptoms. In this chapter, the main clinical features and molecular genetics of the MEN syndromes are discussed.

Multiple Endocrine Neoplasia Type 1 (MEN1)

Clinical features

Parathyroid, pancreatic and pituitary tumours constitute the major components of MEN1. In addition to these tumours, adrenal cortical, carcinoid, facial angiofibromas, collagenomas and lipomatous tumours may also occur in some patients.

Parathyroid tumours

Primary hyperparathyroidism is the most common feature of MEN1 and occurs in more than 95% of all MEN1 patients. Patients may present with asymptomatic hypercalcaemia, or nephrolithiasis, or vague symptoms associated with hypercalcaemia – for example, polyuria, polydipsia, constipation, malaise or occasionally with peptic ulcers. Osteitis fibrosa cystica is now a rare presentation. Biochemical investigations reveal hypercalcaemia usually in association with raised circulating parathyroid hormone (PTH) concentrations. The hypercalcaemia is usually mild, and severe hypercalcaemia resulting in crisis or parathyroid carcinoma is a rare occurrence. Additional differences in the primary hyperparathyroidism of MEN1 patients from that in non-MEN1 patients include an earlier age of onset (20–25 years versus 55 years), and an equal male : female ratio (1 : 1 versus 1 : 3). Primary hyperparathyroidism in MEN1 patients is unusual before the age of 15 years. No effective medical treatment for primary hyperparathyroidism is generally available and surgical removal of the abnormally overactive parathyroids is the definitive treatment. However, all four parathyroid glands are usually affected with multiple adenomas or hyperplasia, although this histological distinction may be difficult, and total parathyroidectomy has been proposed as the definitive treatment for primary hyperparathyroidism in MEN1, with the resultant lifelong hypocalcaemia being treated with oral calcitriol (1,25-dihydroxyvitamin D_3). It is recommended that such total parathyroidectomy should be reserved for the symptomatic hypercalcaemic patient with MEN1, and that the asymptomatic hypercalcaemic MEN1 patient should not have parathyroid surgery but have regular assessments for the onset of symptoms and complications, when total parathyroidectomy should be undertaken.

Pancreatic tumours

The prevalence of pancreatic islet cell tumours in MEN1 patients varies from 30 to 80% in different series. The majority of these tumours produce excessive amounts of hormone – for example gastrin, insulin, glucagon or vasoactive intestinal polypeptide (VIP) – and are associated with distinct clinical syndromes.

Gastrinomas. These gastrin-secreting tumours represent over 50% of all pancreatic islet cell tumours in MEN1, and approximately 20% of patients with gastrinomas will have MEN1. Gastrinomas are the major cause of morbidity and mortality in MEN1 patients. This is due to the recurrent severe multiple peptic ulcers, which may perforate. This association of recurrent peptic ulceration, marked gastric acid production and non-β-islet cell tumours of the pancreas is referred to as the Zollinger–Ellison syndrome. Additional prominent clinical features of this syndrome include diarrhoea and steatorrhoea. The diagnosis is established by demonstration of a raised fasting serum gastrin concentration in association with an increased basal gastric acid secretion. Medical treatment of MEN1 patients with the Zollinger–Ellison syndrome is directed to reducing basal acid output to less than 10 mmol/l, and this may be achieved with high-dose proton pump inhibitors. The ideal treatment for a non-metastatic gastrinoma is surgical excision of the gastrinoma. However, in patients with MEN1 the gastrinomas are frequently multiple or extrapancreatic and the role of surgery has been controversial. For example, in one study, only 16% of MEN1 patients were free of disease immediately after surgery, and at 5 years this had declined to 6%; the respective outcomes in non-MEN1 patients were better, at 45% and 40% . The treatment of disseminated gastrinomas is difficult, and hormonal therapy with somatostatin analogues, chemotherapy with streptozotocin and 5-fluorouracil, hepatic artery embolization and removal of all resectable tumour have all occasionally been successful.

Insulinoma. These β-islet cell tumours secreting insulin represent one-third of all pancreatic tumours in MEN1 patients. Insulinomas also occur in association with gastrinomas in 10% of MEN1 patients, and the two tumours may arise at different times. Insulinomas occur more often in MEN1 patients who are below the age of 40 years, and many of these arise in individuals before the age of 20 years, whereas in non-MEN1 patients insulinomas generally occur in those above the age of 40 years. Insulinomas may be the first manifestation of MEN1 in 10% of patients, and approximately 4% of patients presenting with insulinoma will have MEN1. Patients with an insulinoma present with hypoglycaemic symptoms that develop after a fast or exertion and improve after glucose intake. Biochemical investigations reveal raised plasma insulin concentrations in association with hypoglycaemia. Circulating concentrations of C peptide and proinsulin, which are also raised, may be useful in establishing the diagnosis, as may an insulin suppression test. Medical treatment, which consists of frequent carbohydrate feeds and diazoxide, is not always successful and surgery is often required. Most insulinomas are multiple, and small and preoperative localisation with computed tomography (CT) scanning, coeliac axis angiography and pre-peri operative percutaneous transhepatic portal venous sampling is difficult, and success rates have varied. Surgical treatment, which ranges from enucleation of a single tumour to a distal pancreatectomy or partial pancreatectomy, has been curative in some patients. Chemotherapy, which consists of streptozotocin or octreotide, is used for metastatic disease.

Glucagonoma. These α-islet cell, glucagon-secreting pancreatic tumours occur in <3% of MEN1 patients. The characteristic clinical manifestations of a skin rash (necrolytic migratory erythema), weight loss, anaemia and stomatitis may be absent and the presence of the tumour is indicated only by glucose intolerance and hyperglucagonaemia. The tail of the pancreas is the most frequent site for glucagonomas and surgical removal of these is the treatment of choice. However, treatment may be difficult, as 50% of patients have metastases at the time of diagnosis. Medical treatment of these with octreotide, or with streptozotocin has been successful in some patients.

VIPoma. Patients with VIPomas, which are VIP-secreting pancreatic tumours, develop Watery Diarrhoea, Hypokalaemia and Achlorhydria, referred to as the WDHA syndrome. This clinical syndrome has also been referred to as the Verner–Morrison syndrome or the VIPoma syndrome. VIPomas have been reported in only a few MEN1 patients and the diagnosis is established by documenting a markedly raised plasma VIP concentration. Surgical management of VIPomas, which are mostly located in the tail of the pancreas, has been curative. However, in patients with unresectable tumour, treatment with streptozotocin, octreotide, corticosteroids, indomethacin, metoclopramide and lithium carbonate has proved beneficial.

PPoma. These tumours, which secrete pancreatic polypeptide (PP), are found in a large number of patients with MEN1. No pathological sequelae of excessive PP secretion are apparent and the clinical significance of PP is unknown, although the use of serum PP measurements has been suggested for the detection of pancreatic tumours in MEN1 patients.

Pituitary tumours

The incidence of pituitary tumours in MEN1 patients varies from 15 to 90% in different series. Approximately 60% of MEN1-associated pituitary tumours secrete prolactin, <25% secrete growth hormone (GH), 5% secrete adenocorticotrophic hormone (ACTH) and the remainder appear to be nonfunctioning. Prolactinomas may be the first manifestation of MEN1 in <10% of patients and somatotrophinomas occur more often in patients over the age of 40 years.

Less than 3% of patients with anterior pituitary tumours will have MEN1. The clinical manifestations depend upon the size of the pituitary tumour and its product of secretion. Enlarging pituitary tumours may compress adjacent structures such as the optic chiasm or normal pituitary tissue and cause bitemporal hemianopia or hypopituitarism, respectively. The tumour size and extension are radiologically assessed by CT scanning and nuclear magnetic resonance imaging (MRI). Treatment of pituitary tumours in MEN1 patients is similar to that in non-MEN1 patients and consists of medical therapy or selective hypophysectomy by the trans-sphenoidal approach if feasible, with radiotherapy being reserved for residual unresectable tumour.

Associated tumours

Patients with MEN1 may have tumours involving glands other than the parathyroids, pancreas and pituitary: thus, carcinoid, adrenal cortical, facial angiofibromas, collagenomas, thyroid and lipomatous tumours have been described in association with MEN1.

Carcinoid tumours. They occur in > 3% of patients with MEN1 and may be inherited as an autosomal dominant trait in association with MEN1. The carcinoid tumour may be located in the bronchi, the gastrointestinal tract, the pancreas or the thymus. Bronchial carcinoids in MEN1 patients predominantly occur in women (M : F = 1:4), whereas thymic carcinoids predominantly occur in men, with cigarette smokers having a higher risk of developing tumours. Most patients are asymptomatic and do not suffer from the flushing attacks and dyspnoea associated with the carcinoid syndrome, which usually develops after the tumour has metastasised to the liver.

Adrenal cortical tumours. The incidence of asymptomatic adrenal cortical tumours in MEN1 patients has been reported to be as high as 40%. The majority of these tumours are nonfunctioning. However, functioning adrenal cortical tumours in MEN1 patients have been documented to cause hypercortisolaemia and Cushing's syndrome, and primary hyperaldosteronism, as in Conn's syndrome.

Lipomas. They may occur in > 33% of patients, and frequently they are multiple. In addition, pleural or retroperitoneal lipomas may also occur in patients with MEN1.

Thyroid tumours. They consist of adenomas, colloid goitres and carcinomas and have been reported to occur in over 25% of MEN1 patients. However, the prevalence of thyroid disorders in the general population is high and it has been suggested that the association of thyroid abnormalities in MEN1 patients may be incidental and not significant.

Facial angiofibromas. Multiple facial angiofibromas, which are similar to those observed in patients with tuberous sclerosis, have been observed in 88% of MEN1 patients.

Collagenomas. They have been reported in > 70% of MEN1 patients.

Genetics

The gene causing MEN1 was localised to chromosome 11q13 by genetic mapping studies that investigated MEN1-associated tumours for loss of heterozygosity (LOH) and by segregation studies in MEN1 families. The results of these studies, which were consistent with Knudson's model for tumour development, indicated that the *MEN1* gene represented a putative tumour suppressor gene. Further genetic mapping studies defined a <300 kb region as the minimal critical segment that contained the *MEN1* gene, and characterisation of genes from this region led to the identification of the *MEN1* gene, which consists of 10 exons with a 1830 bp coding region (Figure 19.1) that encodes a novel 610 amino acid protein, referred to as 'MENIN'. Over 250 germline mutations of the *MEN1* gene have been identified, and the majority (>80%) of these are inactivating, and are consistent with its role as a tumour suppressor gene. These mutations are diverse in their types: approximately 25% are nonsense mutations; ≈45% are frameshift deletions or insertions; 15% are in frame deletions or insertions; <5% are donor-splice site mutations; and ≈10% are missense mutations.

More than 10% of the MEN1 mutations arise *de novo* and may be transmitted to subsequent generations. It is also important to note that between 5 and 10% of MEN1 patients may not harbour mutations in the coding region of the MEN1 gene, and that these individuals may have mutations in the promoter or untranslated regions (UTRs), which remain to be investigated. The mutations are not only diverse in their types but are also scattered throughout the 1830 bp coding region of the MEN1 gene with no evidence for clustering as observed in MEN2 (see below).

Correlations between the MEN1 mutations and the clinical manifestations of the disorder appear to be absent. This apparent lack of genotype–phenotype correlations, which contrasts with the situation in MEN2, together with the wide diversity of mutations in the 1830 bp coding region of the MEN1 gene, has made mutational analysis for diagnostic purposes in MEN1 time consuming and expensive. Tumours from MEN1 patients and non-MEN1 patients have been observed to harbour the germline mutation together with a somatic LOH involving chromosome 11q13, as expected from Knudson's model and the proposed role of the MEN1 gene as a tumour suppressor. MENIN has been shown to be located in the nucleus, where it directly interacts with the N-terminus of the AP1 transcriptional factor JunD. MENIN suppresses JunD-activated transcription and, thus, MENIN acts via the transcriptional regulation pathway to control cell proliferation.

Multiple Endocrine Neoplasia Type 2 (MEN2)

MEN2 describes the association of MTC, phaeochromocytomas and parathyroid tumours. Three clinical variants of MEN2 are recognised – MEN2a, MEN2b and familial MTC-only. MEN2a is the most common variant, and the development of MTC is associ-

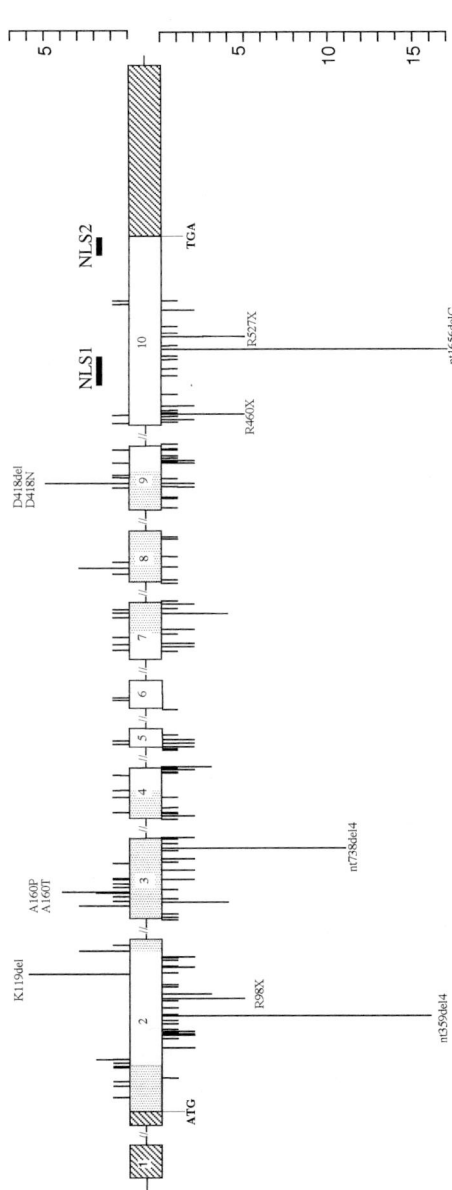

Figure 19.1 Schematic representation of the genomic organisation of the *MEN1* gene illustrating germline mutations. The human *MEN1* gene, which is located on chromosome 11q13, consists of 10 exons that span > 9 kb of genomic DNA and encode a 610 amino acid protein. The 1.83 kb coding region is organised into 9 exons (exons 2–10) and 8 introns (indicated by a line but not to scale). The sizes of the exons (boxes) range from 88 to 1312bp and those of the introns range from 41 to 1564 bp. The start (ATG) and stop (TGA) sites in exons 2 and 10, respectively, are indicated. Exon 1, the 5′ part of exon 2 and 3′ part of exon 10 are untranslated (indicated by the hatched boxes). The locations of the two nuclear localisation sites (NLS), which are at codons 479–497, and 588–608 at the C-terminus, are represented by the thick horizontal lines, and the locations of the three domains, which are formed by codons 1–40 (exon 2), 139–242 (exons 2, 3 and 4) and 323–428 (exons 7, 8 and 9), that interact with JunD are indicated by the grey boxes. The sites of the 262 germline mutations are indicated by the vertical lines; the missense and in-frame mutations are represented above the gene and the nonsense, frameshift and splice site mutations are represented below the gene. Mutations which have occurred more than four times (scale shown on the right) are indicated. (Reproduced with permission from Pannett & Thakker, 1996.)

ated with phaeochromocytomas (50% of patients), which may be bilateral, and parathyroid tumours (20% of patients). MEN2b, which represents 5% of all MEN2 cases, is characterised by the occurrence of MTC and phaeochromocytoma in association with a marfanoid habitus, mucosal neuromas, medullated corneal fibres and intestinal autonomic ganglion dysfunction leading to multiple diverticulae and megacolon (Figure 19.2). Parathyroid tumours do

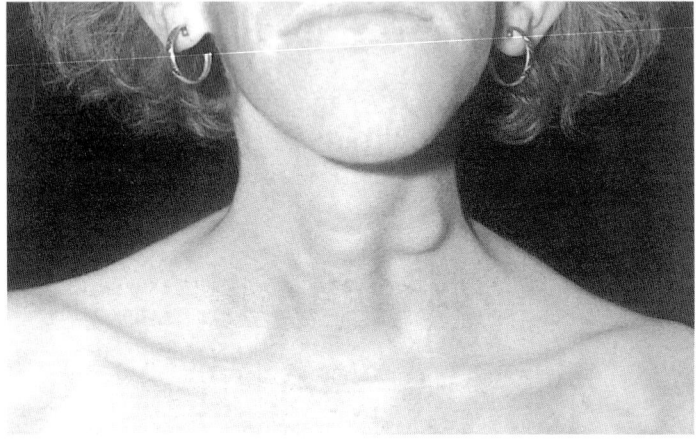

A

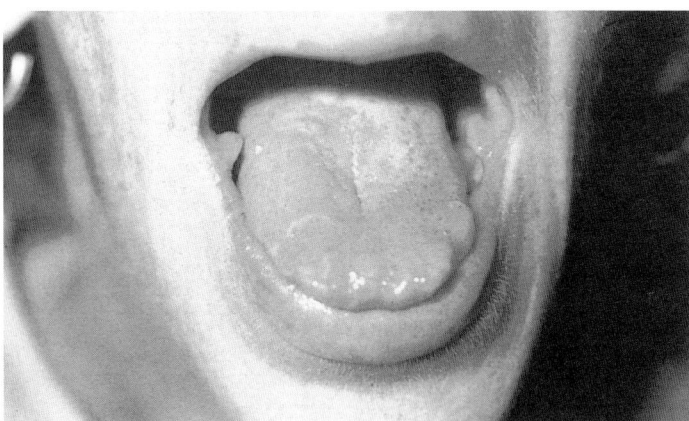

B

Figure 19.2 *For captions, see opposite*

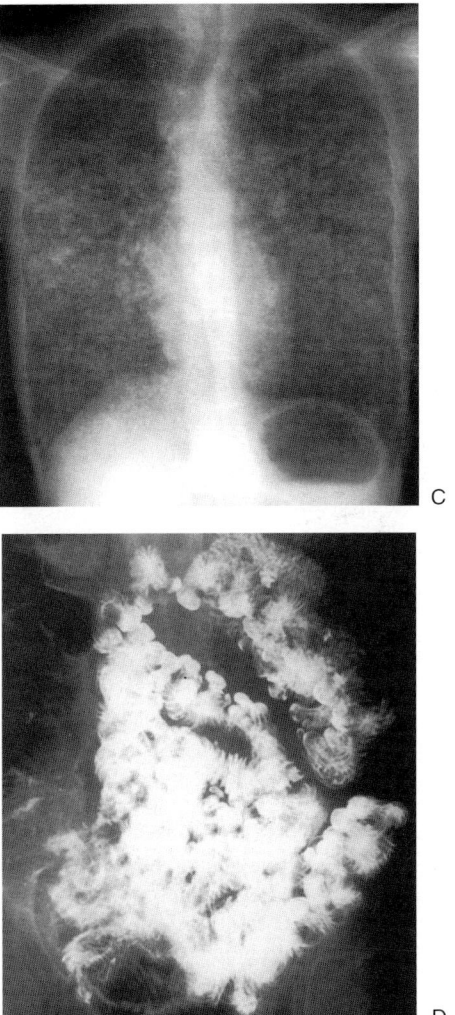

Figure 19.2   Some clinical features in a patient with MEN2b. A, Note thyroidectomy scar and nodule on left side of neck representing metastases of MTC. B, Mucosal neuromas on tongue and lips. C, Bilateral lung metastases of MTC. D, Radiograph of barium meal and follow-through, illustrating the presence of multiple intestinal diverticulae, which are secondary to autonomic ganglion dysfunction. (Reproduced with permission from Thakker, 1997.)

not usually occur in MEN2b. MTC-only is a variant in which medullary thyroid carcinoma is the sole manifestation of the syndrome. The clinical features of MTC, phaeochromocytoma and parathyroid tumours in MEN2 will be reviewed.

Clinical features

Medullary thyroid carcinoma

MTC is the most common feature of MEN2a and occurs in almost 100% of affected individuals. MTC represents 10% of all thyroid gland carcinomas, and 20% of MTC patients have a family history of the disorder. Patients with MTC may be asymptomatic, and the presence of MTC may have been detected by the demonstration of hypercalcitoninaemia at family screening. However, MTC may also present as a palpable mass in the neck, which may be asymptomatic or associated with symptoms of pressure or dysphagia in 16% of patients. Diarrhoea may occur in 30% of patients and is associated either with elevated circulating concentrations of calcitonin or tumour-related secretion of serotonin and prostaglandins. Some patients may also suffer from flushing. In addition, ectopic ACTH production by MTC may cause Cushing's syndrome. Radionuclide thyroid scans reveal MTC tumours as 'cold' nodules.

The diagnosis of MTC relies on the demonstration of hypercalcitoninaemia, either in the basal state (> 90 pg/ml, 0.08 pmol/l) or following stimulation with intravenous pentagastrin (0.5 µg/kg) and/or calcium infusion (2 mg/kg). Metastases of MTC in the early stages usually occur to the cervical lymph nodes, and in later stages to the mediastinal nodes, lung, liver, trachea, adrenal, oesophagus and bone. Radiography may reveal dense irregular calcification within the involved portions of the thyroid gland and the lymph nodes involved with the metastases. However, the presence of metastases does not necessarily lead to a poor prognosis, and in 80% of patients the tumour(s) pursue a relatively indolent course. MTC does pursue an aggressive course with early metastases and death in <10% of patients and there may be a family history of such aggressive MTC or MEN2b (Figure 19.2). Treatment for MTC is total thyroidectomy, with central lymph node resection, followed by replacement thyroxine therapy.

Phaeochromocytoma

These noradrenaline (norepinephrine)- and adrenaline (epinephrine)-secreting tumours occur in > 50% of patients with MEN2a, and are a major cause of morbidity and mortality. Patients may have symptoms and signs of catecholamine secretion (e.g. headaches, palpitations, sweating and poorly controlled hypertension), or they may be asymptomatic and have been detected through biochemical screening because of a history of either familial MEN2a or MTC. The biochemical and radiological investigation of phaeochromocytoma in MEN2a patients is similar to that in non-MEN2 patients, and includes the estimation of urinary free catecholamines, CT (or MRI) scanning and radionuclide scanning with meta-iodo (^{123}I or ^{131}I) benzylguanidine (MIBG). An early biochemical abnormality in MEN2 patients with phaeochromocytoma and medullary hyperplasia is an increase in the adrenaline/noradrenaline ratio to > 0.15. Bilateral adrenomedullary hyperplasia is the precursor to phaeochromocytoma in patients with MEN2. This is associated with the expansion of the medullary tissue into the body and tail of the gland, with a decrease in corticomedullary ratio and nodular hyperplasia. Nodules exceeding 1 cm diameter are designated phaeochromocytomas. The prevalence of bilateral adrenal medullary tumours in MEN2a patients is 70%, compared with a 10% prevalence observed in non-MEN2 patients. In addition, phaeochromocytomas in patients with MEN2a differ significantly in distribution when compared with those in non-MEN2 patients. Thus, extra-adrenal phaeochromocytomas, which occur in 10% of non-MEN2 patients, are rarely observed in MEN2a patients and, similarly, malignancy in MEN2a phaeochromocytoma is much less common. Thus, one suggested treatment for phaeochromocytoma in patients with MEN2a is bilateral adrenalectomy, even in those MEN2a patients in whom only a unilateral tumour has been demonstrated by radiology.

Parathyroid tumours

The incidence of parathyroid tumours in MEN2a patients varies from 40 to 80% in different series. However, more than 50% of these patients do not have hypercalcaemia, and the presence of abnormally enlarged parathyroids, which are usually hyperplastic, is revealed in the normocalcaemic patient undergoing thyroidectomy for MTC. The biochemical investigation and management for the hypercalcaemia MEN2a patients is similar to that of the MEN1 patient.

Genetics

The gene causing all three MEN2 variants was mapped to chromosome 10cen-10q11.2, a region containing the *c-ret* proto-oncogene which encodes a tyrosine kinase receptor with cadherin-like and cysteine-rich extracellular domains, and a tyrosine kinase intracellular domain. Specific mutations of *c-ret* have been identified for each of the three MEN2 variants (Figure 19.3). Thus, in 95% of patients, MEN2a is associated with mutations of the cysteine-rich extracellular domain, and mutations in codon 634 (Cys→Arg) account for 85% of MEN2a mutations. MTC-only is also associated with missense mutations in the cysteine-rich extracellular domain, and most mutations are in codon 618. However, MEN2b is associated with mutations in codon 918 (Met→Thr) of the intracellular tyrosine kinase domain in 95% of patients. Interestingly, the *c-ret* proto-oncogene is also involved in the aetiology of papillary thyroid carcinomas and in Hirschsprung's disease.

Mutational analysis of *c-ret* to detect mutations in codons 609, 611, 618, 620, 634, 768 and 804 in MEN2a and MTC-only, and codon 918 in MEN2b, has been used in the diagnosis and management of patients and families with these disorders. Such testing quickly and reliably identifies the 50% of family members who do not have the mutation and who therefore do have to undergo further screening. For those family members who have inherited the mutation and are at high risk of developing tumours, there are two clinical approaches. In the preferred approach, a total thyroidectomy is recommended, on the sole basis of the abnormal genetic test, at the age of 5 years; this is the earliest age at which metastasis in MEN2a has been identified. In an alternative approach, continued testing of calcitonin release following pentagastrin stimulation is recommended, with total thyroidectomy being reserved until an abnormal pentagastrin test is observed. This usually delays total thyroidectomy until 10–13 years of age but is associated with increased morbidity and mortality. In MEN2b, metastasis at 2 years of age has been reported, and total thyroidectomy at an earlier age has been recommended. The advantages of this approach are that pentagastrin testing is avoided and it is more likely that a cure will be achieved before micrometastases develop. The management of affected families is complicated, and requires careful coordination between the medical team (endocrinologists, geneticists, surgeons and general practitioners) and the family.

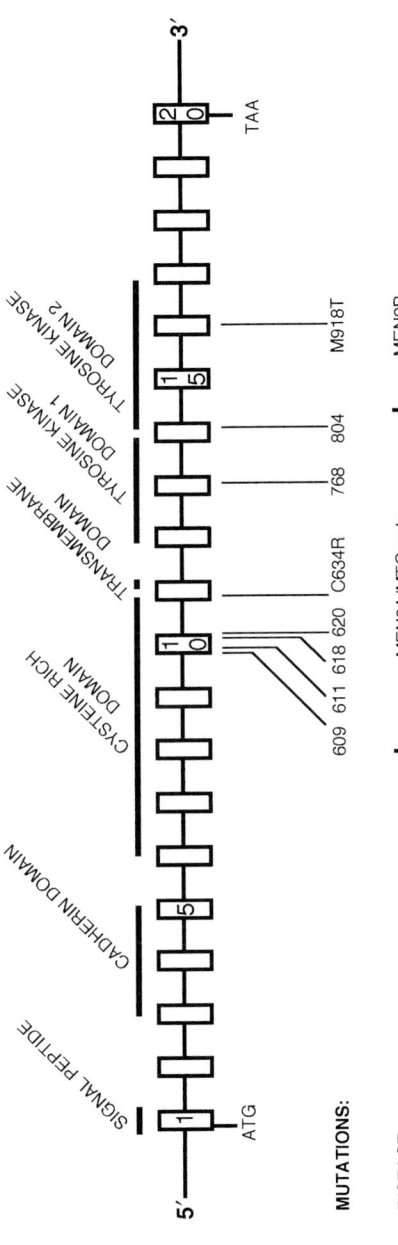

Figure 19.3 Schematic representation of the genomic organisation of the *c-ret* gene illustrating germline mutations causing MEN2. The human *c-ret* (MEN2) gene, which is located on chromosome 10q11.2, consists of 20 (21) exons that span ≈ 30 kb of genomic DNA and encodes a 1114 amino acid membrane-associated tyrosine kinase receptor. The 3342 bp coding region is organised into 20 exons and 19 introns (indicated by a line but not to scale). The sizes of the exons (boxes) range from 70 to 292 bp and those of the introns range from 333 to 2456 bp. The start (ATG) and stop (TAA) sites in exons 1 and 20, respectively, are indicated. The receptor consists of a signal peptide region, cadherin-like domain a region containing several conserved cysteine residues (cysteine-rich domain), a transmembrane domain and two tyrosine kinase domains. The occurrence of MEN2a and MTC-only involves codons 609, 611, 618, 620, 634, 768 and 804, whereas that of MEN2b involves only codon 918. C634R indicates Cys 634 Arg and M918T indicates Met 918 Thr. (Reproduced with permission from Thakker, 2000).

Acknowledgements

I am grateful to the Medical Research Council (MRC), UK for support; to B Harding and J Turner for preparing the figures and to Miss Julie Allen for expert secretarial assistance.

Further Reading

Agarwal SK, Guru SC, Heppner C *et al*. Menin interacts with the AP1 transcription factor JunD and represses JunD-activated transcription. *Cell* 1999;**84:**730–5.

Chandrasekharappa SC, Guru SC, Manickam P *et al*. Positional cloning of the gene for multiple endocrine neoplasia-type 1. *Science* 1997;**276:**404–7.

Darling TN, Skarulis MC, Steinberg SM, Marx SJ, Spiegel AM, Turner M. Multiple facial angiofibromas and collagenomas in patients with multiple endocrine neoplasia type 1. *Arch Dermatol* 1997;**133**:853–61.

Davis JRE. Molecular biology techniques in endocrinology. *Clin Endocrinol*, 1996;**45:**125–133.

European Consortium on MEN1. Identification of the multiple endocrine neoplasia type 1 (MEN1) gene. *Human Molec Gen* 1997;**6:**1177–83.

Gagel RF, Cotes GJ. *Ret* protooncogene mutations in multiple endocrine neoplasia type 2. In: Bilezikian JP, Raisz LG, Rodan GA (eds), *Principles of Bone Biology*. San Diego: Academic Press, 1996:799–807.

Knudson AG. Antioncogenes and human cancer. *Proc Natl Acad Sci USA* 1993;**90:**10914–21.

Lips CJ, Landsvater RM, Hoppener J *et al*. Clinical screening as compared with DNA analysis in families with multiple endocrine neoplasia type 2a. *New Engl J Med* 1994;**331**:828–35.

Marx SJ. Multiple endocrine neoplasia type 1. In : Vogelstein B, Kinzler KW (eds), *Genetic Basis of Human Cancer*. New York: McGraw-Hill, 1998:489–506.

MEN2 CRC UK register, Professor B Ponder, CRC Department of Oncology, Strangeways Research Laboratory, Worts Causway, Cambridge CB1 8RN.

Norton JA, Fraker DL, Alexaxder R *et al*. Surgery to cure the Zollinger–Ellison syndrome. *New Engl J Med* 1999;**341**:635–44.

Pannett AAJ, Thakker RVT. Multiple endocrine neoplasia type 1 (MEN1) gene. *Endocrine-Related Cancer* 1999;**6**:449–73.

Raue F, Frank-Raue K, Graver A. Multiple endocrine neoplasia type 2. Clinical features and screening. In: Gagel RF (ed), *Endocrinology and Metabolism Clinics of North America* 1994;**23**(1):137–56.

Skogseid B, Larsson C, Lindgren PG *et al.* Clinical and genetic features of adrenocortical lesions in multiple endocrine neoplasia type 1. *J Clin Endocrinol Metab* 1992;**75**:76–81.

Skogseid B, Oberg K, Benson L *et al.* A standardized meal stimulation test of the endocrine pancreas for early detection of pancreatic endocrine tumours in multiple endocrine neoplasia type 1 syndrome: five years experience. *J Clin Endocrinol Metab* 1987;**64**:1233–40.

Teh BT, Zedenius J, Kytola S *et al.* Thymic carcinoids in multiple endocrine neoplasia type 1. *Ann Surg* 1998;**228**:99–105.

Thakker RV. Multiple endocrine neoplasia type 1 (MEN1). In: DeGroot LJ, Besser GK, Burger HG et al. (eds), *Endocrinology*. Philadelphia: WB Saunders, 1995:2815–31.

Thakker RV. Multiple endocrine neoplasia. Thakker RV, Wass JAH (eds), *Medicine* 1997;**25**(6):86–8. The Medicine Group (Journals) Limited, Abingdon, Oxon, UK.

Thakker RV. Multiple endocrine neoplasia – syndromes of the twentieth century. *J Clin Endocrinol Metab* 1998;**83**:2617–20.

Thakker RV. Multiple endocrine neoplasia. In Goltzman D (ed), *Metabolic Diseases of Common Inherited Diseases*. Philadelphia: WB Saunders, 2000.

Trump D, Farren B, Wooding C *et al.* Clinical studies of multiple endocrine neoplasia type 1 (MEN1) in 220 patients. *Quart J Med* 1996;**89**:653–69.

Vortmeyer AO, Böni R, Pak E, Pack S, Zhuang Z. Multiple endocrine neoplasia 1 alterations in MEN1-associated and sporadic lipomas. *J Natl Cancer Inst* 1998;**90**:398.

Wells SA Jr, Chi DD, Toshima K *et al.* Predictive DNA testing and prophylatic thyroidectomy in patients at risk for multiple endocrine neoplasia type 2a. *Ann Surg* 1994;**220**:237–50.

Wohllk N, Cote GJ, Bugalho MMJ *et al.* Relevance of RET proto-oncogene mutations in sporadic medullary thyroid carcinoma. *J Clin Endocrinol Metab* 1996;**81**:3740–5.

Wolfe MM, Jensen RT. Zollinger–Ellison syndrome. Current concepts in diagnosis and management. *New Engl J Med* 1987;**317**:1200–9.

20

Lipids

Callum Livingstone and Michael F Laker

Introduction

Lipid disorders can be divided into the hyperlipidaemias, which are common, and the much rarer hypolipidaemias. Hypercholes-terolaemia is associated with a risk of developing atherosclerosis with consequent ischaemic heart disease (IHD), cerebrovascular disease and peripheral vascular disease. Although the association between hypercholesterolaemia and vascular disease has been known about for a long time, we now have evidence-based medi-cine that early treatment of hypercholesterolaemia can reduce the risk of premature cardiovascular death. In severe hypertriglyceri-daemia there is a risk of developing acute pancreatitis.

Hyperlipidaemias are common conditions whose clinical import-ance lies primarily in their association with coronary artery disease. Identification of those at risk is essential if coronary risk is to be reduced by early institution of lipid-lowering treatment.

Definitions

Hyperlipidaemias are defined on the basis of risk of adverse outcome at particular lipid levels rather than by reference ranges. As the cut-off levels are directly related to risk, they influence the decision as to whether to offer treatment. The definitions are shown in Table 20.1.

Clinical Features

Classification of hyperlipidaemias

There are various means of classifying hyperlipidaemias. They can be divided into the primary hyperlipidaemias, where there is a

Table 20.1   Therapeutic classification of hyperlipidaemia

Hypercholesterolaemia		Hypertriglyceridaemia	
Degree	Serum cholesterol (mmol/l)	Degree	Serum triglyceride (mmol/l)
Mild	> 5.2, ≤ 6.5	Moderate	> 2.3, ≤ 4.6
Moderate	> 6.5, ≤ 7.8	Severe	> 4.6
Severe	> 7.8		

genetic predisposition for elevated serum lipid levels, and secondary hyperlipidaemias, where serum lipid levels are elevated as a result of an underlying condition. For the majority of patients with primary hyperlipidaemias encountered in the lipid clinic it is not possible to make a diagnosis of the specific underlying primary hyperlipidaemia with certainty as the clinician is not in a position to carry out family studies: for example, to definitively diagnose the familial disorders. However, it is patients' lipid levels which define their cardiovascular or pancreatitis risk and so, for therapeutic purposes, classification according to the lipid abnormality is more useful than genetic classification (Table 20.2).

Classifying hyperlipidaemias according to the lipid abnormality is relatively simple and convenient for clinical purposes, but it does not identify individual disorders and/or distinguish between primary and secondary disorders. The Fredrickson (phenotypic) classification, based on the appearance on lipoprotein electrophoresis, has been used extensively in the past and is still given in some textbooks.

Table 20.2   Genetic classification of hyperlipidaemias

Lipid abnormality	Genetic (metabolic) classification
Hypercholesterolaemia	Familial hypercholesterolaemia (familial
Hypertriglyceridaemia	defective apolipoprotein B-100)
Combined hyperlipidaemia	Polygenic hypercholesterolaemia
	Familial combined hyperlipidaemia
	Familial dysbetalipoproteinaemia
	Familial hypertriglyceridaemia
	Chylomicronaemia syndrome
	Hyperalphalipoproteinaemia

Although knowledge of the precise nature of the primary hyper-lipidaemia is generally not essential for effective management, there are four hyperlipidaemias that it is important to be able to diagnose definitively as there are specific implications for their management:

- familial hypercholesterolaemia (FH) indicates early and aggressive lipid-lowering treatment and, in addition, screening of family members
- familial dysbetalipoproteinaemia indicates treatment with a fibrate or a statin if unresponsive to diet
- lipoprotein lipase deficiency indicates treatment with a very low fat diet
- hyperalphalipoproteinaemia, not associated with increased coronary risk, is important to identify, as lipid-lowering treatment is not indicated.

Secondary hyperlipidaemias

Secondary hyperlipidaemias are extremely common in clinical practice. Primary and secondary hyperlipidaemias can occur in combination and some of the most severe hyperlipidaemias occur in this way, e.g. a high alcohol intake in a patient with FH. In addition, a mild primary hyperlipidaemia can be 'unmasked' by the development of a secondary component. Secondary hyperlipid-aemias can also occur in patients already on lipid-lowering treatment. The severity of the hyperlipidaemia may provide a clue to the cause. The more severe the hyperlipidaemia, the more likely it is that there is a secondary component.

Secondary causes of hypercholesterolaemia and hypertrigly-ceridaemia are shown in Table 20.3. There is wide variation in the pattern and severity of the actual lipid disorder.

Table 20. 3   Secondary causes of hyperlipidaemias

Hypercholesterolaemia	Hypertriglyceridaemia
Hypothyroidism	Obesity
Nephrotic syndrome	Diabetes mellitus
Cholestasis	Alcohol excess
Anorexia nervosa	Renal failure
Acute intermittent porphyria	Glycogen storage disease
Anabolic steroids	Beta-blockers
Diuretics	Thiazides
Cyclosporin	Retinoids

Stigmata of hyperlipidaemia

These should always be sought in the hyperlipidaemic patient, as the presence of stigmata may point to a specific disorder. The four types of stigmata listed below correlate well with the biochemistry and resolve as the hyperlipidaemia is treated:

- Tendon xanthomata. These are found on extensor tendons of hands and Achilles tendon. Their presence in combination with hypercholesterolaemia usually indicates a diagnosis of FH although they can also occur in some rare disorders.
- Palmar crease xanthomata and tuberous xanthomata are pathognomonic of familial dysbetalipoproteinaemia (type III Fredrickson classification).
- Eruptive xanthomata occur in the chylomicronaemia syndrome.
- Lipaemia retinalis may be observed in severe hypertriglyceridaemia.

Other stigmata correlate less well with the biochemistry, and corneal arcus tends to be present with increasing age. However, their presence points to the possibility of a hyperlipidaemia and should be noted:

- xanthelasmata (lipid deposits in the palpebral fissures)
- corneal arcus.

Other features of hyperlipidaemias

If atherosclerosis is advanced, there may be clinical evidence of vascular disease associated with the hyperlipidaemia:

- carotid bruits
- renal artery/aortic bruits in the abdomen
- impairment of the peripheral pulses.

Patients with acute pancreatitis or chronic pancreatitis with pancreatic insufficiency as a result of severe hypertriglyceridaemia will have the clinical features of these disorders.

Hyperlipidaemias may be accompanied by clinical and/or laboratory evidence of other coronary risk factors (Table 20.4). They should always be considered in the context of these risk factors and not in isolation. The effects of risk factors are multiplicative rather than additive. Obviously, reduction of some of the modifiable risk factors has been shown to reduce cardiovascular risk (e.g. smoking) and for some of those factors (e.g. homocysteine) data are not available.

Table 20.4   Cardiovascular risk factors

Non-modifiable	Modifiable
Age	Cigarette smoking
Male sex	Raised LDL-cholesterol
Family history	Low HDL-cholesterol
Previous MI	Hypertension
	Diabetes
	Sedentary lifestyle
	Obesity
	High fibrinogen levels
	High haematocrit
	Diet
	Hyperhomocysteinaemia

HDL = high-density lipoprotein, LDL = low-density lipoprotein,
MI = myocardial infarction.

Syndrome X

Syndrome X or 'metabolic syndrome' is a collection of modifiable risk factors occurring together in the same patient (Box 20.1). Insulin resistance is believed to be the underlying feature in this disorder and there is good evidence that it precedes hypertension and type 2 diabetes in the pathological process. The occurrence of these risk factors together means that patients with syndrome X are at considerable risk of developing macrovascular disease and should have their hyperlipidaemia treated aggressively as well as having their individual risk factors addressed.

Box 20.1   Components of syndrome X

- Insulin resistance
- Hyperinsulinaemia
- Hypertension
- Hypertriglyceridaemia
- Low HDL-cholesterol
- Obesity

HDL = high-density lipoprotein.

Hypolipidaemias

Hypocholesterolaemia is most commonly secondary to malnutrition, malabsorption or any acute severe illness such as a myocardial infarction (MI). The primary hypolipoproteinaemias are extremely rare (Table 20.5). A full discussion of these disorders is beyond the scope of this chapter.

Investigations

The purpose of carrying out laboratory investigations in patients with hyperlipidaemias is threefold:

- to define the nature and severity of the hyperlipidaemia itself
- to exclude secondary causes of hyperlipidaemia
- to establish baselines prior to starting lipid-lowering treatment.

Defining the nature and severity of the hyperlipidaemia

Lipid levels

Hyperlipidaemic patients referred from primary care to the lipid clinic should have a full fasting lipid profile performed at their first visit – total cholesterol, triglyceride, high-density lipoprotein (HDL)-cholesterol and estimated low-density lipoprotein (LDL)-cholesterol. HDL-cholesterol is assayed in the laboratory after precipitation of apolipoprotein B (ApoB)-containing lipoproteins. The LDL-cholesterol is then estimated using the Friedewald formula, which makes an allowance for the cholesterol content of very-low-density lipoprotein, VLDL (Box 20.2).

Points to watch in assessment of lipid levels:

- Lipid levels show considerable intra-individual variation, and it is preferable to have at least two measurements before making a diagnosis and considering treatment.

Table 20.5   The primary hypolipoproteinaemias

Condition	Defect	Lipids
Hypobetalipoproteinaemia	↑ ApoA-I catabolism	↓ chol ↓ trig
Abetalipoproteinaemia	Absence of ApoB	↓↓ chol ↓↓ trig
Tangier disease	↓ synthesis of ApoB	↓↓ HDL-chol
		↓ LDL-chol

ApoB = apolipoprotein B, chol = cholesterol, trig = triglyceride.

> ### Box 20.2   Friedewald formula for estimating LDL-cholesterol
>
> LDL-cholesterol = Total cholesterol – HDL-cholesterol – Triglyceride/2.2
>
> This formula is only reliable if the plasma triglyceride is below 4.5 mmol/l. At triglyceride levels higher than this, LDL-cholesterol levels cannot be accurately estimated.
>
> HDL = high-density lipoprotein, LDL = low-density lipoprotein.

- Total and HDL-cholesterol are not influenced by recent dietary intake, but triglyceride levels climb markedly after a meal. If these are to be assessed properly, it is essential that the patient is fasted.
- Either serum or plasma can be used to assess lipid levels, although it is important to use the material preferred by the local laboratory.
- Acute illness can cause cholesterol levels to fall, and assessment should not be carried out within 3 months of a major illness. However, cholesterol levels will be reliable until 24 hours after myocardial infarction and can be assessed during this interval.

Fridge test

If a serum or plasma sample is noted to be grossly lipaemic, it is useful to inspect the sample after overnight storage at 4°C; this indicates whether the sample contains predominantly chylomicrons, VLDL or both, and so helps identification of the lipid phenotype. Chylomicrons float on the surface as a creamy layer, and VLDL cause a turbid infranatant.

Other tests which are useful in the investigation of hyperlipidaemias

Apoliproteins.   ApoB levels correlate with LDL-cholesterol, and apoliprotein A-I (ApoA-I) levels with HDL-cholesterol. A high ApoB/ApoA-I ratio suggests increased coronary risk. Unfortunately at present there are problems with standardisation of apoliprotein measurements and there is a lack of prospective evidence on the value of their measurement. At present, their measurement adds little in the assessment of hyperlipidaemias but is useful in assessment of hypolipidaemias.

Lipoprotein lipase (LPL) activity.   This can be measured to confirm a diagnosis of LPL deficiency. Its level in plasma can be measured after a heparin injection. It is unstable and if it is to be measured it is important to adhere to the protocol of the centre providing the assay.

ApoE (apolipoprotein E) phenotyping and genotyping.   These can be determined by isoelectric focussing and DNA testing, respectively. Either of the tests, in combination with ultracentrifugation to determine the VLDL cholesterol concentration, can help confirm a diagnosis of familial dysbetalipoproteinaemia. Patients with this disorder have ApoE2 homozygosity and a VLDL cholesterol/total plasma triglyceride ratio of >0.3, but the dramatic response to a fibrate will usually confirm the diagnosis without the need to resort to further investigations.

Lipoprotein(a).   Serum Lp(a) is associated with coronary atherosclerosis independently of the other risk factors. However, as its metabolism is poorly understood and treatments which lower its levels are not known, its place in risk assessment is still unclear.

Homocysteine.   This is a cardiovascular risk factor and should be measured if premature coronary artery disease has occurred in the absence of other risk factors. Prospective evidence about the value of treatment of mild hyperhomocysteinaemia is lacking at present. Once further studies have been published, the role of plasma homocysteine measurement in coronary risk assessment will become clearer.

How to diagnose specific lipid disorders

Familial hypercholesterolaemia.   Although a monogenic disorder, FH is a heterogeneous condition, with many different LDL receptor defects having been described. As a result, no single genetic test is available, and diagnosis depends on the serum cholesterol level, the presence of tendon xanthomata and the family history (Box 20.3).

LPL deficiency and apolipoprotein C-II (ApoC-II) deficiency.   The possibility of LPL deficiency would be raised by the presence of chylomicronaemia syndrome in a child although partial defects of LPL have also been described. The diagnosis requires measurement of post-heparin LPL activity and measurement of ApoC-II levels.

Box 20.3   Diagnostic criteria for familial hypercholesterolaemia (FH)

Definite FH
Serum cholesterol
> 6.7 mmol/l in children
> 7.5 mmol/l in adults

plus

Tendon xanthomata in the patient or first-degree relative

Possible FH
Cholesterol concentrations as above

plus

Family history of myocardial infarction below 50 years of age in second-degree relative or 60 years in a first-degree relative

or

Family history of hypercholesterolaemia in a first- or second-degree relative

Hyperalphalipoproteinaemia.   This condition can be diagnosed by finding elevated HDL-cholesterol and ApoA-I levels.

Exclusion of secondary causes of hyperlipidaemia

It is important that secondary causes are sought before lipid-lowering treatment is considered, as appropriate treatment of an underlying cause can lead to marked improvement in a secondary hyperlipidaemia without the need for lipid-lowering treatment. The following investigations are essential in seeking secondary components for a hyperlipidaemia:

- urinalysis for protein and glucose for evidence of nephrotic syndrome and diabetes
- serum creatinine for evidence of renal failure
- liver function tests (LFTs), including γ-glutamyl transferase (GGT) for evidence of cholestasis and excessive alcohol consumption
- fasting plasma glucose for evidence of diabetes
- thyroid-stimulating hormone (TSH) to screen for hypothyroidism
- mean cell volume (MCV) for evidence of excessive alcohol consumption.

Investigations required for setting baselines

Serum creatinine.   In renal impairment the doses of statins which can be prescribed are limited and so it is essential to check the renal function beforehand.

Serum creatine kinase (CK).   In the event that the patient develops symptoms suggestive of myositis after commencing lipid-lowering therapy, a raised serum CK level can help confirm the diagnosis. However, there is wide inter-individual variation in serum CK levels and it is difficult to interpret an individual measurement unless a baseline CK has been previously measured.

Serum alanine aminotransferase (ALT).   Measurement of serum ALT as a baseline is essential to check for any disorder of liver function that may result from lipid-lowering therapy. Mild ALT elevations are commonly observed in obese patients and, if a baseline check is not made initially, the elevation noted after commencement of treatment may be wrongly attributed to the lipid-lowering therapy.

Management

The first step in clinical management of the hyperlipidaemic patient is a full clinical history and examination and laboratory investigations. Thereafter, a decision can be made as to how to treat the patient and regular follow-up arranged. The clinical examination must be aimed at assessing the overall coronary risk. It is important to distinguish between primary prevention, where there has been no previous coronary disease, and secondary prevention, where there is established ischaemic heart disease.

The main points to elicit from the history are:

- evidence of other cardiovascular risk factors (see Table 20.4)
- symptoms of vascular disease; i.e. angina, claudication, dyspnoea
- previous MI or revascularisation procedure
- fat content of diet
- alcohol consumption
- amount of exercise taken.

During the physical examination it is essential to:

- record the weight and body mass index (BMI)
- look for stigmata of hyperlipidaemia
- measure the blood pressure

- listen for arterial bruits
- check the peripheral pulses
- waist circumference can be assessed as a simple cardiovascular risk predictor.

Other action to be taken at the initial consultation:

- carry out a metabolic screen (discussed above under Investigations).
- make an assessment of coronary risk
- set targets for body weight and serum cholesterol (see below)
- give dietary advice and initiate a 3-month trial on a low-fat diet
- advise the patient about lifestyle changes if appropriate (stop smoking, take more exercise and moderate alcohol consumption).

Target values for serum cholesterol

The Joint British Recommendations on Prevention of Coronary Heart Disease (1998) recommend the target serum cholesterol values shown in Box 20.4.

Assessment of coronary risk

A careful assessment of coronary risk is important, as it influences the decision as to how aggressively to treat the hyperlipidaemia. The 10-year risk of developing coronary heart disease (CHD) can be determined as described in the Joint British Recommendations either by using a computer program or by using the diagrams given in the publication. Thereafter, the hyperlipidaemia is managed as shown (Table 20.6).

This means of risk assessment does not take account of the family history. The risk can be adjusted up 1.5-fold if a first-degree

---

Box 20.4   Cholesterol goals (Joint British Recommendations 1998)

- **Total cholesterol:** < 5.0 mmol/l
- **LDL-cholesterol:** < 3.0 mmol/l

In cases of secondary prevention, the National Cholesterol Education Programme (NCEP) has recommended a more stringent low-density lipoprotein (LDL)-cholesterol goal of < 2.6 mmol/l.

Table 20.6   Management of hypercholesterolaemia (Joint British Recommendations 1998)

10-year CHD risk	Serum cholesterol (mmol/l)	Action
≥ 15%	≥ 5	Lifestyle changes and lipid lowering treatment
≥ 15%	< 5	Lifestyle changes and reassess annually
< 15%	< 5	Lifestyle changes and reassess after 5 years

CHD = coronary heart dsease.

male relative has developed CHD or another atherosclerotic disease at an age of <55 years or if a first-degree female relative has developed CHD at an age of <65 years. The risk can also be adjusted upwards at the clinician's discretion in the presence of hypertriglyceridaemia, impaired glucose tolerance or premature menopause. Coronary artery disease mortality is higher among South-Asian immigrants in the UK but the above method of risk calculation should be applied with caution in this population as it has not been validated for use in ethnic minorities. Always focus on the patients at highest coronary risk: the greatest benefit in terms of risk reduction will come from treating these patients.

Dietary advice

The total calorie content of the diet should be adjusted so as to achieve the ideal body weight. The total fat content of the diet should be reduced to less than 30% of the caloric intake, with an increase in the ratio of polyunsaturated to saturated fat, and the intake of complex carbohydrate and dietary fibre should be increased. A dietetic consultation should be arranged in order to reinforce this advice.

Some cardioprotection may be obtained from moderate levels of alcohol consumption, but the benefit is probably lost at levels of alcohol consumption exceeding 20 units per week, at which level it starts to contribute adversely to the hyperlipidaemia. Although smoking is the most important risk factor for ischaemic heart disease, it is modifiable, and so the severity of the family history tends to be the main additional factor in deciding whether to treat hypercholesterolaemia.

Lipid-lowering treatment

In the authors' clinic the aim is to achieve as much of the above as possible at or after the first visit so that when the patient returns for the second visit a decision can be made as to whether to commence lipid-lowering treatment.

If the patient has newly diagnosed type 2 diabetes it is reasonable to wait to observe whether the target LDL-cholesterol is achieved once glycaemic control improves before considering lipid-lowering treatment.

Questions to answer before deciding whether to prescribe lipid-lowering treatment:

- What is the coronary risk?
- Can the target be reached by dietary means alone or after treating a secondary cause?
- What is the patient's age? At present there is no evidence from clinical trials to suggest benefit in terms of risk reduction by treating patients over 70 years of age, and so lipid-lowering agents should not routinely be prescribed to patients in this age group.
- How motivated is the patient to comply with treatment?
- Is the patient a woman of child-bearing age? The effect of statins and fibrates on the fetus is unknown and therefore it is difficult to justify their use in women of child-bearing age.

Lipid-lowering agents

The main lipid-lowering agents are shown in Box 20.5.

Box 20.5   Lipid-lowering agents

Statins
Simvastatin
Atorvastatin
Fluvastatin
Pravastatin

Resins
Cholestyramine
Colestipol

Nicotinic acid derivatives
Acipimox

Fibrates
Bezafibrate
Fenofibrate
Ciprofibrate

Fish oils
Maxepa

Statins

Statins work by inhibiting 3-hydroxy-3-methylglutaryl coenzyme A (HMGCoA) reductase in the liver and so reduce endogenous cholesterol synthesis. As a result, the LDL-receptor becomes upregulated and LDL-cholesterol is removed from the circulation by the liver. Their predominant effect is to lower LDL-cholesterol (by 20–35%) but atorvastatin has, in addition, a triglyceride-lowering effect. They are usually prescribed as a single dose at night.

Fibrates

Fibrates have a more complex mechanism of action. They increase LPL activity and reduce hepatic production of VLDL. Their predominant effect on serum lipids is to reduce triglyceride (by 30–60%), but they also lower LDL-cholesterol (by 5–25%) and increase HDL-cholesterol (by 10–30%). They are usually prescribed as a single daily dosage.

Resins

Resins act by binding bile acids and so interrupting their entero-hepatic circulation, which causes hepatic cholesterol to be diverted into bile acid synthesis, thus lowering the serum LDL-cholesterol (by 20–25%). The effect of resins is blunted by a compensatory increase in endogenous cholesterol synthesis; however, as they are not systemically absorbed, they are safe in pregnancy and remain the drug of first choice in young children with FH. Although they are also useful in patients who react adversely to statins and fibrates, patient compliance may be poor as they are unpleasant to take.

Fish oils

The fish oil preparation Maxepa is rich in omega-3-triglycerides. Its effect is to lower serum triglyceride levels. Unfortunately, it also has an LDL-cholesterol elevating effect and, for that reason, is best avoided in patients with diabetes.

Nicotinic acid derivatives

The only drug in common use in this group is acipimox. It lowers both LDL-cholesterol (by around 25%) and triglyceride levels (by

20–50%), as a result of decreasing VLDL synthesis, and also elevates HDL-cholesterol levels (by 15–30%). It tends to cause flushing, which may limit its use, but this effect is less marked than with the parent drug nicotinic acid.

Factors influencing the choice of drug

Nature of the hyperlipidaemia.   As a result of clinical trial evidence, statins are the drug of first choice in isolated hypercholesterolaemia.[2] Fibrates are chosen first for hypertriglyceridaemia. In practice, the choice of drug may be limited by factors such as previous adverse effects. Any drug that can enable the patient to achieve the target cholesterol level and which the patient can tolerate on a long-term basis is to be recommended.

The possibility of drug interactions.   Fibrates and statins (with the exception of cerivastatin) potentiate the action of warfarin.

Severity of the hyperlipidaemia.   If the hyperlipidaemia is severe, a more potent agent may be used from the outset.

Previous adverse effects.   Previous adverse effects to a particular agent or class of agents.

Information to give the patient on starting treatment with a lipid-lowering agent

- The aim is to prevent early ischaemic events and death not to relieve symptoms
- The treatment offers risk reduction not risk elimination
- Long-term compliance is essential if benefit is to be obtained in terms of risk reduction
- Lipid-lowering treatment is not a substitute for dietary treatment or lifestyle measures
- There is a possibility of side effects and any that arise should be reported promptly
- Regular follow-up is important in order to monitor progress.

Long-term compliance with lipid-lowering treatment needs considerable motivation on the part of the patient and, while warning patients about the possibility of adverse effects, it is important to keep the input as positive as possible in order to encourage compliance.

Management of hypertriglyceridaemia

As in the case of hypercholesterolaemia, the priority should be to identify and treat any secondary cause before concluding that there is a genetically determined hypertriglyceridaemia. Isolated hypertriglyceridaemia should be treated conservatively if possible and levels up to 4.5 mmol/l should be treated by dietary means. Levels from 4.5 to 11.3 mmol/l may need drug treatment if persistent, and levels above this need immediate treatment to reduce the risk of acute pancreatitis. The aim should be to reduce the fasting serum triglyceride to below 2.3 mmol/l.

Problems in managing patients with hyperlipidaemias

Side effects of lipid-lowering medication

The majority of patients tolerate lipid-lowering agents well on a long-term basis, but a few suffer adverse effects severe enough to warrant discontinuation of the treatment.

Myositis.   Myositis is a common side effect of statins and fibrates. The symptoms range from mild muscle aches to a more severe sensation of burning in the muscles and rhabdomyolysis with renal failure has also been reported. When symptoms are severe there is no difficulty in making the diagnosis, but occasionally it can be difficult to confirm the diagnosis in patients with milder symptoms. Measuring the serum CK level can help confirm the diagnosis. If the level climbs to more than 10 times the upper reference limit, the drug should be discontinued. Myositis is more likely to occur with large doses, with statin/fibrate and statin/cyclosporin combinations and in the presence of renal impairment. Muscle aches can also occur in the absence of biochemical evidence of myopathy.

Sleep disturbance.   Sleep disturbance can occur with the statins. This side effect can sometimes be cured by giving patients their treatment as a morning rather than an evening dose, although the therapeutic effect of the drug is also likely to be less when it is given at this time as most endogenous cholesterol synthesis occurs at night.

Gastrointestinal side effects.   Gastrointestinal side effect are common. They often settle as the patient gains tolerance to the medication and, if the symptoms are mild, it is worth recommending that the patient perseveres with the treatment initially.

Skin rashes and hair loss. Skin rashes and hair loss are more unusual but require discontinuation of the treatment.

Elevation of serum transaminase levels. These can occur with both statins and fibrates. If the serum ALT climbs to more than three times the upper reference limit of normal, then the drug should be discontinued. Serum ALT should be checked 3 months after starting treatment and thereafter at 6-monthly intervals.

Statins and fibrates are contraindicated in severe renal impairment, active liver disease, pregnancy and breast-feeding. They should be used with caution in patients with a past history of liver disease, excessive alcohol intake and in patients with mild renal impairment.

Poor response to lipid-lowering medication

Patients often respond poorly to lipid-lowering treatment. In dealing with this problem, the authors take the approach shown in Figure 20.1.

Combination therapy

Combinations of lipid-lowering agents should only be considered when monotherapy is considered unlikely to enable the patient to achieve target lipid levels and when the patient is believed to be at considerable coronary risk. It is often required in resistant FH. Patients on combination therapy should be followed up regularly in the lipid clinic and not discharged from care. Note that

- Statin/resin is a potent combination, as the two drugs act synergistically.
- Statin/fibrate is also a potent combination but carries an increased risk of myositis. This risk seems greatest in patients taking immunosuppressive therapy

Lipids and diabetes

Sixty per cent of patients with diabetes will die of IHD; therefore, hypercholesterolaemia should be aggressively treated in patients with diabetes.[3] In the non-diabetic population, the presence of IHD increases the risk of a further vascular event and therefore lowers the threshold for lipid-lowering therapy. It is not yet clear whether all patients with diabetes should be treated as for secondary rather than primary prevention.

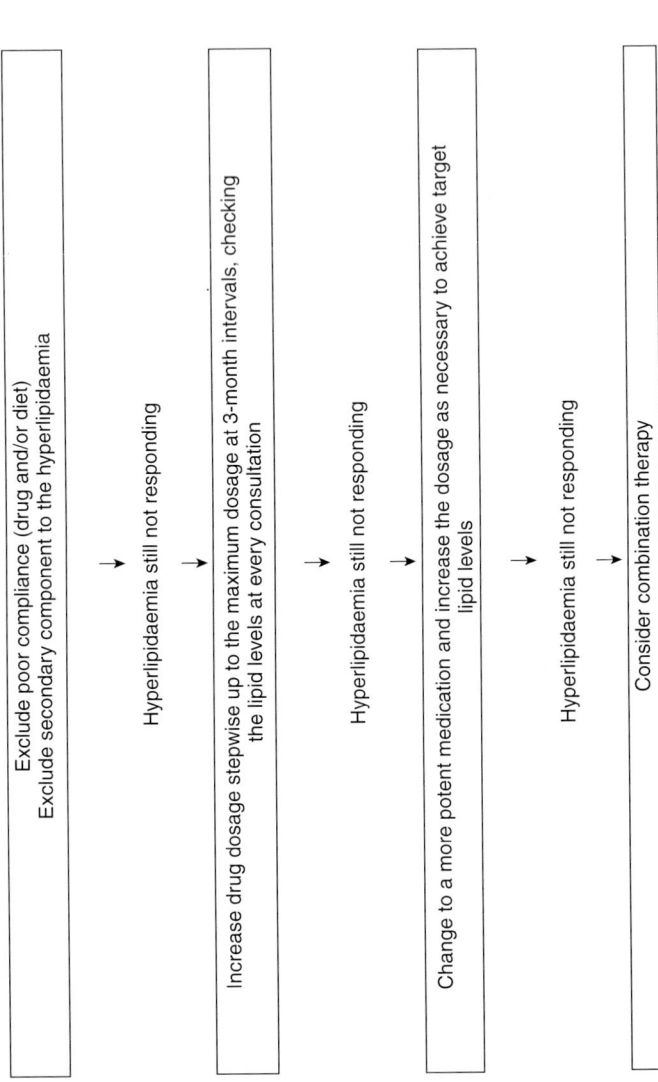

Exclude poor compliance (drug and/or diet)
Exclude secondary component to the hyperlipidaemia

↓

Hyperlipidaemia still not responding

→

Increase drug dosage stepwise up to the maximum dosage at 3-month intervals, checking the lipid levels at every consultation

↓

Hyperlipidaemia still not responding

→

Change to a more potent medication and increase the dosage as necessary to achieve target lipid levels

↓

Hyperlipidaemia still not responding

→

Consider combination therapy

Figure 20.1   Dealing with poor response to lipid-lowering treatment.

In patients with well-controlled type 1 diabetes, the lipids and lipoprotein concentrations are similar to the non-diabetic population; indeed, the HDL-cholesterol may be higher than non-diabetics. Poor glycaemic control is associated with increased concentrations of triglyceride-rich chylomicrons and VLDL. Insulin deficiency and ketosis are associated with lipaemia and chylomicronaemia. Treatment of lipid abnormalities should be aimed at diabetes control, diet and then management similar to that outlined above. The patient is likely to have macrovascular disease and therefore one may be using secondary rather than primary prevention. There is no evidence-based medicine for lipid-lowering specifically in type 1 diabetes mellitus.

Patients with type 2 diabetes have a particularly atherogenic lipoprotein phenotype characterised by small dense LDL particles. This phenotype can be recognised by the combination of:

- hypertriglyceridaemia
- raised LDL-cholesterol
- low HDL-cholesterol.

Treatment is aimed first at diabetes and dietetic control. Many would consider lipid-lowering therapy for all patients with macrovascular disease; there is evidence-based medicine for treatment of those with a cholesterol >5.5 mmol/l. For those without overt macrovascular disease, a high LDL-cholesterol should be treated as in the non-diabetic population. A low HDL-cholesterol should be treated with fibrates. There is evidence-based medicine for the use of fibrates in diabetic dyslipidaemia. In patients who have a serum cholesterol $\geq$5.2 mmol/l or triglyceride $\geq$1.8 mmol/l or HDL-cholesterol <1.1 mmol/l, bezafibrate treatment was associated with less progression of resting ECG (electrocardiographic) changes. There are also data to suggest the use of statins (in the diabetic subgroups of the large statin trials) reduces coronary events in the patients with an LDL-cholesterol >4.5 mmol/l after diet therapy.

Impaired glucose tolerance (IGT)

Impaired glucose tolerance (2-hour glucose after 75 g oral glucose 7.8-11.0 mmol/l) is a risk factor for progression to type 2 diabetes while carrying the same macrovascular risks as diabetes. This is similar to impaired fasting glucose (fasting plasma glucose >6.0 but <7.0 mmol/l) but there is debate whether IFG carries the same macrovascular risk information as the 2-hour glucose in an OGTT.

Clearly, all patients being screened for lipid abnormalities should have a fasting plasma glucose.

Screening

There are clear benefits to secondary prevention; therefore, all patients with an ischaemic event should have lipid estimation and risk factor reduction. The benefits of primary prevention are not so clear; the frequency of screening in particular groups of subjects remains to be delineated.

Further Reading

Detection and management of lipid disorders in diabetes. Consensus statement for American Diabetes Association. *Diabetes Care* 1993,**16**:106–12.

Knopp RH. Drug treatment of lipid disorders. *New Engl J Med* 1999;**341**:498–511.

Scandinavian Simvastatin Survival Study Group. Randomised trial of cholesterol lowering in 4444 patients with coronary heart disease: the Scandinavian simvastatin survival study. *Lancet* 1994,**344**: 633–8.

Shepherd J, Cobbe SM, Ford I *et al.* and WOSCP Study Group. Prevention of coronary heart disease with pravastatin in men with hypercholesterolaemia. *New Engl J Med* 1995;**333**:1301–7.

Wood D, Durrington P, Poulter N *et al.* on behalf of British Cardiac Society, British Hyperlipidaemia Association, British Hypertension Association & British Diabetic Association. Joint British Recommendations on Prevention of Coronary Heart Disease in Clinical Practice. *Heart* 1998;**80** (Suppl 2):S1–S29.

21

Obesity

Shahid T Wahid and Adam CJ Robinson

Introduction

Obesity has been acknowledged as a chronic medical condition with negative health consequences. Currently, 250 million people are regarded as obese, i.e. 7% of the world's population. It is a growing problem in developing countries, as life becomes more sedentary and the diet rapidly undergoes metamorphosis to a 'western style'. Obesity has reached epidemic proportions in childhood, and this can only increase the burden of disease in adulthood. The mainstay of treatment remains dietary and lifestyle modification. Drug treatment has been disappointing, and although surgery can be effective, it is reserved for the very few people where obesity is life threatening in the immediate future.

The pathophysiology of obesity is poorly understood. Adipose tissue is no longer regarded as physiologically inert and is involved in endocrine axes. The discovery of leptin, the cloning of the *ob* gene and the description of cases of isolated leptin deficiency due to genetic mutations, and their subsequent treatment with leptin, have provided valuable insights and stimulated further research into the aetiology of obesity. Figure 21.1 illustrates how leptin is thought to influence body weight: despite the latter, and epidemiological evidence of a strong genetic component to obesity, it is the environmental components that most strongly influence its development. Manipulation of the environment through dietary means and physical exercise are the traditional methods to prevent and treat obesity. At present, pharmacological and surgical interventions should be used in conjunction with the other modalities. We are spectacularly unsuccessful in obesity prevention or treatment.

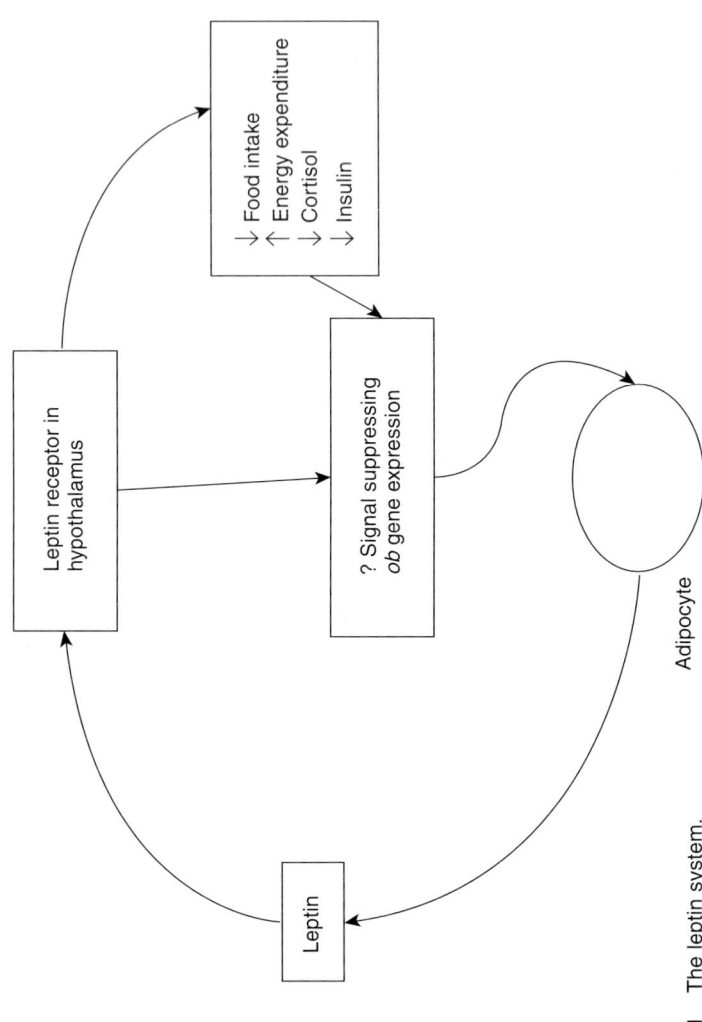

Figure 21.1 The leptin system.

Definition of Obesity

Obesity can be defined clinically as the excess storage of body fat or adipose tissue that leads to a degree of increased mortality and morbidity. The concept of an 'ideal body weight' originated from the Metropolitan Life Insurance studies. These studies demonstrated a j-curve relationship between body weight and mortality. More recently, data from the Nurses Health Study and Harvard Alumni Study suggest a linear relationship between body weight and mortality after correction for pre-existing illness and smoking.

A number of measurements can be used to statistically define obesity (Table 21.1). The original ideal body weight tables were found to be cumbersome, and most clinicians now use the body mass index (BMI) to diagnose obesity. Quetelet, a Belgian astronomer, was the first to note that the weight of adults of normal build was proportional to their height squared, so the index (kg/m^2) is a convenient measure of obesity. A BMI of 20–24.9 is normal; 25–29.9, overweight; 30–34.9, moderately obese; 35–39.9, severely obese; and >40, morbidly obese. An individual who has one other risk factor, for example diabetes or hypertension, and a BMI >27 should be considered moderately obese not overweight.

The distribution of fat can determine the health risks of obesity. Numerous studies have demonstrated that central adipose tissue deposition is associated with more adverse health consequences than peripheral adipose tissue deposition. Commonly used indirect measures of central obesity (Table 21.1) include waist circumference, waist-to-hip ratio (WHR) and the ratio of waist circumference to height (waist/height). These proxy measures have been compared to more direct measures of intra-abdominal visceral fat made by computed tomography (CT) and magnetic resonance imaging (MRI). Waist circumference and WHR are good predictors of intra-abdominal visceral fat, whereas waist : height ratio is better. In the Asian population, BMI underestimates the health risks of obesity, and measures of central obesity should be utilised instead.

Morbidity and Mortality

Large, good-quality studies (Box 21.1) have now demonstrated with certainty an increased mortality in those patients who are not within the ideal BMI of 20–25 kg/m^2. It is still controversial as to whether this relationship is J-shaped, especially since the recently

Table 21.1 Definitions of obesity

Measurement	Definition	Value
1. Body mass index (BMI)	Weight (kg)/height (m²)	> 30 = obese
2. Waist circumference	Mid-point between lower costal margin and the superior iliac crest after a gentle expiration	Men > 92 cm = obese Women > 84 cm = obese
3. Waist-to-hip ratio (WHR)	Waist circumference/hip circumference at level of greater trochanters	Men > 0.95 = obese Woman > 0.8 = obese
4. Waist-to-height ratio	Waist circumference/height	> 0.5 = obese
5. C-index	Abdominal girth (m)/(0.109) $\sqrt{}$ weight (kg)/height (m)	Men > 0.8 = obese Women > 0.7 = obese
6. Skin-fold thickness	Middle of triceps muscle, callipers	Men > 21 mm = obese Women > 31 mm = obese

---

Box 21.1   Studies on obesity

American Cancer Society Study in 1980	760,000 subjects followed for 13 years
The Framingham Study in 1983	5070 subjects followed for 26 years
The Norwegian Experience in 1984	1.7 million subjects followed for 10 years
Hoffmans et al. in 1988	78,612 men followed for 32 years
Rissanen et al. in 1989	22,995 men followed for 12 years
Nurses Health Study in 1990	116,000 nurses followed for 8 years
Calle et al. in 1999	1 million subjects followed for 14 years

---

published findings of Eugenia Calle et al. [1] in one million subjects from the USA have demonstrated a J-shaped relationship not in keeping with the previously cited studies. Some investigators have suggested that this relationship only occurs with respect to cardio-vascular deaths, but is linear when only cancer deaths are considered. Table 21.2 illustrates disease-specific mortality risk due to obesity.

Box 21.2 lists the consequences of obesity that contribute to morbidity. The clustering of hypertension, diabetes, dyslipidaemia and increased procoagulant factors may be explained by the deposition of excess abdominal visceral adipose tissue, i.e. central

Table 21.2   Disease-specific mortality risk due to obesity

Condition	Increased mortality risk	
	Men	Women
Diabetes mellitus	5.2	7.9
Digestive system diseases	4.0	2.3
Coronary heart disease	1.9	2.1
Cerebrovascular disease	2.3	1.5
Malignancy[a]	1.3	1.6

[a]This includes carcinomas of the prostate, colon, rectum, gallbladder, biliary tree, endometrium and cervix.

Box 21.2   Consequences of obesity that contribute to obesity

Hypertension
Diabetes mellitus
Impaired glucose tolerance
Raised serum triglyceride
Low high-density lipoprotein (HDL)-cholesterol
Hyperinsulinaemia and insulin resistance
Raised plasma fibrinogen levels
Raised plasma plasminogen activator inhibitor 1 (PAI-1) levels
Menstrual disturbances
Sleep apnoea

obesity, leading to increased delivery of free fatty acids to the liver via the portal circulation (Figure 21.2).

There is no direct evidence that a reduction in weight into the ideal range results in a reduction in mortality, but co-morbid conditions such as hypertension, diabetes and dyslipidaemia do significantly improve. Indirect evidence that weight loss results in reduced mortality risk is provided by life insurance studies (Table 21.3), which demonstrate that subjects who maintain a weight loss have a lower mortality risk compared with subjects who maintain a weight gain from when the policy was initiated. Surgical results of vertical gastric banding for obesity – the mortality in 787 vertically banded treated patients was one-fifth the mortality of 200 conventionally treated patients in one study – also provide evidence that weight loss is beneficial.

Table 21.3   Mortality ratios and obesity

| | Mortality ratios by duration of policy years | | | |
	1–5	6–10	11–15	16–22
Men 15–69 years				
> 25% underweight	1.27	1.19	1.14	1.05
15–25% overweight	1.06	1.14	1.23	1.31
Women 15–69 years				
> 25% underweight	1.67	1.28	1.34	0.90
15–25% overweight	1.06	1.03	1.13	1.12

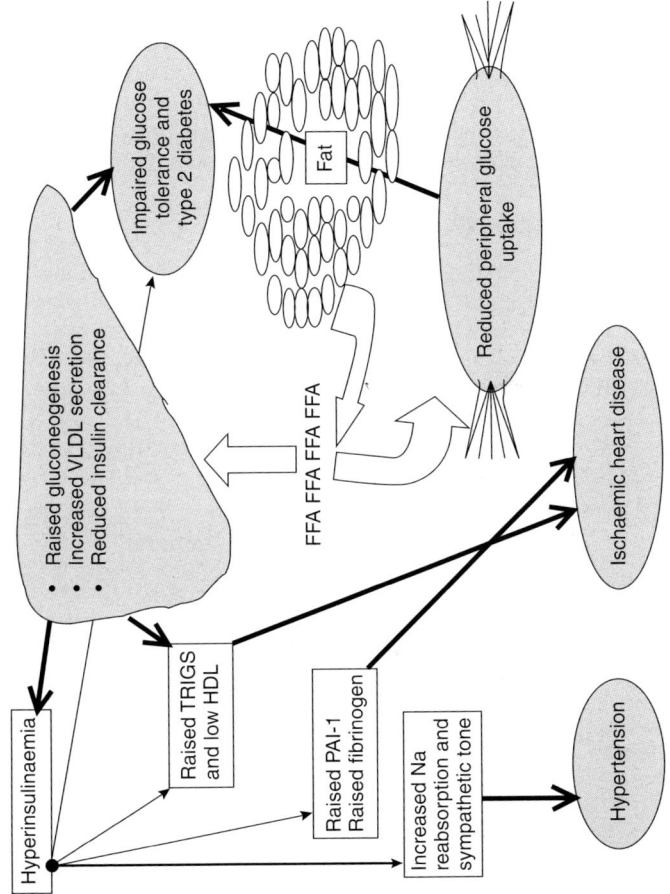

Figure 21.2 Pathophysiological consequences of increased central adiposity.

Epidemiology

Obesity has reached epidemic proportions, with one-third of adults in the USA with a BMI >30 kg/m². In the UK, since 1980 there has been a greater than 100% increase in the prevalence of obesity in the adult population: from 6 to 16% in men and from 8 to 17.5% in women. This trend is mirrored in other countries. The increase in prevalence of obesity has resulted in an increase in co-morbid conditions such as type 2 diabetes mellitus and dyslipidaemia. Health professionals should be very concerned about the increasing prevalence of obesity in childhood, with figures as high as 25% from the USA. This can only have detrimental consequences for the future.

Clinical Aspects

As well as concentrating on weight reduction for obese patients, it is important that a multiple risk factor treatment approach is used (Box 21.3). All patients should be seen and regularly assessed by an experienced dietician. Figure 21.3 suggests an approach to managing patients with obesity. One should be vigilant for any secondary causes of obesity; these are outlined in Box 21.4

Box 21.3   Multiple risk factor treatment

- Regular blood pressure monitoring: aim for systolic < 140 and diastolic < 80 mmHg
- Annual lipid screen: aim for total cholesterol < 5.0, LDL < 3.0, HDL > 1.1 and TRIGS < 2.0 mmol/l
- Discourage smoking: apply active methods such as counselling or nicotine patches
- Encourage moderate alcohol intake: in those with heart disease encourage abstinence
- Be vigilant for diabetes: in those who develop diabetes aim for an HbA_{1c} < 7%
- Be vigilant for ischaemic heart disease: consider an annual ECG, with at least a baseline ECG
- Be vigilant for any psychological complications: actively treat depression
- Discourage added salt to diet: consider salt restriction if hypertension exists

ECG = electrocardiogram; HDL = high-density lipoprotein; LDL = low-density lipoprotein; TRIGS = triglycerides

First consultation
- Calculate BMI and acceptable weight range to achieve a BMI of 20–25
- History & examination: *be vigilant for any complications of obesity and for any secondary causes of obesity (Box 21.4)*
- Initial investigations: *plasma glucose, urea & electrolytes, lipid screen, thyroid function tests and ECG*
- Discuss the importance of weight loss with the patient: *What have they already attempted? Concentrate on positive points*
- Discuss lifestyle measures: *smoking, exercise, alcohol, dietary salt intake*
- Give simple dietary advice: *reduce saturated fats, increase carbohydrates, increase fibre, etc. (Figure 21.4)*

Dietician
- Calculate daily energy expenditure (*Box 21.4*)
- Construct a food diary to assess eating pattern *and modify it if necessary*
- Apply standard dietary guidelines (*Figure 21.4*)
- Arrange a diet whereby the patient reduces daily calorie intake by 500 kcal
- Advise patient that weight loss will be gradual: *1–2 kg per month*
- Arrange regular follow up

Follow up
- Calculate weight and BMI
- Treat any complications uncovered from previous visit (*Box 21.3*)
- Discuss any positive points: *e.g. exercise, stopped smoking, etc.*
- Discuss any negative points: *e.g. binge eating, alcohol, etc.*
- Detailed dietician review: *encourage above points*

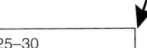

1 BMI 25–30
- Continue to encourage above points: *concentrate on positive points*
- Adapt a multiple risk factor approach (*Box 21.3*)
- Reduce daily calorie intake by 1000 kcal
- Continue regular dietary review

2 BMI 30–40 or BMI 27–35 and any complication
- As in Table 21.1
- Attempt using a very low calorie diet: *this can be alternated with the standard 1000 kcal per day reduction*
- Consider treatment with orlistat: *only if there has been a 2.5 kg weight loss in the previous 4 weeks*
- Consider behavioural therapy

3 BMI >40 or BMI >35 and any complication
- As in Table 21.1 and Box 21.1
- Consider surgical treatment: *vertical gastric banding, gastric balloon, gastrointestinal bypass techniques, jaw wiring*
- Maintain regular review

Figure 21.3 Managing patients with obesity.

Box 21.4   Secondary causes of obesity

Hereditary/congenital
- Prader–Willi syndrome
- Laurence–Moon–Biedl syndrome

Endocrine
- Hypothyroidism
- Cushing's syndrome
- Stein–Leventhal syndrome

Drug-induced
- Corticosteroids
- Phenothiazines: *haloperidol, chlorpromazine, thioridazine*
- Antiepileptics: *sodium valproate*
- Lithium
- Tricyclic antidepressants: *amitriptyline, clomipramine*
- Monoamine oxidase antidepressants: *phenelzine, tranylcypromine*

Hypothalamic damage
- Trauma
- Tumour
- Radiation

Dietary Therapy

Dietary manipulation is the cornerstone of treatment for obesity. All health professionals should be aware of the general dietary guidelines, as illustrated in Figure 21.4, and be able to offer simple advice to patients using these guidelines. Input from an experienced dietician is essential. It is important to note that obese subjects have a raised basal metabolic rate, necessitating a large intake of food to satisfy their raised energy requirements. It has been shown that a steady weight loss of 1–2 kg/month can be achieved by reducing an obese subject's daily calorie intake by 500 kcal, and a higher rate of weight loss can be achieved by targeting a 1000 kcal/day reduction. A very low calorie diet (VLCD) targets a total daily calorie intake of 1000 kcal, but used alone this can be dangerous and often leads to rapid weight gain – after cessation. VLCDs can be alternated with the standard 500 kcal/day reduction – for example, the first 3 weeks of every month – and this often achieves reasonable results. It is essential to calculate an obese patient's daily energy requirements (Box 21.5), and tailor a diet to suit the individual that achieves her

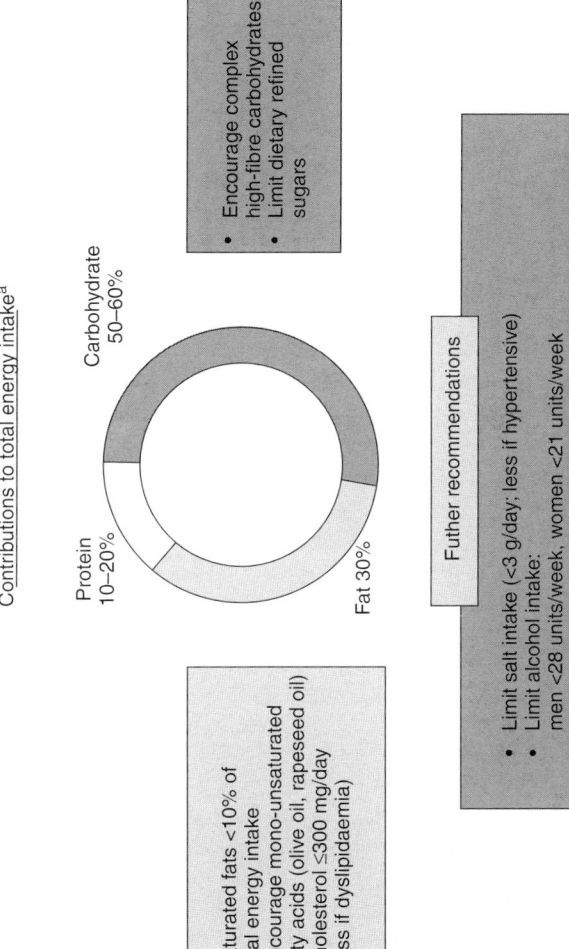

Contributions to total energy intake[a]

Carbohydrate 50–60%

Protein 10–20%

Fat 30%

- Encourage complex high-fibre carbohydrates
- Limit dietary refined sugars

- Saturated fats <10% of total energy intake
- Encourage mono-unsaturated fatty acids (olive oil, rapeseed oil)
- Cholesterol ≤300 mg/day (less if dyslipidaemia)

Futher recommendations

- Limit salt intake (<3 g/day; less if hypertensive)
- Limit alcohol intake: men <28 units/week, women <21 units/week less if hypertensive or dyslipidaemic
- If diabetic avoid 'diabetic foods'

Figure 21.4 General dietary guidelines. [a]Endorsed by Diabetes UK and American Diabetes Association.

Box 21.5 Formulae for estimating basal metabolic rate (BMR) and total 24-hour energy expenditure

Basal metabolic rate (MJ/day)

Men

Age (years)

18–30 (weight x 0.063) + 2.896

31–60 (weight x 0.048) + 3.653   } x

> 60   (weight x 0.040) + 2.459

Women

Age (years)

18–30 (weight x 0.062) + 2.036

31–60 (weight x 0.034) + 3.538   } x

> 60   (weight x 0.038) + 2.755

Physical activity multiplier

Activity

Light   1.55

Moderate   1.79   } = 24-hour energy

Heavy   2.10   expenditure (MJ/day)

Activity

Light   1.56

Moderate   1.64   } = 24-hour energy

Heavy   1.82   expenditure (MJ/day)

Weight is in kilograms. 10 MJ = 2400 kcal. The physical activity multiplier assumes that at least light activity is undertaken. A reduction of 15% in total 24-hour energy expenditure should be made for those who are very sedentary. Adapted from FAO/WHO/UNO. Energy and protein requirements. Technical report series, Vol. 724. Geneva: WHO, 1985.

target weight. It is at this point that a dietician is invaluable, and Figure 21.4 illustrates a standard approach that is used in managing obesity by dieticians. It is often useful that a doctor is able to give sound dietary advice based on foodstuffs and not just based on calories (Box 21.6). Finally, it should be made clear that the patient may feel hungry and that the changes to diet are for life.

The causes of non-compliance in dietary therapy are complex, and include:

1. poor education and insufficient explanation about the importance and rationale of dietary changes
2. unrealistic expectations and disappointment about the rate of weight loss and the time required to reach the target weight
3. prescription of a diet that the patient finds unpalatable, unsatisfying or too expensive
4. overeating and craving for sweet foods in patients who are trying to stop smoking at the same time.

Box 21.6   Practical food recommendations for patients with obesity

- Quench thirst with water or other sugar-free drinks
- Eat regular meals: avoid fried and very sugary foods
- Eat plenty of vegetables
- Have cereals, bread, pasta, potato, pasta, rice or chapattis as the main part of each meal
- Eat meat, egg, cheese as a small part of each meal
- Encourage fruit and vegetables, including pulses
- Eat double helpings of vegetables as part of every main meal
- Bread, cereal, pasta or potatoes should form the largest part of each meal or snack
- Meat, fish, cheese or eggs should form only a small part of main meals (e.g. one-quarter of the area of the plate)
- Fish and pulses (e.g. beans) are good alternatives
- For snacks between meals, avoid convenience foods such as biscuits, cake or confectionery (which are high in saturated and *trans*-fatty acids, glucose and salts)
- Use fats and oils that are low in saturated and *trans*-fatty acids (e.g. olive oil), or reduced fat dairy products
- Avoid spreads on bread
- Drink water, tea, coffee, milk and low-calorie beverages and avoid sugary drinks and alcohol, especially between meals

The management of non-compliance is difficult and often unsuccessful. Direct confrontation and accusations of cheating should be avoided, but the patient is not helped by the bland acceptance by the health professional that slimming instructions are being rigidly followed. Dietary advice should be simplified rather than made more detailed once the patient has 'failed to comply'. It is more constructive to concentrate on the steps that a patient has already taken, rather than those not taken, with a view to encouraging further action. Various behavioural approaches can be attempted, such as a 'contract' or 'cash payment and reward'.

Exercise

The role of exercise in the treatment of obesity must not be under-estimated. A structured exercise programme along with dietary therapy is a lot more effective than dietary treatment alone. In mild exercise, skeletal muscle uses plasma non-esterified fatty acids (NEFA) to provide fuel but, with moderate exercise, its metabolism switches to utilise the muscle's own triglyceride. Glycogen becomes the major fuel, as exercise becomes more strenuous. In humans, 30 min of exercise at half-maximum capacity will consume about 0.8 MJ (200 kcal) of energy. Obese individuals preferentially preserve their fat stores, as they tend to rely more on carbohydrate oxidation to fuel exercise than do lean individuals. Exercise training increases the proportion of insulin-sensitive fibres in muscle as well as increasing fat oxidative enzyme activity, and both these changes favour the utilisation of fat as fuel. Exercise enhances lipolysis by improving tissue sensitivity to cate-cholamines, and this provides more NEFA for skeletal muscle use. Exercises also alter food selection, in that preference for carbohy-drates over fat increases as energy expenditure increases. This physiological explanation of the benefits of exercise for weight loss does not help the patient. All obese patients should be advised to undertake half an hour of moderate exercise per day, via simple activities such as walking to work or 'walking the dog'. More stren-uous activity such as swimming should also be encouraged. As the severity of obesity increases, common sense needs to be applied; exercise is of most benefit when BMI <35, due to the physics involved in exercising with a large amount of weight. Clearly, co-morbidity must be taken into account when advising on exercise programmes: precautions may be indicated, for instance, in the presence of ischaemic heart disease.

Pharmacological Therapy

The pharmacological treatment of obesity can be classified by the mechanism of drug action (Box 21.7), or it can be categorised into whether the drug reduces energy intake (dexfenfluramine), increases energy expenditure (β_3-adrenoreceptor agonists) or reduces absorption of nutrients (orlistat). Currently, only orlistat (tetrahydrolipstatin) and sibutramine are licensed for use in treating obesity.

Box 21.7 Mechanism of drug action

1 **Central serotonergic appetite suppressants**
 • Dexfenfluramine
 • Fenfluramine ⎤ Recently withdrawn because of
 • Phentermine ⎦ increased risk of heart valve fibroses

2 **Central serotonergic and noradrenergic appetite suppressants**
 • Sibutramine

3 **Thermogenic agents**
 • β_3-Adrenoreceptor agonists, e.g. CL 316, 243:
  Initial promising results from animal studies have not been duplicated in human subjects, but with the recent cloning of the β_3-adrenoreceptor gene more highly selective compounds can be produced

4 **Intestinal lipase inhibitors**
 • Tetrahydrolipstatin: see text (orlistat)

5 **Bulking agents**
 • Guar gum ⎤ Ineffective
 • Methylcellulose ⎦

Orlistat

Orlistat is a fungal-derived specific long-acting intestinal lipase inhibitor that reduces intestinal fat absorption by one-third. Recent randomised, double-blind, placebo-controlled trials have demonstrated the benefit of orlistat used in conjunction with a hypocaloric (low-fat) diet in facilitating weight reduction and the long-term maintenance of this weight loss. Orlistat resulted in a 5% weight loss compared with 3.5% in those patients receiving placebo ($p = 0.009$) in the short term, and this weight loss was maintained after 2 years in 74% of those patients receiving orlistat compared with 57% of those receiving placebo ($p = 0.039$). Orlistat also has beneficial effects on the lipid profile compared with placebo: total cholesterol and low-density lipoprotein (LDL)-cholesterol reduced by 6.5% and 9.7%, respectively ($p = 0.002$) vs placebo. It should be noted that the beneficial effects of orlistat are only observed at its top dose of 120 mg three times a day Approximately 7% of patients do not tolerate this dose because of severe gastrointestinal side effects, which include abdominal pain, flatus with discharge, fatty/oily evacuation and faecal incontinence. These side effects can be reduced by reducing dietary fat content to 60 g/day, administering the tablet 2 hours before food or encouraging perseverance as the side effects diminish in severity by 6 months in the majority of patients. Malabsorption of fat-soluble vitamins may occur and, indeed, diabetic patients receiving orlistat should be prescribed multivitamins. Currently, orlistat should only be prescribed to obese patients with a BMI >30, or >27 and at least one risk factor, who have managed to lose at least 2.5 kg in weight (or 5% of their initial body weight) over a preceding period of 4 consecutive weeks while on a hypocaloric diet. It can be continued for up to 2 years. It is important that the latter is used in conjunction with a hypocaloric diet, and that regular dietetics follow-up is maintained.

Sibutramine

Sibutramine inhibits the re-uptake of neurotransmitters that control food intake (serotonin and noradrenaline). This has shown to be an effective aid to weight reduction and weight maintenance by helping patients to feel satisfied with smaller portions of food, so they eat less. Sibutramine may have effects on increasing energy expenditure through stimulation of the sympathetic nervous system and increased thermogenesis. This has been demonstrated in rodents, but not confirmed in humans. Sibutramine has no effect on adrenaline-induced energy expenditure; therefore, the effect is probably central rather than peripheral. Sibutramine, unlike dexfenfluramine, does not enhance neural release of noradrenaline or serotonin.

Change in absolute weight, percentage and BMI at both 10 and 15 mg of sibutramine combined with diet and exercise are demonstrated to be statistically superior to placebo combined with diet and exercise. These effects have been demonstrated for periods up to and including 24 months. Clinically, relevant weight loss of between 5 and 10% of baseline is achieved in long-term trials. Weight loss after dieting can also be maintained. Studies have also been performed in patients with co-morbid conditions, dyslipidaemia, type 2 diabetes and hypertension.

Weight loss is not essential before treatment, unlike orlistat. A concern is with an increase in blood pressure, which has now been further investigated in a meta-analysis. At 10 mg dose, there is no significant change in blood pressure. At 15 mg dose, there is an average 1 mmHg increase in blood pressure. However, in patients who lose weight, blood pressure is decreased: e.g. in those who have lost 10% of weight, the blood pressure falls 2.7/1.0. Therefore, one would recommend that all patients starting sibutramine have blood pressure checks. However, this is not a long-term concern, because sibutramine would not be continued if patients do not lose weight. If patients are losing weight, they can expect a significant fall in blood pressure.

Surgical Treatment

Surgical treatment should be offered to those patients with very severe obesity: BMI > 40, or BMI > 35 and at least one risk factor. Over the years a number of surgical options have been utilised:

1. *Jaw wiring and nylon waist cord.* Both of these techniques should be used in tandem. Jaw wiring can result in effective initial, waist loss: in one trial of 101 patients, an average weight loss of 52.6 kg over 1 year was achieved. But, once the wiring is removed, weight is rapidly regained, and to prevent this rebound a nylon waist cord, which tightens as weight is regained – reminding the patient to eat less – can be utilised.

2. *Gastric volume reduction procedures.* A balloon can be inserted into the stomach, reducing gastric volume and resulting in the patient eating smaller amounts to avoid feeling 'full'. But complications such as balloon puncture, stomach ulceration and stomach wall erosion are not uncommon. Vertical banded gastroplasty can be used to provide the same mechanism of weight loss, but with lower rates of complications. This involves the construction of a small stomach pouch with a volume of 10–15 ml using vertical stapling and restricting the outlet to 9–12 mm diameter, reinforced with non-absorbable mesh. In one trial, which utilised the latter, an average 36 kg in

weight was lost over 1 year, with only 5 kg regained by 3 years. Gastric banding has also been used in the past. This involves pinching off a small part of the upper stomach with a Dacron-type band.

3. *Gastric bypass (Roux-en-Y).* This involves bypassing the distal stomach, duodenum and upper jejunum by creating a stomach pouch with a volume <30 ml by stapling across the stomach and then connecting a piece of small intestine as a conduit for food. This procedure results in the most effective weight loss compared with other procedures, with up to 92% of excessive weight lost at 18 months. But, this has to be balanced with this operation's higher risk of nutritional deficiencies.

4. *Laparoscopic banded gastroplasty (LBG)* has emerged as the safest most effective technique in the treatment of, especially, morbid obesity. The stomach volume is effectively reduced to 10 ml with an inflatable cuff. This is re-filled with an external catheter port: the procedure is reversible without additional surgery. Dietetic advice through the treatment is essential. The largest series from France has had no postoperative deaths; 11 of 300 subjects needed conversion to laparotomy. After the first 50 procedures, the complication rate was 5%. Eighty per cent of patients lost up to 60% of their excess weight.

Surgery should not be taken lightly because of the high peri-operative mortality risk associated with obesity and its related conditions, and informed consent by an experienced physician, surgeon and anaesthetist is essential. Long-term outcomes from pharmacological or surgical treatment of obesity are not available.

Conclusion

Obesity is now widely accepted as a chronic disease with genetic and neurological associations rather than a state resulting from lack of will power. The prevention of obesity may require more novel approaches on a nationwide basis, whereas pharmacological treatment of obesity is likely to change considerably over the next decade.

Further Reading

Calle EE, Thun MJ, Petrelli JM, Rodriguez C, Heath CW Jr. Body-mass index and mortality in a prospective cohort of U.S. adults. *New Engl J Med* 1999;**341**:1097–105.

Garfinkel L. Cancer mortality in on-smokers: prospective study by the American Cancer Society. *J Natl Can Inst* 1980;**65**:1169–73.

Hoffmans MD, Kromhout D, de Lezenne Coulander C. The impact of body mass index of 78,612 18-year-old Dutch men on 32-year mortality from all causes. *J Clin Epidemiol* 1988;**41**:749–56.

Hubert HB, Feinlab M, McNamara PM, Castelli WP. Obesity as an independent risk factor for cardiovascular disease: a 26-year follow-up of participants in the Framingham Heart Study. *Circulation* 1983;**67**:968–72.

James WPT, Astrup A, Finer N *et al.* Effect of sibutramine on weight maintenance after weight loss: a randomised trial. *Lancet* 2000;**356**:2119–25.

Kopleman PG. Investigation of obesity. *Clin Endocrinol* 1994;**41**:703–8.

Mallarkey G. *Managing Obesity.* Auckland (NZ): Adis International, 1999.

Manson JE, Colditz GA, Stampfer MJ *et al.* A prospective study of obesity and risk of coronary heart disease in women. *N Engl J Med* 1990;**322**:882–9.

Rissanen A, Heliovaara M, Knekt P *et al.* Weight and mortality in Finnish men. *J Clin Epidemiol* 1989;**42**:781–9.

Schauer PR, Ikramuddin S. Laparoscopic surgery for morbid obesity. *Surg Clin North Am* 2001;**81**:1145–79.

Sjostrom L, Rissanen A, Andersen T *et al.* Randomised placebo-controlled trial of orlistat for weight loss and prevention of weight regain in obese patients. *Lancet* 1998;**352**:167–72.

Stunkard JA, Wadden TA. *Obesity, Theory and Therapy.* Philadelphia (USA): Lippincott-Raven, 1998.

Waaler HT. Height, weight and mortality. The Norwegian experience. *Acta Med Scand* 1984;**679**(suppl):1–56.

22

Hyperaldosteronism

Miles J Levy and Karim Meeran

Introduction

Hypertension is a common disorder affecting up to 25% of the general population. The prevalence depends on the definition used: indeed the normal distribution for blood pressure demonstrates no clear cut-off for normality and abnormality. There is uncertainty regarding which hypertensive patients should be screened for endocrine disease. The incidence of hypertension due to known secondary endocrine causes is between 2 and 5%, although many endocrine causes may be undiagnosed. The combination of an adrenal tumour with hypertension may require further investigation. If an adrenal tumour is found by chance in the absence of hypertension (e.g. when scanning the chest or abdomen in search of malignancy or to document lung pathology), the probability of it being functional is small. To exclude a functioning adrenal tumour, Cushing's syndrome (Chapter 5), Conn's syndrome (this chapter) and a phaeochromocytoma (Chapter 23) must be excluded. This can be most easily performed by sending 24-hour urine samples for catecholamines, urinary-free cortisol and urinary aldosterone.

Aldosterone

Aldosterone is a mineralocorticoid steroid produced by the zona glomerulosa of the adrenal gland. Glucocorticoids are secreted predominantly by the zona fasciculata. Aldosterone acts on type 1 mineralocorticoid receptors to promote sodium transfer across epithelial cells. An increase in aldosterone production or action causes hypertension by increased sodium and water retention by the kidney, and expansion of the extracellular fluid compartment.

The production of aldosterone is mainly kept under control by the renin–angiotensin (R–A) system (Figure 22.1). Activation of the R–A system is a normal physiological response to low sodium intake or hypovolaemia, and results in the production of angiotensin II. Angiotensin II causes release of aldosterone from the zona glomerulosa of the adrenal. Pharmacological disruption of this system with angiotensin-converting enzyme (ACE) inhibitors and angiotensin II receptor antagonists is widely used in antihypertensive treatment.

Changes in sodium and potassium concentration have a direct effect on the responsiveness of the adrenal gland to angiotensin II. Andrenocorticotrophic hormone (ACTH) also stimulates secretion of aldosterone, but the main physiological stimulus is angiotensin II.

Mineralocorticoids are secreted in far smaller quantities than glucocorticoids; the daily secretion of cortisol from the zona fasciculata is approximately 10–20 mg compared with 100–150 µg of aldosterone from the zona glomerulosa. The mineralocorticoid receptor itself is non-selective. Specificity of mineralocorticoids for their receptor is based on metabolism of cortisol to cortisone by 11β–hydroxysteroid dehydrogenase type 2 of target tissues such as the distal convoluted tubule, allowing aldosterone to be the major agonist at the receptor. This mechanism is overwhelmed in the presence of excess glucocorticoid (e.g. Cushing's syndrome).

Hyperaldosteronism

Mineralocorticoids cause hypertension by increasing sodium and water retention by the kidney, thereby expanding the extracellular fluid compartment and suppressing the plasma renin activity (PRA). The first step in investigating the cause of hyperaldosteronism is to determine if the hyperaldosteronism is primary or secondary. PRA must be assessed with aldosterone in order to describe the appropriateness of the aldosterone (Figure 22.1). PRA is a good marker of fluid status, and is used in both the diagnosis and surveillance of therapy in both hypoadrenalism and hyperaldosteronism. A low PRA indicates hypervolaemia and vice versa.

Secondary hyperaldosteronism (Table 22.1) occurs in conditions where renin production is increased as a physiological response to the underlying pathology, and the subsequent increase in aldosterone is appropriate. Examples include renovascular hypertension and renal artery stenosis. In this situation, aldosterone production is driven by a high plasma renin and is suppressed by volume expan-

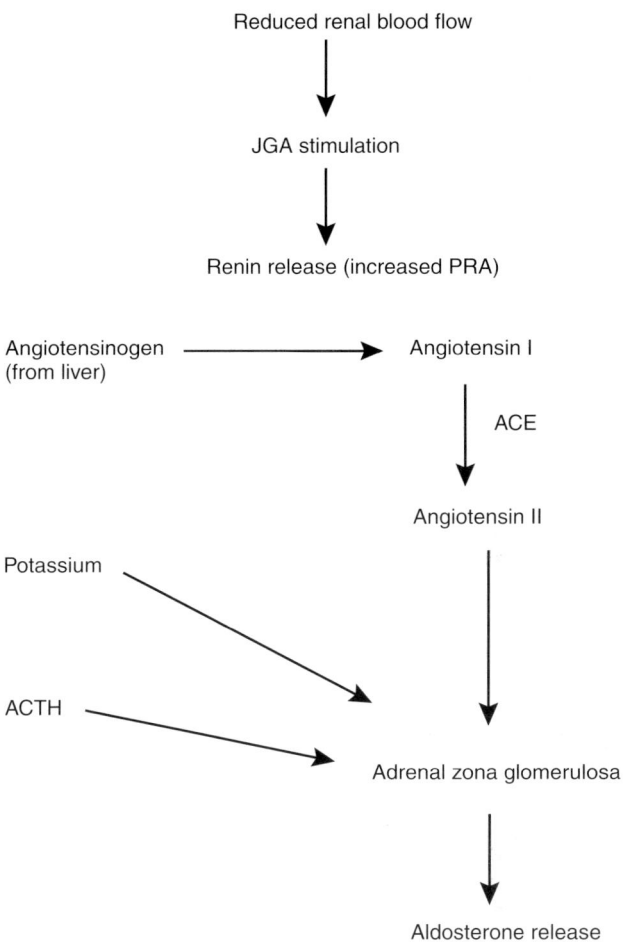

Figure 22.1 Aldosterone secretion is mainly controlled by the renin–angiotensin (R–A) system. Activation of the R–A system is a normal physiological response to low sodium intake or hypovolaemia, and results in the production of angiotensin II. Angiotensin II causes release of aldosterone from the zona glomerulosa of the adrenal. This then affects osmolality through sodium retention. Changes in osmolality do not directly affect aldosterone secretion. Antidiuretic hormone causes water retention (Chapter 18). ACE = angiotensin-converting enzyme; ACTH = adrenocorticotrophic hormone; JGA = juxta glomerular apparatus; PRA = plasma renin activity.

Table 22.1   Secondary vs primary hyperaldosteronism

Secondary hyperaldosteronism (PRA high), causes	Primary hyperaldosteronism (PRA low), causes
Renovascular disease	Aldosterone-producing adenoma (APA)
Congestive cardiac failure (CCF)	Idiopathic hyperaldosteronism (IHA)
Cirrhosis	Adrenal carcinoma
Nephrotic syndrome	Ovarian carcinoma
	Genetic causes

sion. The presence of high aldosterone and high renin may also be seen in patients with CCF, cirrhosis or nephrotic syndrome.

Primary hyperaldosteronism is due to the presence of autonomous aldosterone synthesis. As a result, PRA is low. Unlike secondary hyperaldosteronism, increased sodium intake or volume expansion does not suppress aldosterone secretion.

Primary Hyperaldosteronism

Aldosterone-producing adenoma (APA)

The most common cause of primary hyperaldosteronism results from an aldosterone-producing adenoma (APA) as described by Conn in 1955: they account for approximately 60–70% of mineralocorticoid-induced hypertension. APAs are usually small (0.5–2.0 cm), benign, and have a yellow colour macroscopically. The adenoma gives rise to autonomous aldosterone secretion, which usually fails to respond to an increase in PRA, during either upright posture or infusion of angiotensin II; thus, aldosterone is secreted independently from the R–A system.

Idiopathic hyperaldosteronism (IHA)

Idiopathic hyperaldosteronism (IHA), mostly related to bilateral hyperplasia, is less common and is characterised by non-adenomatous hyperplasia and low PRA. The adrenal gland usually responds to angiotensin II. IHA accounts for approximately 30–40% of primary hyperaldosteronism. The cause of IHA is unknown, but genetic analysis of these patients shows an increase in aldosterone synthase activity secondary to altered regulation of this enzyme. The syndrome of IHA has much phenotypic variation, and represents a spectrum of disease. In a minority of cases, the typical R–A responsiveness is not seen and a subgroup of IHA mimics an APA because it is independent of the R–A system. Conversely, 20% of APAs are responsive to small increases in angiotensin and are therefore affected by changes in posture. The clinical and biochemical diversity of this syndrome is important to recognise as it has implications in deciding on medical or surgical treatment. Generally, R–A unresponsive lesions are best treated surgically, and R–A responsive lesions are best treated medically.

The remaining causes of primary hyperaldosteronism include adrenal carcinoma, ovarian carcinoma and specific genetic conditions which, although rare, provide an important insight into the molecular basis for hypertensive disease and are therefore discussed at the end of the chapter.

Clinical features

The clinical features of primary hyperaldosteronism are generally nonspecific. Some patients are completely asymptomatic: others complain of tiredness, muscle weakness, thirst, polyuria, and nocturia due to hypokalaemia. APAs are more common in females, whereas IHAs are more common in males. APAs occur in a younger age group than IHAs.

Biochemical features

Routine laboratory data are rarely diagnostic of primary hyperaldosteronism. Up to 40% of patients with surgically confirmed primary hyperaldosteronism will have had a normal serum potassium concentration: therefore, only screening for the condition when the potassium concentration is low will miss many cases. Patients with APAs tend to have a lower potassium than IHA, although there is considerable overlap. In one study the mean pre-treatment potassium was 3.0 mmol/l and 3.5 mmol/l in APA and IHA, respectively. Hypokalaemia can be accentuated or induced in normokalaemic patients by oral sodium loading. Often, severe diuretic-induced hypokalaemia is a presentation of hyperaldosteronism. Increased urinary potassium excretion (> 30 mmol/day) in the presence of hypokalaemia is suggestive of the presence of primary hyperaldosteronism.

Screening

Hypertensive patients with spontaneous or profound diuretic-induced hypokalaemia, young hypertensive subjects, patients with a strong family history of hypertension and those with refractory hypertension should be screened.

The random aldosterone/renin ratio can be used in the outpatient setting. The posture is not important to the screening test, but in order to help differentiate APA from IHA the supine/ambulant test is used (see below). Spironolactone should be discontinued 6 weeks prior to the investigation and calcium channel blockers 2 weeks before. Alpha-blockers are ideal therapy during this investigation. The patient should be potassium replete before investigation.

An aldosterone: PRA ratio of >2000 is highly suggestive of primary hyperaldosteronism, a ratio of >1000 is suggestive and a ratio <800 excludes primary hyperaldosteronism (PHA). For the diagnosis of PHA, the PRA should be <0.5 pmol/ml/h (reference range 0.5–3.1 pmol/ml/h) and aldosterone >250 pmol/l (reference range 100–800 pmol/l).

Once the diagnosis of primary hyperaldosteronism has been confirmed, the main differential diagnosis is between APA and IHA (Table 22.2). Because of the increasing incidence of adrenal 'incidentalomas', it is preferable to make a biochemical diagnosis first. Moreover, the biochemical behaviour has more implications on the appropriate subsequent management than the radiological appearance. Box 22.1 illustrates the investigation of adrenal incidentalomas.

The postural test

Patients with APAs secrete aldosterone autonomously and do not respond to the R–A axis, whereas IHAs are typically R–A responsive. In normal individuals, the change from supine to erect posture causes activation of the R–A system and a subsequent increase in aldosterone concentration.

Table 22.2   Differences between IHA and APA

Idiopathic hyperaldosteronism (IHA)	Aldosterone-producing adenoma (APA)
Bilateral	Unilateral
R–A responsive	R–A unresponsive
Medical management	Surgical management

IHAs may behave like APAs.

Box 22.1. Adrenal incidentalomas

With increasing use of abdominal imaging, incidental adrenal adenomata are reported, resulting in referral to an endocrinologist. In general, if the mass is greater than 5 cm in diameter, then the risk of malignancy would encourage surgical removal. Minimum endocrine investigations include:

- 24-hour catecholamines (essential prior to surgery)
- 24-hour urine free cortisol (to exclude Cushing's syndrome)
- Testosterone
- Electrolytes and further full Conn's syndrome investigations only if indicated by low potassium concentration and hypertension. We DO NOT recommend full Conn's syndrome investigations in all adrenal incidentalomas

---

The postural test (Figure 22.2) involves keeping the patient in bed overnight or after 30 min supine in the morning and measuring serum aldosterone concentration, PRA and cortisol at 09.00. The tests are repeated at 12.00 after patient ambulant for at least 60 min. If aldosterone levels decrease, or fail to increase, a lack of R–A responsiveness is indicated, which suggests the presence of an APA. The change in aldosterone in these cases will be parallel with changes in serum cortisol concentration and, therefore, it is essential to measure the latter concurrently. This is important as aldosterone levels may be increased due to a rise in ACTH as part of the stress response, rather than as a response to the R–A axis and may lead to false-positive results if not considered.

In patients with IHAs, the change from lying to standing leads to a physiological increase in aldosterone, in keeping with the typical response to the R–A axis. The postural test is reported to have approximately 85% sensitivity and 80% specificity. Unfortunately, approximately 20% of IHAs are R–A unresponsive, mimicking APAs. In these cases, further investigation is required.

The 3-day sodium loading test is used in some units in order to confirm a diagnosis suspected on screening.

C18-oxymetabolites

Levels of C18-oxymetabolites of cortisol are the most abundant urinary free steroid in patients with primary hyperaldosteronism.

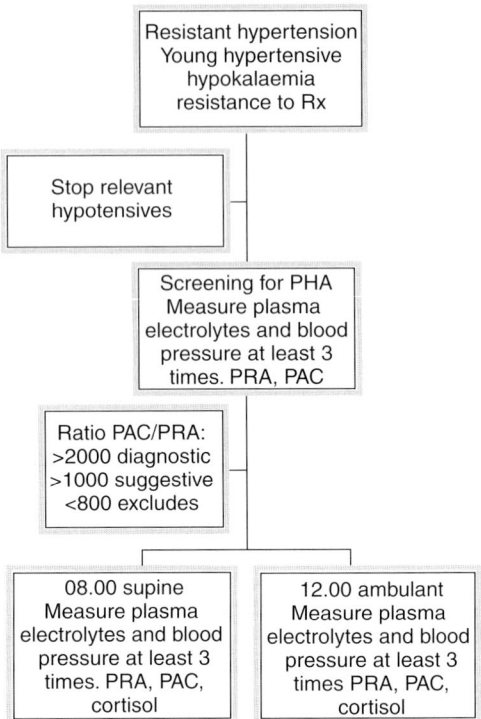

Figure 22.2   Screening for primary hyperaldosteronism and differential diagnosis of APA and IHA. (For abbreviations, see list on pages xv–xviii.)

Both plasma and urine levels are high in APAs, and higher in cases of glucocorticoid-suppressible hyperaldosteronism.

The 18-hydroxylase enzyme is usually found exclusively in the zona glomerulosa, and does not usually act on cortisol. It is thought that the loss of normal functional zonation of the enzyme is responsible for its action on cortisol in these conditions. Urinary excretion of 18-oxocortisol of >18 μg/day and 18-hydroxycortisol of >60 μg/day is thought to distinguish APAs from IHAs with a high degree of sensitivity. 18-Oxymetabolites are not uncommonly raised in secondary hyperaldosteronism, so it is important to exclude this by showing a suppressed PRA.

Imaging

Biochemical data should give a strong indication of the cause of primary hyperaldosteronism. Radiological investigations are used as an attempt to localise the site of mineralocorticoid excess. Although it is essential in the management of mineralocorticoid hypertension, imaging does not confirm primary hyperaldosteronism or its cause. Up to 10% of normal individuals may have adrenal incidentalomas.

Computed tomography (CT) scanning can detect most APAs, which will typically show a unilateral lesion although bilateral nodules may be present. Further confusion arises from the fact that IHAs, although typically showing bilateral enlarged adrenal glands, may occasionally have unilaterally dominant nodules. If imaging shows a particularly large lesion (>3 mm diameter), then the possibility of adrenal carcinoma should be considered. Magnetic resonance imaging (MRI) can also be used but does not have distinct advantages over CT in imaging of cortical, as opposed to medullary, adrenal lesions.

Some centres also use adrenal scintigraphy studies using radiolabelled iodocholesterol or selenium, which may be particularly useful for demonstrating unilateral uptake in an adenoma. Selenium has recently (July 2001) been withdrawn from commercial synthesis.

Selective adrenal vein sampling

This technique is useful in the differential diagnosis of primary hyperaldosteronism. Studies suggest approximately 95% sensitivity and specificity. Selective adrenal vein sampling can be performed in order to localise the site (i.e. left or right) of the lesion in primary hyperaldosteronism. Most unilateral lesions will be APA but occasionally IHA. Cortisol and aldosterone are measured to confirm adrenal vein cannulation. It may be technically difficult to cannulate the left adrenal vein, as it drains into the left renal vein. The right adrenal vein drains directly into the inferior vena cava, and so is easier to cannulate.

Treatment

The most important decision to be made is whether surgical or medical management is most appropriate. Generally, patients with APAs are treated surgically and IHAs are treated medically.

However, the subset of IHAs which show functional lateralisation may be treated surgically; this is true even when an adrenal tumour is not apparent radiologically. Laparoscopic adrenalectomy is generally accepted as the optimum procedure in experienced hands.

Potassium replacement should be given in an attempt to normalise plasma potassium concentrations. Patients should be given at least 2–3 weeks of spironolactone therapy preoperatively. This helps potassium replacement and reduces postoperative hypoaldosteronism.

Surgery alone cures hypertension in less than 50% of cases, and subsequent medical therapy is often required. Previous studies have shown that curative surgery is more likely in younger patients with higher preoperative aldosterone levels and lower PRA. Following surgery, most patients will not need potassium replacement.

The optimum medical treatment for IHA is spironolactone, an aldosterone antagonist. Spironolactone has dose-dependent side effects, which may preclude its use. These include gynaecomastia, menstrual irregularities, impotence and fatigue. If side effects are not tolerated, then other potassium sparing agents, such as amiloride or triamterene, should be used. Calcium antagonists and ACE inhibitors may be useful alone, or in combination with potassium sparing agents.

Glucocorticoid-suppressible hyperaldosteronism (GSH)

GSH is an autosomal dominant condition characterised by primary hyperaldosteronism, which is controlled by the corticotrophin axis rather than the R–A system. This lack of negative feedback of aldosterone on the R–A system leads to an uncontrolled elevation of aldosterone. Normal control in the R–A system is regained when ACTH is suppressed with the exogenous administration of steroids.

The mechanism of GSH has been well described at the molecular level: 11β-hydroxylase (P450c11) catalyses the final pathway in cortisol synthesis (see Chapter 7), converting 11-deoxycortisol into cortisol in the zona fasciculata. Aldosterone synthase (also P450c11) catalyses the conversion of corticosterone to aldosterone in the zona glomerulosa. These two enzymes catalyse essentially the same reaction, but have different substrates. The genes responsible for these enzymes are *CYP11B1* and *CYP11B2*, located on chromosome 8. The two genes are structurally very similar (95%

homology), but are under different control mechanisms. The 11β-hydroxylase gene is under the control of ACTH via cyclic adenosine monophosphate (cAMP); the aldosterone synthase gene is under control by angiotensin II via intracellular calcium. These different control mechanisms lead to the functional zonality of the adrenal gland: i.e. the production of aldosterone in the zona glomerulosa and cortisol in the zona fasciculata.

In GSH, a hybrid gene is formed by crossover at meiosis. The proximal component consists of the 11β-hydroxylase gene and the distal component consists of the aldosterone synthase gene. This hybrid gene has the combined properties of being under control of ACTH rather than angiotensin II, and stimulating the production of aldosterone rather than cortisol. The result is that normal concentrations of ACTH stimulate inappropriate amounts of aldosterone synthesis. Suppression of ACTH secretion with low-dose dexamethasone will thus result in a fall in aldosterone, and hence a fall in blood pressure. Patients with suspected GSH should be given 2 mg dexamethasone daily for 3 days. Aldosterone, PRA and blood pressure are measured before and after steroid administration. Once the diagnosis is confirmed, GSH responds to 0.25–0.5 mg dexamethasone daily. It is important to show normalisation of blood pressure and aldosterone before committing the patient to long-term steroid treatment.

As the genetic sequence of the mutation is known, testing is available in the form of Southern blotting and polymerase chain reaction (PCR). The condition has phenotypic variation in terms of the effect on mineralocorticoid level and blood pressure. Most patients are normokalaemic.

Apparent mineralocorticoid excess

This condition is characterised by cortisol acting as a potent mineralocorticoid. Aldosterone levels are low in these patients.

The mechanism of the disease is based on the fact that cortisol and aldosterone compete for the mineralocorticoid receptor *in vivo*. In the renal tubule, aldosterone has priority over cortisol to the mineralocorticoid receptor through the inactivation of cortisol to cortisone by 11β-hydroxysteroid dehydrogenase. In apparent mineralocorticoid excess, there is a mutation in this enzyme, which results in an increase in the concentration of cortisol around the mineralocorticoid receptor. This leads to cortisol-mediated mineralocorticoid hypertension.

The condition is inherited in an autosomal recessive fashion and has phenotypic heterogeneity. Treatment is usually with spironolactone or amiloride, although dexamethasone is sometimes used. Dexamethasone is specific to the glucocorticoid receptor, and will suppress ACTH cortisol synthesis, again resulting in resolution of hypertension with hypokalaemia.

The inhibition of 11β-hydroxysteroid dehydrogenase may also result from metabolites of liquorice or carbenoxolone. These two substances are often quoted as being causes of hypertension with hypokalaemia (Table 22.3).

Liddle's syndrome

This condition is inherited as an autosomal dominant. It is a paediatric disease characterised by early-onset hypokalaemia and hypertension (Table 22.4). Mutations in the genes coding for the β and γ subunits of the sodium transport channel, located on chromosome 16, are associated with increased sodium channel activity. There is excessive sodium and water reabsorption, leading to hypertension

Table 22.3 Mineralocorticoid hypertension

Cause	Mineralocorticoid
Primary hyperaldosteronism Aldosterone-producing adenoma/rarely carcinoma Idiopathic hyperaldosteronism Glucocorticoid-suppressible hyperaldosteronism	Aldosterone
Congenital adrenal hyperplasia 11β-hydroxylase deficiency 17α-hydroxylase deficiency	Deoxycorticosterone
Deoxycorticosterone-secreting tumour	Deoxycorticosterone
Glucocorticoid receptor resistance	Deoxycorticosterone
Liddle's syndrome	Increased sensitivity to mineralocorticoids
11β-hydroxysteroid dehydrogenase (11-HSD) deficiency Apparent mineralocorticoid excess Liquorice or carbenoxolone inhibit this enzyme Cushing's syndrome with ectopic adrenocorticotrophic hormone (ACTH)	

Table 22.4 Genetic causes of hyperaldosteronism

Glucocorticoid-suppressible hyperaldosteronism	Apparent mineralocorticoid excess	Liddle's syndrome
Autosomal dominant	Autosomal recessive	Autosomal dominant
Crossover of genes for adrenocorticotrophic hormone (ACTH) receptor and angiotensin II receptor	Mutation 11OHS dehydrogenase	Mutation sodium transport genes
Hyperaldosteronism under ACTH control	Cortisol-mediated hyperaldosteronism	Increased Na/H_2O absorption

and hypokalaemia. Spironolactone, acting on the mineralocorticoid receptor, is ineffective whereas epithelial sodium transport blockers such as triamterene are more useful.

Summary

Primary hyperaldosteronism is underdiagnosed and requires a high index of clinical suspicion. If the condition is suspected, the patient should be taken off all antihypertensive medication or changed to an α-blocker if this is not possible. The best screening test is an aldosterone/PRA ratio and a value >2000 suggests the diagnosis. The combination of postural testing, measurement of 18-oxosteroids and radiological appearance should lead to the diagnosis in most cases. Malignancy should be considered in tumours >3 cm diameter. A strong family history and early onset of hypertension should lead one to consider the genetic aetiologies. Treatment depends upon the underlying pathology and is medical or surgical. Surgical treatment is usually confined to unilateral APAs or IHAs which show functional laterality. Primary aldosteronism is an important condition to diagnose, as prompt diagnosis and treatment can prevent the morbidity and mortality associated with long-standing hypertension.

Further Reading

Amirlak I, Dawson KP. Bartter syndrome: an overview. *QJM* 2000;**93**(4):207–15.

Dluhy RG, Lifton RP. Glucocorticoid-remediable aldosteronism. *J Clin Endocrinol Metab* 1999;**84**(12):4341–4.

Foo R, O'Shaughnessy KM, Brown MJ. Hyperaldosteronism: recent concepts, diagnosis, and management. *Postgrad Med J* 2000;**77**(912):639–44.

Gordon RD, Stowasser M, Rutherford JC. Primary aldosteronism: are we diagnosing and operating on too few patients? *World J Surg* 2001;**25**(7):941–7.

Schurman SJ, Shoemaker LR. Bartter and Gitelman syndromes. *Adv Pediatr* 2000;**47**:223–48.

Stewart PM. Mineralocorticoid hypertension. *Lancet* 1999;**353**(9161):134–7.

23

Phaeochromocytomas and Paragangliomas

Pierre-Marc Gilles Bouloux

Catecholamine-Secreting Tumours

Phaeochromocytomas and paragangliomas are rare cate-cholamine-secreting tumours that account for about 1% of all cases of diastolic hypertension. Occurring at all ages, and in both sexes, they are most commonly diagnosed in the 4th and 5th decades. The annual incidence of these tumours is around 2–8 per million of the population, an incidence similar to that of newly diagnosed Cushing's disease and acromegaly. Several post-mortem studies have established an incidence for phaeochromo-cytoma of about 0.1%, suggesting that the usually quoted incidence may represent an underestimate. Although many tumours thus appear inactive and relatively asymptomatic in life, the hazard of missing the diagnosis is emphasised by a report of 54 autopsies on patients with phaeochromocytomas in whom the tumour was unsuspected in 75% of patients, but in whom it con-tributed to death in 55%. Unlike essential hypertension, cate-cholamine-secreting tumours produce a conglomeration of symptoms and signs that are bewildering to the patient; unrecog-nised, the condition is potentially fatal. A sharp index of suspicion remains the cornerstone of diagnosis.

Catecholamine-secreting tumours originate from within the adrenal medulla (phaeochromocytoma) or from extra-adrenal neural crest derivatives (paraganglioma) such as the sympathetic ganglia. A tumour classification is given in Table 23.1. Tumours

Table 23.1   Classification of catecholamine-secreting tumours

Tumour	Cell or origin
Phaeochromocytoma	Chromaffin cell
Paraganglioma	Chromaffin cell
Ganglioneuroma	Ganglion cell
Ganglioneuroblastoma	Ganglion cell
Sympathoblastoma	Sympathogone
Neuroblastoma	Sympathoblast

are neuroectodermal in origin, and the extensive distribution of neural crest derivatives underlies the diverse localisation of paragangliomas, which can occur at many sites from the base of the skull, the pericardium, the atria, the para-aortic area (classically the organ of Zuckerkandl) to more remote locations such as the urinary bladder and even the testicle. Given the potential multicentric origin of paragangliomata, as well as their metachronicity, malignant behaviour may be difficult to predict from histology alone, and depends upon the demonstration of metastases, such as within lymph nodes, liver and bone. Multiple and extra-adrenal tumours are more common in children (35% of cases) than in adults (8%), reflecting the greater abundance of extra-adrenal chromaffin tissue in children. Malignancy in paragangliomas (30–40%) is reported at 3–15 times that of the incidence in phaeochromocytomas.

A useful aide-memoire, the 'rule of 10,' usefully summarises many features of chromaffin tumours (Table 23.2). Although mainly sporadic, hereditable lesions are recognised in association with the multiple endocrine neoplasia (MEN) type 2a and 2b, and such neurocutaneous syndromes as neurofibromatosis and von Hippel–Lindau disease (Table 23.3). In familial cases, there is a higher incidence of bilaterality, multiplicity and multicentricity. Rarely, the metachronous association of gastric leiomyosarcoma, pulmonary chondroma and extra-adrenal paraganglioma has been reported ('Carney's triad'). It occurs in young women and is not familial.

Pathology

The term 'phaeochromocytoma' (*phaios*: dusky colour) was first proposed by Ludwig Pick in 1912 after the tumour's chromaffin

Table 23.2   Aide-memoires to important features of phaeochromocytomas

Aide-memoire	Feature
Six Hs	Hypertension
	Headache
	Hyperhidrosis
	Hypomotility of gut
	Hyperglycaemia
	Hypermetabolism
Rule of 10	10% hypermetabolism
	10% hyperglycaemia
	10% malignant
	10% extra-adrenal
	10% occur in children
Four Cs	Cholelithiasis
	Cutaneous lesions
	Cerebellar haemangioblastoma
	Cushing's syndrome

Table 23.3   Disorders associated with phaeochromocytomas

Multiple endocrine neoplasia syndromes (MEN) 2a
    Medullary carcinoma of thyroid
    Hyperparathyroidism (hyperplasia)
    Phaeochromocytoma

MEN2b
As above +
Marfanoid phenotype
Visceral neuromas

Neurocutaneous syndromes
Neurofibromatosis
von Hippel–Lindau disease
Ataxia telangiectasia
Tuberose sclerosis
Sturge–Weber syndrome
Multiple neoplasia triad syndrome
    extra-adrenal paraganglioma
    gastric epithelioid leiomyosarcoma
    pulmonary chondromas

reaction. Usually slow growing, these tumours vary in size from a few grams to over 3 kg, are solitary, spheroid or ovoid in shape, and are often sharply circumscribed. The cut surface is usually greyish pink, with central areas of haemorrhage and necrosis. Microscopically, neoplastic cells may be arranged in cords, a trabecular pattern, an alveolar pattern (*zellballen*), a solid or diffuse pattern or a mixture of these patterns. Angiomatoid foci with prominent endothelial cells in some phaeochromocytomas can be quite striking.

Neither tumour ploidy nor histological features are reliable predictors of biological and clinical behaviour of phaeochromocytomas. Cellular and nuclear polymorphism, nuclear 'pseudo-inclusions', increased mitotic indices, and even bizarre giant cells may be seen in both benign and malignant lesions. Cells are neurone-specific enolase, synaptophysin and chromogranin A positive, reflecting their neural crest origin. Electron microscopy reveals typical dense core noradrenaline-containing granules with a 'blister-like' halo, somewhat larger (270 nm) than those found in normal chromaffin cells. Adrenaline-containing granules, because they do not react with glutaraldehyde, are less electron dense and are finely granular.

Genetics, cytogenetics and molecular biology

The genetic predisposition to phaeochromocytoma is complex, but at least three genes are known to be involved. Although most tumours are sporadic, phaeochromocytomas can occur as part of well-defined genetic syndromes such as MEN2a and b, neurofibromatosis type I (NF) and the von Hippel–Lindau syndrome. Familial phaeochromocytoma can also occur independently of the above syndromes.

Tumour catecholamine synthesis and release

Tumour chromaffin granules do not differ significantly from those of the normal adrenal medulla. However, in some tumours the intravesicular catecholamine : ATP ratio exceeds the normal 4 : 1. Catecholamine synthesis is substantially greater than normal; the activities of tyrosine hydroxylase, aromatic amino acid decarboxylase and dopamine β-hydroxylase are markedly increased, whereas the activities of the enzymes involved in catecholamine catabolism – monoamine oxidase (MAO) and catecholamine-O-methyl transferase (COMT) – are reduced. Therefore, excess newly synthesised catecholamines that cannot be stored in the filled vesicles may not be degraded, and freely diffuse into the circulation. The size of the tumour may be an important determinant of the catecholamine secretory products. Small tumours (<50 g) have rapid turnover rates with small catecholamine content, releasing largely unmetabolised catecholamines into the circulation. Larger tumours have slow turnover rates, releasing mainly metabolites into plasma, which may explain the frequently observed clinical paradox wherein small tumours cause disproportionately severe symptoms. The mechanism of tumour catecholamine release has not been fully elucidated. Whereas slow leakage of catecholamine release undoubtedly occurs from these tumours, it is possible that foci of tumour infarction and necrosis also play a role as well as release of catecholamines from increased peripheral sympathetic nervous stores.

Catecholamine biosynthesis and adrenergic receptors

It is useful to review the physiology of catecholamines prior to discussing the pathophysiology of catecholamine hypersecretion. Noradrenaline, adrenaline, dopamine and DOPA have important neural and endocrine functions, exerting profound metabolic, physiological and pharmacological effects. Biosynthesis occurs in certain brain nuclei, sympathetic neurones and chromaffin cells. Certain cells in the brain, adrenal medulla and chromaffin cells express the phenylethanolamine-N methyl transferase (PNMT) essential for conversion of noradrenaline to adrenaline neurones. Catecholamines cause their effect by binding to specific plasma membrane binding sites, designated alpha (α), beta (β) and dopaminergic receptors, which have been characterised pharmacologically on the basis of rank order of potency of their responses to agonists and antagonists. When stimulated by noradrenaline, α_1-receptor activations effect vasoconstriction and glycogenolysis; α_2-receptors are predominantly located on the presynaptic terminals and mediate inhibition of catecholamine release at the sympathoeffector junction. Postsynaptic α_2-stimulation causes smooth muscle vasoconstriction, whereas central α_2-postsynaptic stimulation reduces sympathetic tone peripherally. Stimulation of α_2-receptors in the pancreatic islet cells reduces insulin secretion, reduces lipolysis in adipocytes and, in the intestine, induces smooth muscle relaxation.

When stimulated, β_1-receptors have a positive inotropic and chronotropic effect on the heart, induce lipolysis and increase renin secretion. By contrast, β_2-receptor stimulation leads to bronchodilatation, vasodilatation in skeletal muscle, activation of muscle sodium–potassium ATPase (with uptake of extracellular potassium), sensitisation of muscle spindle afferents, glycogenolysis, myometrial and intestinal smooth muscle relaxation and increased noradrenaline release from sympathetic nerves. Adrenaline and noradrenaline are equipotent in eliciting β_1-responses, whereas adrenaline is a more potent β_2-agonist. Stimulation of dopamine receptors (DA1) in renal vasculature causes vasodilatation, whereas DA2 receptor stimulation presynaptically inhibits noradrenaline release.

Prolonged exposure of receptors to catecholamines decreases responsiveness to these amines. The process of desensitisation is associated with a loss of adrenoceptor numbers, whereas absence of agonist leads to upregulation of receptor numbers. The regulation of adrenoceptors by agonists is a multistep process involving several discrete events: these include rapid phosphorylation of receptors, receptor sequestration in a cellular compartment not readily accessible from outside the cell and uncoupling of the receptor so that ligand binding still occurs but secondary messenger formation is decreased. Loss of receptors can also occur with persistent exposure to agonists, through degradation, but this is a relatively slow process.

Clinical features of catecholamine-secreting tumours

Pathophysiological considerations

Hypertension is intermittent in 50% of patients (when it can occur on a background of normotension) and constant in the remainder, and is ascribed to tumour secretion of free catecholamines. Surprisingly, there is poor correlation between the plasma catecholamine concentration and the height of arterial pressure, and some patients are normotensive even in the presence of elevated plasma catecholamine levels. In those patients with persistent hypertension, the normal circadian blood pressure variation (with nocturnal falls, caused largely by decreased sympathetic tone to resistance vessels and a fall in cardiac output) is retained in some but by no means all patients, strongly suggesting that despite pathological circulating catecholamine levels, underlying sympathetic nervous regulation – and by inference noradrenaline release at the sympathoeffector junction – within the cardiovascular system is still operative. The unexpected fall in blood pressure following the centrally acting α_2-adrenoceptor agonist clonidine in patients with phaeochromocytoma further supports this contention. These discrepancies can be explained by the confounding effects of inherent reactivity of vascular smooth muscle, receptor sensitivity, as well as the underlying sympathetic tone at the sympathoeffector junction. Of all these mechanisms, receptor desensitisation is likely to play a particularly important role, and may involve both downregulation of α_1-adrenoceptors as well as postreceptor (signal-transduction) mechanisms. Desensitisation of β-receptors has also been demonstrated, and it has been shown that adipocytes and lymphocytes from phaeochromocytoma patients are relatively resistant to the effects of β-adrenoceptor stimulation by isoprenaline.

Occasionally, a paradoxical rise in blood pressure occurs on introducing a β-blocker in the treatment regimen (presumably exposing unopposed α-adrenergic stimulation of resistance vessels), thus alerting the physician to the possibility of underlying phaeochromocytoma (see below).

Symptoms and signs of phaeochromocytoma and paraganglioma

Patients with phaeochromocytoma usually present with a history of poorly controlled and occasionally accelerated hypertension; detailed history then reveals superimposed 'crises', comprising episodes of headache, palpitations (with or without tachycardia), pallor and profuse sweating occurring during the paroxysms of hypertension at which point blood pressure can rise in excess of 250/150 mmHg; other presentations are listed in Table 23.4. Other features include tremor, nervousness and anxiety, weakness, nausea, vomiting and chest or abdominal pain. Occasionally, patients present with acute myocardial infarction, or acute renal failure and stroke due to massive catecholamine release; presentations with pseudo-obstruction of the bowel and chronic constipation are well recognised. The 'crises' are usually of uniform composition in individual patients, although they may vary in duration and intensity.

The onset is usually sudden, and the peak severity is reached within a few minutes, with a slower offset and a total duration usually less than 15 min, and shorter than 60 min in 80% of cases. An episode may begin with a sensation of something about to happen deep inside the chest, and a drive to deeper breathing is

Table 23.4   Clinical features of catecholamine-secreting tumours

Symptoms
Headache
Hyperidrosis
Palpitations
Anxiety
Tremulousness
Nausea, vomiting
Chest and abdominal pain
Weight loss
Dyspnoea
Heat intolerance
Constipation
Acroparaesthesiae
Seizures

Signs
Hypertension (sustained and/or paroxysmal)
Orthostatic hypotension
Bradycardia, tachycardia
Postural tachycardia
Pallor and flushing
Tremor
Raynaud's phenomenon
Thyroid swelling (intermittent)
Pyrexia

Signs of complications
Left ventricular failure
Pulmonary oedema
Circulatory shock
Cerebrovascular accident
Paralytic ileus

noted. Awareness of a pounding or forceful heartbeat is then noted. The throbbing sensation may then affect the rest of the trunk and head, causing headache or a pounding sensation in the head. Alpha-mediated vasoconstriction causes peripheral vasoconstriction, cool moist hands and feet and pallor. The combination of a β_1-inotropic effect on the heart with intense peripheral α-adrenoceptor stimulated vasoconstriction leads to the rise in blood pressure and subsequent reflex baroreflex-mediated bradycardia.

Cardiac tachyarrhythmias resistant to treatment and reversible changes of transmural myocardial infarction on electrocardiography (ECG) may also suggest the presence of phaeochromocytoma.

Chronic symptoms of phaeochromocytoma

In between attacks, the patient may feel perfectly well. However, increased metabolic rate may cause heat intolerance, increased sweating and occasionally weight loss. The effects on glycogenolysis and insulin release can cause hyperglycaemia and glucose intolerance. Occasional patients have presented with a pyrexia of unknown origin (PUO) and hypertension. Tumour production of interleukin-6 may play a role in these presentations.

Early diagnosis of phaeochromocytoma is of considerable importance. Patients harbouring such tumours are at risk of severe hypertensive crises, often unpredictable, the result of massive tumour catecholamine release. The mechanism of such uncontrolled catecholamine release is uncertain, but it is episodic in some individuals and continuous in others. The pressor crises have a significant morbidity and occasional mortality. Although frequently spontaneous, they may be precipitated by a number of stimuli, such as a twisting motion, massage or pressure over the tumour, postural changes, exercise, ingestion of certain foods or alcoholic drinks, hyperventilation, Valsalva manoeuvre, coitus, laughing, sneezing, coughing, defaecation and micturition (Table 23.5). In most of the above situations, direct pressure over the tumour may be responsible. Certain procedures may induce paroxysms of hypertension in patients, including the administration of intravenous contrast media (e.g. for IVU or arteriograms), tracheal intubation, induction of anaesthesia, hypoxia and parturition. A number of conditions may mimic phaeochromocytomas clinically; these are referred to as pseudophaeochromocytoma and are listed in Table 23.6.

Atypical presentation of phaeochromocytomas abound and are probably overrepresented in the literature. They include transient cortical blindness, gangrene, polycythaemia without hypertension, rhabdomyolysis and acute myoglobinuric renal failure. Constipation and a paralytic ileus-like picture with abdominal pain may occur.

The dominant tumour secretory products are noradrenaline, adrenaline, dopamine and their precursor dihydroxyphenylalanine (DOPA). These vasoactive biogenic amines produce their effect by

Table 23.5   Factors known to precipitate catecholamine release from phaeochromocytomas

Spontaneous secretion
Exercise
Bending over
Urination
Defecation
Pressure on the abdomen
Induction of anaesthesia
Tumour palpation
Straining, as during parturition
Drugs, injection of:
    histamine
    tyramine
    guanethidine
    glucagon
    naloxone
    metoclopramide
    droperidol
    ACTH (adrenocorticophic hormone)
    cytotoxic drugs
    saralasin
Tricyclic antidepressants
Phenothiazines

interacting with α_1, α_2, β_1 and β_2 or dopamine (D1 and D2) receptors, which are widely distributed in vascular tissues.

Biological actions of catecholamines account for the characteristic symptoms and signs of phaeochromocytoma. The manifestations in individual cases depend to some extent on the dominant type of catecholamine released, the site and size of the tumour, as well as the amount and pattern of release. Predominantly, noradrenaline-secreting tumours (e.g. extra-adrenal tumours) activate peripheral (α_1 and α_2) receptors with widespread cutaneous effects (pallor) and splanchnic vasoconstriction, territories dense in α-receptors. Associated pressor crises are accompanied by baroreflex-mediated bradycardia. Adrenaline-secreting tumours (usually, although not invariably, of intra-adrenal origin), cause both α- and β-stimulation; pressor crises are associated with increased pulse pressure and tachycardia. Glucose intolerance is associated with adrenaline-secreting tumours. Dopamine and DOPA secretion may contribute to occasional cases of hypotension seen in phaeochromocytoma. Postural hypotension is more usually

Table 23.6 Differential diagnosis: causes of 'pseudophaeochromocytoma'

Anxiety state
Hyperadrenergic essential hypertension
Menopausal vasomotor instability
Hyperventilation
Excess caffeine intake
Alcohol withdrawal syndrome
Diencephalic seizures (autonomic epilepsy)
Autonomic hyper-reflexia
Thyrotoxicosis

Other causes of paroxysmal hypertension
Acute intermittent porphyria
Acute or chronic lead poisoning
Tabetic crisis
Clonidine, methyldopa withdrawal
Tetanus
Guillain–Barré syndrome
Cord section

due to shrinkage of the intravascular volume secondary to vasoconstriction, with concomitant failure to compensate fully on orthostatic stimulation.

There is no correlation between tumour size and symptomatology. Indeed, the larger tumours are characterised by intratumour catecholamine metabolism, and thus release proportionately fewer active amines. Paradoxically, small tumours are capable of producing devastating pressor crises.

Cardiac manifestations of phaeochromocytoma

In a proportion of cases cardiac manifestations predominate, with chest pain, angina pectoris, myocarditis and myocardial infarction not associated with coronary artery disease (presumed intense coronary vasospasm). The ECG may show nonspecific ST-T wave changes and prominent U waves (sometimes seen with hypokalaemia induced by β_2-adrenoceptor stimulation). Sinus tachycardia, sinus bradycardia, supraventricular tachycardia (SVT) and ventricular premature beat (VPB) can be associated with palpitations. Major bundle branch blocks may be present, and cardiomyopathy of the congestive or hypertrophic type may be present, usually reversible following successful surgery. Massive noncardiogenic pulmonary oedema may be present, due to massive venoconstriction (both peripheral and pulmonary venous constriction) that shifts volume towards the central veins.

Physical examination of the patient with suspected phaeochromocytoma

In 50% of cases, the patient is normotensive, and there may be no physical signs. A history of weight loss is sometimes seen in patients who have persistent weight loss because of hypermetabolism. Other physical signs occasionally seen include fine tremor of the outstretched hands, inappropriate perspiration and features of anxiety. The tumour is rarely large enough to be palpated per abdomen. Hypertensive retinopathy may be present. Stigmata of neurocrestopathies should be sought – e.g. features of neurofibromatosis, and von Lippel-Lindau syndrome (VHL).

Special considerations in childhood phaeochromocytoma

Phaeochromocytomas account for 0.5–2% of cases of childhood secondary hypertension. Boys appear to be affected twice as commonly as females, and two-thirds of the tumours are in the adrenal medulla. The most common extra-adrenal site is at the bifurcation of the aorta. Hypertension is sustained in 88% and clinical symptoms include headache (75%), sweating (67%), nausea and vomiting (48%), visual disturbance (37%), abdominal pain (32%), polydipsia and polyuria (31%), convulsions (22%), and acrocyanosis (22%). Sustained hypertension is therefore more common in childhood tumours, where the frequency of multiple lesions and bilaterality is greater. Hypertensive encephalopathy, with fitting, is more common than in adults.

Dopamine-secreting tumours

Pure dopamine-secreting tumours are rare; most are malignant and not associated with hypertension. All patients had an 'inflammatory syndrome' with high erythrocyte sedimentation rate, weight loss and fever. They were being investigated for suspected hypernephromas. Mixed noradrenaline- and dopamine-secreting tumours are commoner, but also tend to portend malignancy. A variety of other neuropeptides have been described to be co-secreted from phaeochromocytoma.

Prognostic features

Malignant tumours (3–14%) are difficult to diagnose because there are no specific histological appearances, and diagnosis relies therefore on the demonstration of unequivocal metastatic disease. Even local invasion is not a reliable marker. It has been stated that tumour aneuploidy can help predict malignant potential; however, while a normal histogram seems to be indicative of a benign lesion, an abnormal histogram (aneuploidy and tetraploidy) can be seen both in tumours that have metastasised and in tumours with more benign behaviour.

Diagnosis

Patients requiring investigation

There is considerable controversy as to which hypertensive patients should be investigated biochemically for exclusion of phaeochromocytoma. Young hypertensives, those with a positive family history of phaeochromocytoma or MEN2, or those with refractory or extremely labile hypertension (especially if accompanied by phaeochromocytoma-associated symptomatology) clearly require investigation. Similarly, patients with hypertension and a neurocutaneous syndrome such as neurofibromatosis, Sturge–Weber syndrome or von Hippel–Lindau disease should be screened for catecholamine-secreting tumours. Hypertension with evidence of glucose intolerance should also prompt an investigation for a phaeochromocytoma. Indications for investigation are listed in Box 23.1.

Box 23.1 Indications for screening for catecholamine-secreting tumours

- Episodic attacks of headache with hypertension
- Adrenal coincidentaloma
- Adverse cardiovascular manifestations in response to anaesthesia, to a surgical procedure or to certain medications known to predispose to phaeochromocytoma crisis
- Difficulty in controlling blood pressure with conventional antihypertensive agents, and paradoxical rise in blood pressure following administration of β-blockers

Diagnosis of phaeochromocytoma

Measurement of urinary catecholamines and their metabolites

Urinary catecholamines are a sensitive indicator of phaeochromocytoma, and may be determined on a 24-hour, a 12-hour overnight or a timed collection during crisis. A correction for renal function is required. Measurement of urinary noradrenaline, adrenaline and dopamine by reversed-phase high-performance liquid chomatography (HPLC) coupled with electrochemical detection has increased the sensitivity of phaeochromocytoma diagnosis to 95%, but with some loss of specificity. In general, only ~70% of tumours produce elevated adrenaline levels, whereas 85% produce elevated noradrenaline levels. The measurement of urinary adrenaline levels is of greatest value in the screening of families for MEN2 and adrenomedullary hyperplasia. Urine collection must be undertaken in an acidified container (20 ml 6N HCl), to retain stability of the metabolites.

Plasma catecholamine estimations

Highly sensitive and specific plasma catecholamine estimations are available in many laboratories. Blood samples need to be taken under standardised conditions (venous cannulation 30 min before sampling supine), and heparinised blood separated by cold centrifugation and plasma stored at −80°C prior to assay. Plasma noradrenaline levels consistently exceeding 10 nmol/l (normal range 1.0–3.07 nmol/l) and adrenaline levels exceeding 1.5 nmol/l (normal range 0.05–1.07 nmol/l) give a diagnostic specificity of about 95%, and a sensitivity of 85%, particularly when other causes of plasma catecholamine elevation have been ruled out. When blood is sampled during a crisis, plasma catecholamine levels are usually diagnostic.

Elevated plasma adrenaline or increased urinary metanephrine excretion generally suggests a tumour of adrenal origin, whereas exclusively noradrenaline-secreting tumours suggest either a very large adrenal tumour or a paraganglioma. This is because large adrenal tumours tend to outstrip their blood supply (cortico-medullary blood flow), and have a direct arterial inflow. Tumour tissue gaining a direct blood supply will not be exposed to the high cortisol levels that are essential for induction of the PNMT enzyme that converts noradrenaline to adrenaline, and will therefore preferentially release noradrenaline.

Diagnosis of small lesions

Suppression tests

Very small lesions pose a problem, and minor elevations of circulating plasma adrenaline under basal conditions may be the only indicator of the presence of small intra-adrenal tumours. Catecholamine levels may be sited in an intermediate 'grey' zone, and therefore are not 'diagnostic'. A suppression test can be used to physiological elevations from genuinely autonomous adrenaline tumour secretion. Oral clonidine (0.3 mg) suppresses plasma noradrenaline into the low normal range in normal and essential hypertensive individuals but not in patients with tumorous noradrenaline secretion. A further hazard during performance of the clonidine test is hypotension, which can occur in patients receiving antihypertensive medication, particularly those associated with volume depletion. Beta-blockers should be discontinued 48 hours before the test. This is because clonidine has a potent vagotonic effect, and concomitant propranolol could lead to severe bradycardia. Furthermore, β-adrenergic antagonists can prevent the plasma catecholamine-lowering effect of clonidine in patients without phaeochromocytoma, because of the ability of such agents to interfere with hepatic clearance of catecholamines. As is the case with pentolinium, clonidine testing should not be performed in a patient with normal plasma catecholamines as, in this instance, false-positive tests may result. Pentolinium suppression testing (pentolinium 2.5 mg i.v. and plasma catecholamines at 0', 5', 10' min.) is probably superior to clonidine suppression testing in patients with renal impairment.

By contrast, plasma catecholamines are invariably raised in hypertensive patients harbouring a phaeochromocytoma. This is because in the presence of persistently raised catecholamines, adrenergic receptors downregulate (desensitisation); in order to produce hypertension under these circumstances, plasma catecholamines have to be elevated several-fold.

Episodic catecholamine secretors

Episodic catecholamine secretors with a background of normotension pose a difficult problem. If sampling is carried out during normotension, plasma catecholamines may be normal;

although 24-hour urinary catecholamine metabolites or timed urinary samples may be elevated under these instances, definitive biochemical assessment of catecholamine secretion in such cases may require sampling during a symptomatic crisis. Where symptomatology strongly suggests the presence of an underlying phaeochromocytoma, and repeated biochemistry is normal, a provocative test with pharmacological agents such as intravenous tyramine (1 mg), histamine (10 mg), glucagon (1 mg) or naloxone (10 mg) may be justified, although this should only be carried out under effective α- and β-blockade with plasma catecholamine measurement rather than blood pressure as the response parameter. The glucagon test (1 mg i.v.) using blood pressure and plasma catecholamine measurement is generally considered to be the least dangerous of the provocation tests. Even this test is not recommended for routine use.

Trial of phenoxybenzamine and propranolol

In occasional patients in whom there is strong clinical suspicion of a catecholamine-secreting tumour, but in whom biochemical investigations are nondiagnostic, a diagnostic trial of phenoxybenzamine and propranolol may be warranted. If hypertension and the 'crises' settle on this combination, further reappraisal of the patient may be warranted.

Localisation

Computed tomography (CT) scanning

Initially, the adrenal glands alone should be scanned, but if this is negative the rest of the abdomen including the pelvis, chest and neck should be included. The resolution of the most advanced scanners is currently in the order of 5 mm. Because intravenous contrast media can precipitate pressor crises, the examination (as indeed any invasive radiographic procedure) should be conducted only after adequate α- and β-blockade.

Magnetic resonance imaging

Magnetic resonance imaging (MRI) allows some degree of tissue characterisation. Most phaeochromocytomas give high T2-weighted signal intensity. The technique is particularly useful in the imaging of tumours in close proximity to major vessels, because of the signal void from flowing blood, and has been of especial value in detecting tumours near or associated with cardiac structures.

Venous catheterisation

Venous catheterisation with contrast may rarely be of use but inter-pretation is difficult and it is not without danger.

Radionuclide scanning

MIBG

The radionuclide meta-iodo (^{123}I or ^{131}I) benzylguanidine (MIBG), a guanethidine analogue is taken up by chromaffin cells and incor-porated into vesicles. The current model of MIBG action is one of so-called type 1 specific, high-affinity, energy- and sodium-dependent uptake into the intravesicular compartment. It has been used to assist in tumour localisation, and is of especial value in the localisation of extra-adrenal paragangliomata and metastases. Normal adrenomedullary tissue can also be visualised in 80–90% of cases using ^{123}I-MIBG. About 10% of tumours are not demon-strable (false negative) by this technique, but false positives are rare (1–3%), but have been shown in cases of benign adrenocortical adenomas. Specificity is 100% in malignant lesions and in familial tumours. Not only is MIBG capable of showing multiple lesions simultaneously but it can also show up a variety of tumours arising from APUD (amine precursor uptake and decarboxylation) cells, such as chemodectomas, carcinoids and medullary carcinoma of the thyroid. In all tissues, there is some nonspecific uptake of MIBG which is diffusional and nonenergy dependent, contributing to the general background activity, but tissue retention is transient and diminishes over time more rapidly than in tissues with specific uptake and storage.

Procedure. Following intravenous MIBG, the patient is scanned at both 24 hours and again at 48–72 hours, to distinguish between early physiological uptake (early scans), and later uptake (tumour tissue). Drugs which interfere with uptake, such as imipramine (tri-cyclic antidepressants) and labetolol should be discontinued for several weeks prior to the scan. Other drugs known to interfere with uptake include reserpine, cocaine, phenylpropanolamine-containing drugs and calcium channel blockers. Within 24 hours, 55% of the injected radioactivity is excreted in the urine, rising to 90% by 4 days, except in renal failure where clearance is markedly reduced. The prominent hepatic uptake appears to be due to metabolism and not to uptake. The prolonged and intense uptake of ^{131}I-MIBG into tumour cells – and their retention – has formed the basis of the application of ^{131}I-MIBG therapy in malignant phaeochromocytomas.

Octreotide scanning

Octreotide scanning has been used but the spleen may confound good adrenal imaging.

Intraoperative localisation with ^{123}I-MIBG

Where there are discrepancies between CT scanning of the abdomen and radionuclide imaging (e.g. MIBG shows uptake, but there is no corresponding mass on CT scanning), a preoperative 4 mCi dose of MIBG may be administered and direct measurement of tissue activity carried out intraoperatively, allowing surgical removal of labelled tumour tissue. A flow chart giving a strategy for the diagnosis, localisation and treatment of suspected phaeochromocytoma is given in Figure 23.1.

Treatment

Medical protocol

Most phaeochromocytomas are benign; complete excision leads to normotension in 75% of cases. However, because of the unpredictable nature of these secretory tumours, it is as well to prepare patients carefully for surgery and, traditionally, oral phenoxybenzamine and propranolol have been given to stabilise blood pressure and heart rate for some weeks prior to elective surgery, supplemented by preoperative phenoxybenzamine infusions (Box 23.2).

Premedication

Droperidol (inhibition of catecholamine reuptake) and phenothiazines, morphine (release of histamine) and atropine (vagolytic effect, causing tachycardia) should be avoided; benzodiazepines are the drugs of choice.

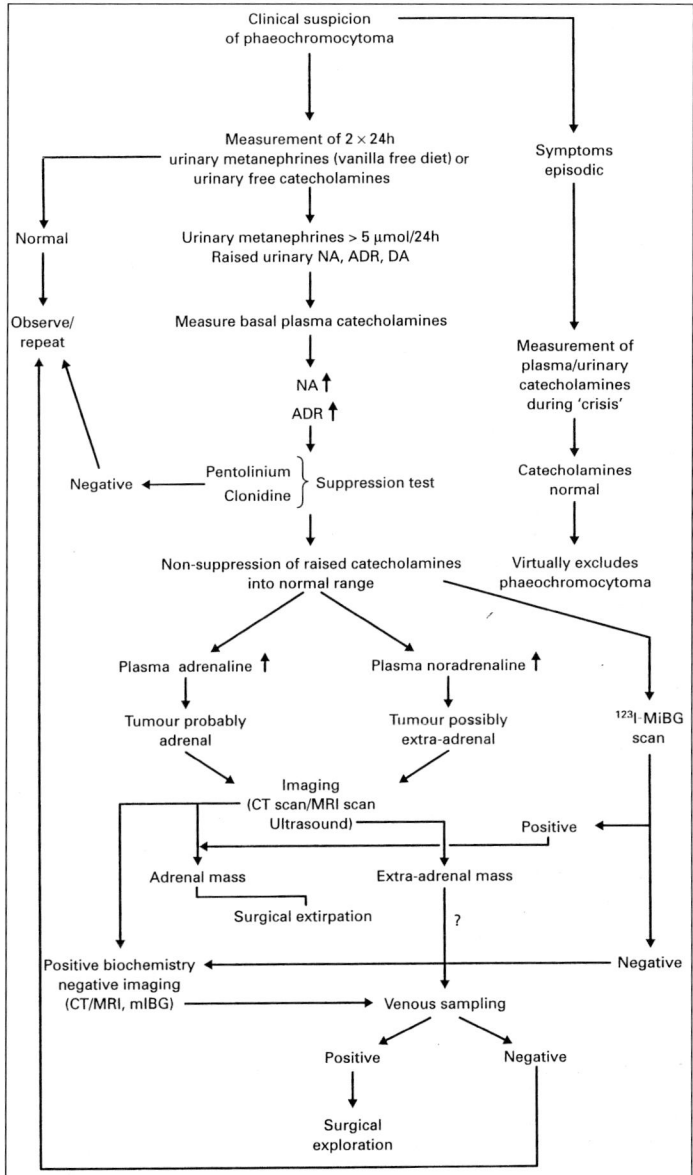

Figure 23.1. A suggested strategy for the diagnosis and treatment of phaeochromocytoma. NA, noradrenaline; ADR, adrenaline; DA, dopamine.

> ### Box 23.2 Medical treatment of phaeochromocy-
> ### tomas
>
> 1. This is a medical emergency; patients must be admitted for α- and β-blockade
> 2. These patients may be dehydrated but vasoconstricted; therefore, initiation of α-blockade can cause life-threatening hypotension
> 3. Phenoxybenzamine, 10 mg, increasing o.d., then b.i.d., then t.i.d.
> 4. Then β-blockade within 48 hours of starting α-blockade. (Nadolol, a once daily non-selective β-blocker, may be useful.)
> 5. Three days of intravenous phenoxybenzamine (0.5 mg/kg) will totally α-block the patient prior to surgery

Intraoperative

Surgery should be elective wherever possible, and should not use anaesthetic agents or manoeuvres known to provoke catecholamine release. Vecuronium appears to be the muscle relaxant of choice, as it has no autonomic effects and does not provoke catecholamine release directly or indirectly through histamine release. Hypoxia, which sensitises the myocardium to the effects of catecholamines, is to be avoided. Isoflurane or enflurane are the inhalational agents of choice as they are associated with a smaller arrhythmogenic risk. Continuous intraoperative blood pressure and ECG monitoring is mandatory. Even with complete α-blockade with this noncompetitive inhibitor, pressor crises may still be precipitated by induction of anaesthesia and tumour manipulation. These usually respond to bolus doses of phentolamine or sodium nitroprusside infusions. Phenoxybenzamine has the advantage that it is an antagonist at both α_1- and α_2-sites. Intravenous propranolol and lignocaine should be available in the event of cardiac arrhythmias. Noradrenaline infusion (for hypotension) should not be necessary if the patient has been prepared by preoperative α-blockade, which allows plasma volume re-expansion. Preoperative blood transfusions are occasionally required if haematocrit falls excessively during preparatory treatment.

General principles of phaeochromocytoma surgery

Certain rules apply to lesions irrespective of the site. There should be wide exposure of tumours, meticulous attention to haemostasis, early isolation of vascular supply, minimal tumour manipulation, delivery of tumour with capsule intact and exploration of all access-ible sites of second primary or metastatic lesions.

Phaeochromocytoma during pregnancy

If the diagnosis is made in early pregnancy, termination is recom-mended. Should the condition be discovered late in the pregnancy, α-blockade with phenoxybenzamine is recommended, and elective Caesarean section should be performed via a vertical lower abdom-inal incision. This may then be extended, and the abdomen explored at the time of delivery. There have been reports of successful laparo-scopic exeresis of phaeochromocytomas in pregnancy.

Postoperative management

Particular attention needs to be paid to volume status following resection. Hypovolaemia may ensue, particularly in the presence of α-blockade and blood loss. Central venous pressure measurement will assist in fluid repletion therapy. Preoperative blood transfusions, given if the haematocrit has fallen significantly following α-block-ade, significantly lessen the severity of hypovolaemia. Complete normalisation of plasma and urinary free catecholamines may take several days after the operation. This presumably reflects the uptake of and storage of catecholamines of phaeochromocytomal origin in sympathetic neurones. Residual hypertension is present in up to 33% of patients, but this is not paroxysmal and is 'essential'.

Follow-up of patients with phaeochromocytoma

It is recommended that patients who have had phaeochromocy-tomas successfully resected should have periodic blood pressure measurements, and when appropriate, urinary catecholamine estimations, at yearly intervals. Follow-up is particularly impor-tant in patients with paragangliomas and MEN2 and neurocuta-neous syndromes where tumours may be metachronous and multicentric. Where there is suspicion of recurrence, MIBG may be a useful early investigation to locate the lesion.

Screening of family members at risk

Familial phaeochromocytoma is rare and may occur as part of an autosomal dominant condition, in which first-degree relatives should be screened by blood pressure and urinary catecholamine estimations. In patients with MEN2 and relatives, the use of adrenaline estimation appears to be the best indicator as to the presence of adrenomedullary hyperplasia, the precursor to phaeochromocytoma in these patients. The use of provocative testing with glucagon in asymptomatic normotensive at-risk subjects has also been advocated. Newer molecular genetic testing is likely to be increasingly available.

Treatment of inoperable or metastatic lesions

The occurrence of tumour deposits in sites normally devoid of chromaffin tissue is diagnostic of metastatic disease. This may occur from apparently benign primary lesions. Seeding during the resection of the primary tumour may occur. The overall mortality rate at 5 years is 40–50%, but a significant proportion of patients with overt metastatic disease survive for many years with good quality of life.

While good control of blood pressure with long-term α- and β-blockade and the tyrosine hydroxylase inhibitor α-methylparatyrosine is usually possible, external beam irradiation continues to have a role in the relief of pain from osseous metastases. The results of single- or multiple-agent chemotherapy have in general been disappointing. The radioisotope [131] I-MIBG is used for malignant phaechromocytoma. The patient must be monitored in terms of blood pressure and in terms of radioisotope retention for several days: this may be repeated. A quarter of patients will develop myelosuppression. Complete response after therapy is the exception, and more commonly partial remissions occur which may last for many years. This treatment must still be considered experimental, although it is doubtful if a controlled trial will ever be conducted in malignant phaeochromocytoma.

Ganglioneuromas

These may be both secretory and non-secretory, and reach enormous sizes with relatively few symptoms. They tend to behave in a relatively benign manner and can occur in the chest and abdomen.

Further Reading

Bouloux P-M G, Fakeeh M. Investigation of phaeochromocytoma. *Clin Endocrinol* 1995;**43**:657–64.

Bravo EL, Gifford RW. Phaeochromocytoma: diagnosis, localisation and management. *N Engl J Med* 1984;**311**:1298–303.

Col V, de Canniere L, Collard E, Michel L, DoncKier J. Laparoscopic adrenalectomy for phaeochromocytoma: endocrinological and surgical aspects of a new therapeutic approach. *Clin Endocrinol (Oxf.)* 1999;**50**(1):121–5.

Crout JR, Sjoerdsma A. Turnover and metabolism of catecholamines in patients with pheochromocytoma. *J Clin Invest* 1964;**43**:94.

Dahia PLM, Grossman AB. The molecular pathogenesis of adrenal tumours. *Endoc Rel Cancer* 1995;**2**:267–79.

Liggett SB, Raymond JR. Pharmacology and molecular biology of adrenergic receptors. *Baillière's Clin Endocrinol Metab* 1993;**7**:279–306.

Manger WM, Gifford RW Jr, Hoffman BB. Phaeochromocytoma: a clinical and experimental overview. *Curr Probl Cancer* 1985;**9**:1.

Neumann HP, Berger DP, Sigmund G *et al.* Phaeochromocytomas, multiple neoplasia type 2, and Von Hippel–Lindau disease. *N Eng J Med* 1993:**329**:1531–8.

Pattarino F, Bouloux PMG. Diagnosis of malignant phaeochromocytoma. *Clin Endocrinol* 1996;**44**:239–41.

Thomas JE, Rooke ED, Kvale WF. The neurologist's experience with phaeochromocytoma: a series of 100 cases. *JAMA* 1966,**197**:754–8.

Young WF Jr. Phaeochromocytoma: 1926–1993. *Trends Endocrinol Metab* 1993:**4**:122.

24

Paediatric Endocrinology

Nicola A Bridges

Introduction

This chapter will deal with the main areas that differentiate paediatric from adult practice – disorders of growth and puberty and endocrine disorders that present in the neonatal period. Growth distinguishes paediatric from adult endocrine practice – a child with a normal growth pattern is not likely to have a significant endocrine defect.

Growth charts

Updated height and weight centile charts for the UK population were published in 1995. These used cross-sectional data and included some children from ethnic minorities. These charts are included in the parent-held child health record.

Growth can be divided into a number of different phases and the first step in assessing problems is to decide during which phase of growth the problem has occurred. Problems in one phase may not be made up later – for example, a low birth-weight child can be expected to grow normally in childhood but will not catch up the antenatal loss.

Antenatal growth. The most rapid phase of growth. The placenta or maternal health and nutrition are the most important influences at this stage.

Infancy – up to about 2 years.   Many normal babies change their weight and height centile position between birth and about 2 years, adjusting their position between that determined by the intrauterine environment and their childhood centile. Nutrition is the most important influence on growth. Poor growth in infancy may be due to inadequate intake, malabsorption or excessive metabolic requirements (for example, in infants with cardiac or respiratory disease). Growth hormone (GH) does not become an important mediator of linear growth until the 2nd year of life.

Childhood growth – from 2 years to the pubertal growth spurt. Growth hormone and other endocrine factors are the most important mediators of growth in childhood. Normal growth maintains the child on almost the same height centile position between 2 and 3 years of age and puberty. If the child has lost growth in infancy or antenatally, they can be expected to grow normally in childhood, but the loss of height potential may not be regained. The centile a child grows along is determined by genetics (how tall the parents are), preceding events (birth weight and events in infancy), and chance (the same parents may produce children with a range of different heights). A child who is growing normally will have fluctuations but maintain an average height velocity sufficient to keep on the same height centile. The velocity required to remain on the top centile is not much faster than that required for the bottom centile.

The pubertal growth spurt.   The rise in sex steroid secretion at puberty stimulates an increase in GH secretion, and both sex steroids and GH are responsible for the pubertal growth spurt. In girls the pubertal growth spurt commences at breast stage 2 or 3 and in boys at testicular volume of 10 to 12 ml. Endocrine disease (hypothyroidism or GH insufficiency), poor nutrition (as in anorexia nervosa) and illnesses such as inflammatory bowel disease may reduce pubertal growth. The growth chart for the pubertal age range represents the average both for timing of onset of puberty and also pace of development, so many children do not follow the same centile through puberty.

The end of growth.   Skeletal maturation occurs during puberty and growth ceases – fusion of the epiphyses is mediated by oestrogen in both girls and boys. In girls most of the pubertal growth spurt is complete before menarche. The axial skeleton fuses before the spine and pelvis – bone age (from the hand) will be mature when there is still spinal growth to come.

Growth Problems – Short Stature in Childhood

There is no standard definition for short stature. The further below the 0.4th centile a child is, the more likely they are to have a pathological cause for their short stature. Very short adults are disadvantaged socially and in employment but there is limited evidence for psychological disadvantage for short children before puberty.

The investigation of short stature (see Figure 24.1)

In the history, ask for birth weight and any significant illnesses, and on examination include assessment of pubertal status (Tanner stages). Height measurement is the only mandatory investigation in the assessment of a short child. There is no evidence that lists of routine baseline investigations for short stature are helpful. Mid-parental height should be interpreted with caution. Illness may have influenced the parents' final height, and they are often not accurate in their estimates of their own or their partner's height.

Base initial investigations on clinical assessment, such as the following:

- *Chromosomes* – physical signs of Turner's syndrome can be extremely subtle and this should be considered in any short girl, particularly if she seems very short for her parents.
- *Thyroid function* – if there is a characteristic appearance, a family history, or the bone age is very delayed.
- *Coeliac antibodies,* if there is a history of diarrhoea or abdominal pain.
- *Look for inflammatory bowel disease* if there is a history of abdominal pain, weight loss or bloody diarrhoea.
- *Bone age* – this gives an estimate of future growth potential. In very young children (under 3 years) there is a limited amount of ossified bone to score, so results may not be helpful. There is a wide range of normal bone age at any chronological age and children frequently do not age a bone age 'year' per chronological year. Adult height can be predicted from bone age but accuracy is limited, particularly if the pattern of growth is abnormal or there has been a therapeutic intervention. Bone age scores are based on the normal skeleton and do not apply to children with skeletal dysplasia.

After initial assessment, further investigation depends on the pattern of growth. Height velocity fluctuates and this must be mon-

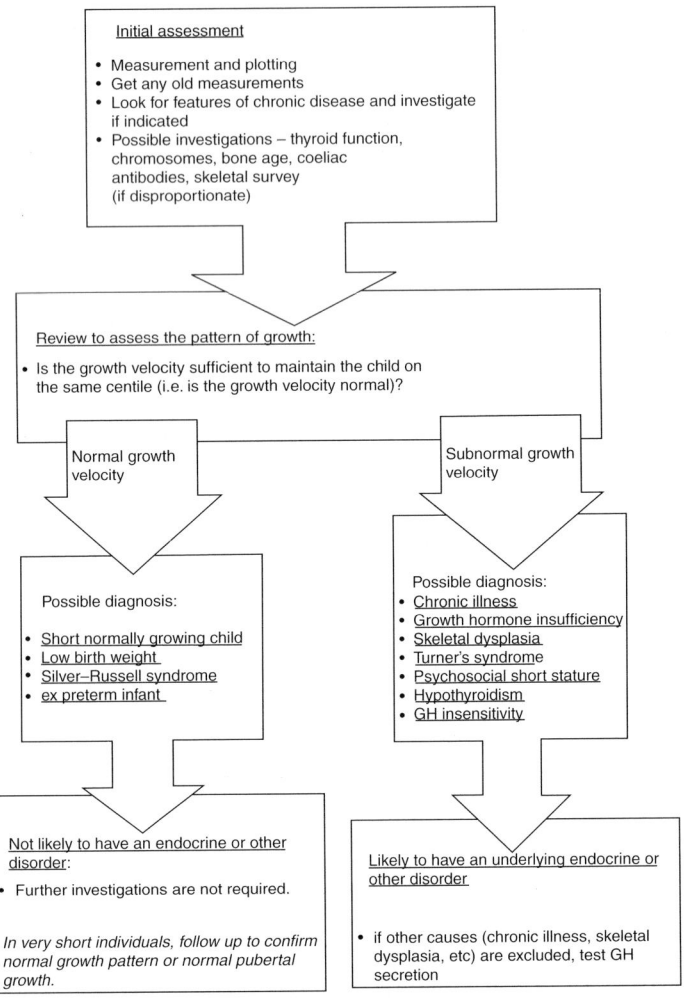

Figure 24.1 The assessment of short stature in childhood.

itored over sufficient time – charts of height velocity are based on a year of measurement and in most circumstances observation over about 1 year is needed. Exceptions to this are children who have stopped growing completely (rare and suggestive of severe underlying illness – investigate at once) or those who are so short that it is highly unlikely they are normal.

Children who are growing at a normal rate do not need further investigations. An explanation should be sought if a child is not growing at a normal rate (see below). With other causes excluded, consider checking GH secretion.

In those in the pubertal age range, assess whether the growth rate is appropriate for the stage of puberty. If the onset of puberty is delayed, growth rate and spontaneous GH secretion falls. A trial of sex steroid treatment may demonstrate a normal growth response. If GH secretion is to be tested, these children should be 'primed' with sex steroids before testing.

Causes of short stature with normal growth velocity in childhood

Children whose growth rate in childhood maintains their relative position on the centiles (however low) are not likely to have an endocrine defect. Likely explanations for their position are given below.

Short normal children.   Most short children fall into this category – the normal children of short parents; those who by chance fall at the bottom of the normal range.

Low birth weight.   Impaired growth due to antenatal factors may be carried through to adult stature. Not all infants catch up in their growth and this catch up is largely complete by the start of childhood growth. Childhood growth rate is normal.

Preterm infants.   Birth weight may be appropriate for gestation but few significantly preterm infants are an appropriate weight by the time they reach term. They then grow in the same pattern as a low-birth-weight infant, although catch-up growth has been reported over a longer period than in low birth weight. Growth in infancy may be compromised because of sequelae of prematurity such as chronic lung disease.

Problems in infancy.   Impaired nutrition in infancy (e.g. malabsorption or diarrhoeal disease) can result in loss of growth potential.

Causes of short stature with a reduced growth velocity in childhood

If height velocity is too slow to maintain the child on the same centile, there is likely to be an endocrine or other abnormality.

Chronic illness. Malabsorption, poor intake, chronic inflammation and steroid treatment can contribute to poor growth in conditions such as renal failure, inflammatory bowel disease, rheumatoid arthritis and cystic fibrosis. In asthma, poorly controlled disease and frequent courses of oral steroids are more likely to contribute to poor growth than inhaled steroids.

GH insufficiency. Growth velocity is slow and the bone age usually delayed. Most have some GH secretion but not enough to maintain normal growth. Severely GH-deficient children present with growth failure at the end of the infancy phase of growth (about 2 years) but growth failure can manifest at any age.

Skeletal dysplasia (achondroplasia, hypochondroplasia, spondylo-epiphyseal dysplasia, etc.). There is reduced birth length and poor growth velocity in childhood followed by a reduced pubertal growth spurt. GH secretion is normal. Disproportion may not be obvious at birth. Diagnosis should be confirmed with a skeletal survey, because it can be difficult to reliably distinguish different diagnoses on examination. Other syndromes associated with short stature such as Down's syndrome, Noonan's syndrome and Turner's syndrome have a similar pattern of growth.

Turner's syndrome. Abnormal growth is associated with a skeletal dysplasia and GH secretion is normal. Even with appropriate oestrogen treatment or spontaneous puberty the pubertal growth spurt is diminished.

Hypothyroidism. Thyroxine is important for the normal secretion of GH and in hypothyroidism growth velocity slows.

Psychosocial short stature. A child in unhappy surroundings can suppress GH secretion even if they are adequately nourished. These children are endocrinologically identical to children with GH insufficiency and diagnosis is based on demonstrating that growth and endocrinology rapidly return to normal when surroundings are changed.

Following radiotherapy and chemotherapy. After treatment for malignancy, growth may be affected by hypothalamic/pituitary damage or because of the impaired growth of irradiated bone (particularly the spine).

GH insensitivity (Laron syndrome). This syndrome comprises a group of rare autosomal recessive defects of the GH receptor or insulin-like growth factor-1 (IGF-1) generation, resulting in extreme short stature.

Growth-promoting agents

GH has been demonstrated to increase final height in GH-insufficient children, and there is limited evidence of an effect on final height in Turner's syndrome and renal failure. GH has been demonstrated to increase height velocity (but not necessarily final height) in a number of other conditions (see below). Oxandrolone has been used in Turner's syndrome and increases height velocity but not final height. Trials of recombinant IGF-1 in Laron syndrome are under way but there are no final height data.

Current evidence on the effect of GH in short stature

Recombinant GH was introduced in 1985, and the timescale of growth trials to final height means that our understanding of the value of GH remains incomplete. Most trials have demonstrated increased height velocity and improved height prediction, but this has not always been translated to improved adult height.

GH insufficiency.   Early trials with pituitary GH demonstrated a benefit in terms of final height, and results have improved over the years because of more generous and efficient dosing regimens and earlier diagnosis and treatment. An analysis of more recent trials demonstrated a height improvement of 1.5 SD score over prediction at the start of treatment. Final height is low compared with parental target height, but most have adult height within the normal range. Treatment is given as a daily subcutaneous injection of 0.7–1 mg/m^2/day (2–3 units/m^2/day). There is evidence that GH given daily is more effective than the same dose given three or four times a week.

Turner's syndrome.   Most (but not all) studies have demonstrated an increase in final height with GH treatment. Doses greater than those for GH insufficiency are required. An analysis of recent studies found an average increase in final height of 5.7 cm, and an average final height of 150 cm. Comparison of results is difficult because of variations in dose, age at starting treatment and age of inducing puberty. Height gain in most studies is calculated against a height prediction based on historical controls. There is a very wide range of outcome, with some individuals getting no benefit or a loss of height. The pubertal growth spurt is still diminished despite growth hormone treatment.

Chronic renal failure. Abnormal GH handling, poor nutrition, steroid treatment and acidosis result in poor growth. Studies of GH treatment have demonstrated an increase in height velocity and there is limited evidence of increased final height.

Short, normally growing children. There have been a number of trials of GH in short children with normal GH secretion (and probably many more children started on treatment outside of trials). There is an increase in velocity with treatment and an increase in predicted final height. Data on adult height give an increment of 2–3 cm over height prediction at the start of treatment. Currently, it seems that the gains do not justify treatment.

Low birth weight. There are currently very limited data on final height which do not suggest a worthwhile final height increase.

Skeletal dysplasia and short stature associated with syndromes. Trials of growth hormone have commenced in a wide range of conditions, including Noonan's syndrome, Prader–Willi syndrome and achondroplasia. Most trials have demonstrated an increase in height velocity but no final height data are available.

Hypothyroidism in childhood

Hypothyroidism in childhood is usually autoimmune and may be diagnosed because of reduced height velocity or typical appearance. Bone age is usually significantly delayed. School performance is rarely affected, and hypothyroidism after the neonatal period does not result in intellectual impairment. Treatment with thyroxine (T_4) often causes a deterioration in behaviour and attention span, which resolves with time. Replacement dose of thyroxine is approximately 100 $\mu g/m^2$ thyroxine and this should be adjusted to allow for growth. Growth velocity should be normal in treated children. Children with significantly impaired growth will have an initial period of rapid catch-up growth.

Follow-up of children referred with short stature

In most cases of short stature, assessment does not demonstrate any pathology. Discussion of the likely pattern of growth and final height may be helpful. It is important to follow children long enough to confirm a normal velocity. Some children should be measured regularly throughout growth:

- those with a chronic illness

- after radiotherapy or chemotherapy
- extremely short or an unexpected height for parents
- high levels of family concern (averting repeat referrals).

Tall Stature

Social changes have made this a rare problem. In the same way as in short stature, the pattern of growth is important – most tall children are growing at a normal height velocity and are the normal children of tall parents. In Klinefelter's syndrome, Marfan syndrome and other syndromes of overgrowth, the height gain is usually in antenatal life or infancy and velocity in childhood is normal. Tall stature with increased height velocity is associated with precocious puberty and (extremely rare) GH-secreting pituitary adenomas.

The established treatment is to induce epiphyseal fusion early with sex steroids. Older treatment regimens involved very large doses of oestrogen (up to 500 μg of ethinyloestradiol), but concerns about the risks of high-dose oestrogen mean most current protocols use doses similar to those used for the induction of puberty.

Endocrine Disorders Presenting in the Neonatal Period

Congenital hypothyroidism

All infants in the UK are screened for elevated thyroid-stimulating hormone (TSH) levels at about 1 week. Those with pituitary hypothyroidism missed by this screening are usually picked up for other reasons (see below). The hypothyroid fetus is relatively protected because of passage of maternal thyroxine across the placenta. Follow-up of children picked up by screening and treated from birth has demonstrated normal outcome in terms of growth and development. Before screening was undertaken, diagnosis was often delayed up to 1 year of age and intellectual outcome was poor. Physical signs of hypothyroidism may be absent at birth, with neonatal jaundice being the most common early manifestation. Children who develop hypothyroidism later in childhood do not develop intellectual impairment: school performance is maintained, although they become rather slow and placid.

Most cases of congenital hypothyroidism are due to developmental defects of the thyroid – the gland is absent, hypoplastic or has not descended normally in the neck (e.g. lingual thyroid).

Defects of thyroxine synthesis such as organification defects are less common.

Investigation

In congenital hypothyroidism, the TSH is often so high as to leave no doubt as to the diagnosis. Thyroid scintigraphy can be helpful in determining if the problem is likely to be permanent and may help by demonstrating anatomical defects in borderline cases with lower TSH and/or normal thyroxine. Goitre is rare and suggests an organification defect. Because of the vital role of thyroxine in brain development, it is important not to delay treatment because of investigation, and if there is doubt it is safest to treat and reassess at a later stage. To confirm that the need for treatment is lifelong, thyroxine may be stopped briefly after the age of 2 years and TSH monitored.

Treatment

A dose of 100 $\mu g/m^2$ surface area corresponds to about 25 μg thyroxine in a newborn. Elevated TSH levels may not suppress into the normal range immediately, and the dose should be adjusted to keep the thyroxine levels normal and maintain a gradual fall in TSH. Recent studies have suggested that long-term intellectual outcome may be better if higher initial doses are used with rapid suppression of TSH levels. Frequent monitoring is needed initially, because rapid growth requires dose adjustments.

Congenital hyperthyroidism

Approximately 1% of the infants of mothers with Graves' disease develop hyperthyroidism because of placental passage of antibodies. Clinical features include exophthalmos, poor weight gain, diarrhoea, tachycardia and cardiac failure.

The problem resolves by approximately 3 months of age, but treatment may be required until this stage – a significant mortality rate was reported in some older series. There is no evidence that placentally transferred antibodies cause hypothyroidism, and the infants of hypothyroid mothers do not need investigation unless there is a history of previous hyperthyroidism.

Hypopituitarism

Pituitary disorders may present in the newborn period with hypoglycaemia secondary to reduced cortisol secretion. Infants may also have conjugated hyperbilirubinaemia (which is related to low cortisol) or micropenis. Congenital hypopituitarism is caused by abnormalities of development or differentiation of the anterior pituitary, and may be isolated or associated with other central nervous system (CNS) developmental abnormalities (holoprosencephaly, absence of the corpus callosum, optic nerve hypoplasia).

Transient low blood glucose measurements are not uncommon in the neonatal period and infants at high risk are routinely screened (low birth weight, preterm, ill or septic, infants of diabetic mothers). When hypoglycaemia does not resolve or requires high concentrations of glucose, further investigations are required. The differential diagnosis includes:

- low cortisol – hypopituitarism or adrenal hypoplasia
- hyperinsulinism – as well as the infants of diabetic mothers, there are a number of genetic defects of insulin regulation with inappropriately elevated insulin levels for the blood glucose
- inborn errors of metabolism – may be accompanied by acidosis or elevated lactate.

Management of hypopituitarism in the newborn

Preventing hypoglycaemia is the most important aspect of management, because even asymptomatic hypoglycaemia in the newborn can result in permanent neurological deficit. Check other aspects of pituitary function – TSH and serum thyroxine, GH and adrenocorticotrophic hormone (ACTH). Luteinising hormone (LH) and follicle-stimulating hormone (FSH) are usually elevated in the newborn period, and low levels suggest an abnormality. Cranial ultrasound can demonstrate absent corpus callosum, although magnetic resonance imaging (MRI) is advisable later to demonstrate hypothalamic–pituitary anatomy.

Elixirs of steroids have a short shelf life and tend to precipitate out, so many clinicians give crushed tablets of hydrocortisone at a dose of 15 mg/m^2 body surface. (The most practical way is to use the smallest tablets, 2.5 mg given 8-hourly.)

Growth failure secondary to GH insufficiency may not present until the 2nd year. Replacement doses need to be constantly reviewed during childhood to keep pace with growth. Parents should be instructed to increase steroid cover during illness. The pituitary problem may progress, with other hormone deficiencies developing during childhood.

Diabetes insipidus in the newborn

In the newborn, increased thirst or dilute urine may not be obvious, and diabetes insipidus may present with failure to thrive. The diagnosis may be obvious without a formal water deprivation test (dilute urine with an elevated plasma osmolality). In X-linked nephrogenic diabetes insipidus there is insensitivity to antidiuretic hormone (ADH) and to DDAVP. Pituitary diabetes insipidus may be related to developmental abnormalities of the pituitary. In sick preterm infants, confirming a diagnosis of diabetes insipidus can be extremely difficult. Wide fluctuations in electrolyte balance are not uncommon, generous fluid replacement may mask the effects of diabetes insipidus, and the preterm kidney does not have the same concentrating ability as in an older child (this can be further impaired if the child is sick).

Congenital adrenal hyperplasia (CAH)

Deficiency of 21-hydroxylase is the commonest cause of ambiguous genitalia in the UK (see below). Other adrenal enzyme defects (11β-hydroxylase, 3β-hydroxysteroid dehydrogenase, etc) are rarer in northern European populations. There are a number of different clinical presentations of 21-hydroxylase deficiency:

- Girls have virilisation or ambiguous genitalia because of antenatal exposure to androgens. A few are so virilised that they are thought to be boys at birth.
- Boys who are 'salt losers' present with a salt-losing crisis.
- Non-salt-losing boys may present with virilisation (genital growth, pubic hair with no testicular enlargement) and rapid growth in the first few years of life.
- Non-classical CAH occasionally presents in adolescent girls.

Salt-losing crises

Infants with significant mineralocorticoid deficit present in the first few weeks of life with salt loss. The child can present acutely unwell and collapsed. There may be a history of poor feeding and floppiness over the days before the child presents. Serum sodium concentration is low and potassium elevated. Salt-losing crisis in infancy is strongly associated with later neurodevelopmental problems, so it is vital to avert this if possible.[6] Infants must not be left untreated while blood results are awaited or observed to see what happens.

The infant should be treated with fluid replacement and intravenous hydrocortisone (for a sick neonate, 25 mg hydrocortisone, 6-hourly). There is a large sodium deficit by the time of presentation and it may take time to correct this. Infants who present with significant salt loss will require permanent mineralocorticoid replacement and should be given sodium supplements while on formula or breast milk (which has a low sodium content).

Investigation of a child with possible congenital adrenal hyperplasia

Check serum electrolytes and 17-hydroxyprogesterone. Urine should be collected for steroid profile: 17-hydroxyprogesterone is elevated in both 21-hydroxylase deficiency and 11β-hydroxylase deficiency. Serum cortisol level at presentation may be within the normal range (because of the elevated ACTH). Clarifying the enzyme defect (urine steroid profile) is important both in predicting outcome and for genetic counselling.

Management of 21-hydroxylase deficiency

Patients should be commenced on 20–25 mg/m^2/day of hydrocortisone and 125–150 μg/m^2/day fludrocortisone, the dose adjusted to keep pace with growth. The aim is to give sufficient hydrocortisone to suppress ACTH secretion but without growth suppression. Discussion continues over the size and timing of dose and monitoring of treatment, and there is considerable variation in practice.

There may be variations in the degree of suppression of 17-hydroxyprogesterone through the day. Checking at different times may provide more information, and some centres measure 17-hydroxyprogesterone on dried blood spots taken throughout the day at home. Plasma renin activity will indicate if mineralocorticoid replacement is adequate, but can be difficult to interpret in infants.

Height and weight should be monitored – changes in height velocity are a sensitive measure of treatment adequacy and some clinicians rely on this and do not routinely check 17-hydroxyprogesterone levels. Inadequate hydrocortisone dose (the child growing out of the dose or poor compliance) results in increased growth velocity followed by advancing bone age and virilisation. Increased androgen secretion can have a maturational effect on the hypothalamus and results in true central precocious puberty, which does not resolve when hydrocortisone dose is increased. Obesity is a common problem in adolescent girls with CAH and the physical features of PCOS frequently develop at this stage.

Adrenal hypoplasia

This is a developmental defect of the adrenal gland – most are X-linked, although autosomal recessive cases are reported. Infants present in the first few weeks of life with signs of adrenal insufficiency – salt loss, jaundice and hypoglycaemia. In the X-linked type there is an associated gonadotrophin deficiency.

Ambiguous genitalia

Infants with ambiguous genitalia should be assessed by a unit with the appropriate specialist surgical and medical skills. It is a great shock for parents if the gender of a newborn infant is unclear, and the immediate reactions of medical and nursing staff can add to problems. Useful rules for the immediate management of the situation are:

- Reassure the parents that the child's gender will be sorted out as soon as possible – the baby will be a he or a she.
- Advise them not to choose a name yet or register the baby.
- Don't guess about a gender.
- The assigned gender of the child may not be the same as the chromosomal sex. Many people know about sex chromosomes and it is helpful to make sure that the parents understand this.
- Take action to assure privacy for the family and discuss how they will deal with relatives and friends.

Causes of ambiguous genitalia

The commonest cause in the UK is 21-hydroxylase deficiency (virilised female infant) which means that an infant with ambiguous genitalia may be at risk of salt-losing crisis. Fetal, placental, maternal and exogenous sources of androgen have all been reported as causes of virilisation of female fetuses. Reduced virilisation of the XY fetus may result from reduced testosterone secretion (developmental or enzyme defects of the testis) or abnormalities of the androgen receptor. Total androgen insensitivity presents as a female phenotype with no ambiguity (previously called testicular feminisation). If there is testicular tissue, secretion of anti-müllerian hormone during development results in regression of the developing uterus and fallopian tubes. The remaining group of infants with ambiguous genitalia have both testicular and ovarian tissue – either 'true' hermaphrodites (who usually have a 46XX karyotype) or XO/XY or XX/XY mosaic.

Disorders of Puberty

The endocrinology of normal puberty

The hypothalamo–pituitary–gonadal axis is active in the neonatal period with pulsatile LH and FSH secretion. There is then a gradual decrease in activity during the first year of life. During childhood, the system is relatively inactive with occasional nocturnal pulses of LH and FSH. In the years preceding puberty, there is a gradual increase in pulsatile gonadotrophin secretion. There is a progressive increase in the number and amplitude of LH and FSH pulses. These occur mainly at night in early puberty, with pulses throughout the whole 24 hours by the end of puberty. The timing of onset of puberty is determined by the hypothalamic secretion of gonadotrophin-releasing hormone (GnRH), although the factors triggering this in the human are not clear: nutrition is important, although there does not seem to be a fixed 'target weight' for the onset of puberty.

Because of the consistent pattern of endocrine changes, the physical changes of puberty are relatively consistent. In girls, the first sign of puberty is breast development, which is followed by pubic hair growth. Menarche does not normally occur until breast stage 4 or 5 is reached (and vaginal bleeding before this should be investigated). In boys, the first sign of puberty is testicular enlargement to over 4 ml, followed by pubic hair and genital growth. Testicular growth is required for the secretion of pubertal concentrations of testosterone – this is important in distinguishing situations where androgens are being secreted by sources other than the testes (e.g. untreated CAH). The pubertal growth spurt occurs at the start of puberty in girls (breast stage 2–3) and is relatively later in boys (10–12 ml testicular volume).

Preceding the onset of puberty, there is a change in the function of the adrenal gland. The growth of the zona reticularis at about 6–9 years of age produces an increase in secretion of adrenal androgens – androstenedione and dehydroepiandrosterone sulphate (DHEAS). This change is called adrenarche.

The pelvic ultrasound in puberty

The uterus and ovaries can usually be visualised even in infants. The uterus grows throughout childhood but remains tubular, with the cervix the same diameter or greater than the fundus. Pubertal concentrations of oestrogen are required for a change to a pear shape (accompanied by an increase in length and width) and the development of a clear endometrial echo. There is growth of the ovaries through childhood and the normal prepubertal ovary will have visible follicles, which can be up to about 10 mm across. In the years before puberty, the ovaries grow and there is an increase in the number of follicles visible.

Pelvic ultrasound can be of value in a number of situations:

- in sexual precocity, progress through centrally mediated puberty includes progression of pelvic ultrasound appearances
- an endometrial thickness of approximately 5 mm is needed for menstruation, so it is unlikely if the endometrium is thin
- ultrasound is not helpful in predicting the likely onset of puberty in pubertal delay but a normal ultrasound may be reassuring for the patient
- visualising (or not) of a uterus can be of value in the investigation of a baby with ambiguous genitalia.

Problems of puberty – pubertal delay

Individuals with pubertal delay will present complaining of short stature or lack of puberty. Growth continues at the same rate as in childhood until the growth spurt, so an individual who is late in puberty will feel increasingly short compared with his pubertal schoolmates. The problem is commoner in boys: almost all will catch up in time, but the problem can cause considerable psychological and social problems.

Causes of pubertal delay

Abnormalities of timing.　　Most individuals with pubertal delay are simply at the end of the normal range for the onset of puberty. Before the development of signs of puberty, it is not possible to reliably distinguish individuals with severe delay from those who have a permanent central defect. Spontaneous pubertal development has been described well after 20 years, but a central defect becomes increasingly likely the older a subject becomes without development.

Gonadal failure. Turner's syndrome should be considered in pubertal delay if a girl seems very short for her parents, if there is a history of some breast development but then progress halts or if there is pubic hair but no breast development. Gonadal failure should be considered in boys with a history of torsion, testicular surgery or undescended testes. Chemotherapy or radiotherapy can cause gonadal failure. Radiotherapy protocols for some brain tumours and leukaemia may include spinal (and therefore possibly gonadal) irradiation.

Assessment and investigation

Every patient should have height and pubertal rating checked. Further investigations should be performed if gonadal failure seems a possibility, if there is a risk factor for a central defect (such as a history of trauma or anosmia) or the individual has reached an age where it becomes less likely that they are normal. There is no clear cut-off age, but this should be considered if there are no signs of puberty and no obvious explanation after 16 years.

Investigation can diagnose gonadal failure but may not predict the onset of puberty, or reliably rule out a central defect:

- *Bone age* may be of value in predicting final height.
- *Gonadotrophin levels* – FSH and LH are likely to be unequivocally elevated in gonadal failure. One-off levels taken during the day are likely to be low in both prepuberty and early puberty.
- *Pelvic ultrasound* cannot predict the onset of puberty but may reassure that all is well.
- *GnRH test* – there is an increase in LH and FSH response to GnRH in early puberty but the test may not help in predicting future development.
- *MRI scan* to rule out structural defects should be considered if the individual is a long way outside the normal age range for puberty or has a risk factor for a central defect.

Management of pubertal delay

In most cases no cause is found and one can either wait and see, or treat to accelerate progress. Individuals with pubertal delay may be excluded from sports and social activities, and can be bullied, or disadvantaged in looking for jobs or college places. There may be very significant psychological benefits in treatment. The feelings of parents about treatment may be very different from their off-spring, and it is important to get the opinion of the patient.

Treatment to accelerate pubertal growth and development. The options are either anabolic steroid (oxandrolone) or low-dose sex steroids. Trials of GH have demonstrated that it is no better than sex steroid treatment in pubertal delay.

Oxandrolone is a synthetic steroid with both anabolic and weak androgenic effects. Low doses accelerate height velocity without advancing bone age or the appearance of secondary sexual characteristics. Final height is unchanged. The treatment is particularly helpful for boys with some signs of puberty but not yet at the pubertal growth spurt (6–8 ml testicular volume). The response is better than in prepubertal boys, and pubertal growth often continues after treatment has stopped. For those with no signs of puberty, low-dose sex steroids may be a better option.

Oxandrolone can be used in females with pubertal delay (and is used in Turner's syndrome), but in practice it is mainly given to boys because it provides an oral alternative to testosterone; 2.5 mg or 1.25 mg oxandrolone is given daily for 3 months. This can be repeated if necessary, but repeated courses carry the potential risk of bone age advance.

Sex steroids provide an increase in height velocity and devel-opment. Sex steroids may be given for a brief period to stimulate some development in those with delay or to take someone all the way through puberty (in gonadal failure or very significant delay). Ethinyloestradiol is available in a range of low-dose tablets. Oestrogen patches have not been studied because of the low dose required. Oral testosterone undecanoate and testosterone patches have both have been studied, but unreliable intestinal absorption and problems with dose mean that intramuscular testosterone esters are the most commonly used treatment in boys. While there is considerable variation in the protocols used, the basic principle is to start at a low dose of sex steroids and then gradually increase the dose to complete development and reach adult doses over about 2–3 years. A more rapid increase may compromise final height and will give poor breast development in females.

In prepubertal individuals, treatment should be started with testosterone esters (Sustanon), 50 mg intramuscularly every month, or oral ethinyloestradiol, 5 µg daily. This should be reviewed at 3 months and the same dose continued for 6 months if required. This should accelerate growth, and provide the gradual onset of secondary sexual characteristics. Development that is more than expected indicates the onset of endogenous puberty and treatment can be stopped. If the patient is happy with the changes when reviewed, there is no harm in stopping and observing. If longer treatment is needed, carry on as described below.

Sex steroid treatment to complete pubertal development

This is needed if there is gonadal failure or a central defect, or if you have given a short course of sex steroids to accelerate development and decide to carry on because no endogenous development is apparent.

Females. If the problem is recognised well before puberty becomes delayed, a dose of 2 µg/day of ethinyloestradiol for 6 months can be used to provide a more 'physiological' start, then giving successive doses of 5 µg, 10 µg, 15 µg and 20 µg ethinyloestradiol/day in 6-month steps. Progesterone (e.g. levonorgestrel 30 µg) should be added in if there is a vaginal bleed, if ultrasound demonstrates an endometrium of over 5 mm or when 15 µg dose is reached. This can be given on days 14–21 of the cycle. Note that 25 µg or 30 µg of ethinyloestradiol may be needed to give regular cycles in larger girls.

Males. Treatment should be started at 50 mg testosterone esters (Sustanon, Organon, Cambridge, UK) every month for 6 months, then 100 mg every month, 100 mg every 3 weeks, then 100 mg every 2 weeks in 6-month steps. More may be needed to maintain adult testosterone levels. If the problem is recognised before puberty is delayed, a starting dose of 50 mg every 6 weeks can be given for 6 months to provide a more 'physiological' start.

Delayed puberty in individuals with severe intellectual or physical disabilities. These patients have an increased prevalence of problems of puberty – pubertal delay and failure are more common and may be picked up very late. The potential benefits of sex steroid treatment should be assessed on an individual basis. There may be concern about inducing difficult or inappropriate behaviour, an increase in the size of a child who relies on parents to lift them or difficulties in managing periods in girls who may not be continent. While sex steroid treatment occasionally induces behaviour problems in adolescents with learning disability, puberty can also produce a more mature personality. The risks associated with osteoporosis may depend on the level of physical activity, and may be less if the adolescent is very immobile.

Sexual Precocity

Introduction

Sexual precocity is conventionally defined as any sign of puberty appearing before 8 years of age in a girl or before 9 years of age in a boy. There is considerable confusion of terminology in this area and I will use the term 'precocious puberty' only for central precocious puberty. The majority of cases of sexual precocity are benign variations of normal sexual development with a normal outcome and most do not need treatment. These disorders provoke great anxiety in parents who may be concerned about malignancy or future fertility problems. The aim of assessment is to identify the small proportion of cases who need treatment, reassure the family and give an assessment of the likely outcome (e.g. in girls the likely timing of menarche).

The source of sex steroids in sexual precocity

The most helpful clinical approach is to first identify the source of steroid production and then to look at the pattern and pace of development.

Gonadal sex steroids. The gonads either secrete sex steroids in response to gonadotrophin stimulation, or rarely have autonomous secretion (McCune–Albright syndrome or testotoxicosis). Gonadotrophin stimulation results in gonadal growth. If virilisation occurs in a boy without testicular growth, the source of androgens is not likely to be testicular (and likely to be adrenal). Breast development implies ovarian activity.

Adrenal sex steroids. Adrenal steroids are responsible for the growth of pubic and axillary hair and the development of 'adult' smelling sweat. This can result from the normal maturation of the adrenal in mid-childhood (adrenarche), or much more rarely from adrenal tumours or CAH.

Tumours. Sexual precocity has been described secondary to adrenal and gonadal tumours, most of which secrete androgens. Gonadotrophin secretion has been described in rare hepatic and cerebral tumours (almost all outside the pituitary). Intracranial tumours can provoke the premature secretion of hypothalamic GnRH, resulting in centrally mediated precocious puberty (Box 24.1).

Box 24.1   CNS lesions associated with central precocious puberty

Tumours:
  Optic nerve glioma
  Pinealoma
  Astrocytoma
  Hypothalamic hamartoma
  Ependymoma
  Pituitary adenoma

Other CNS lesions:
  Following CNS surgery or irradiation
  Hydrocephalus (even if the period of raised intracranial pressure was brief)
  Neurofibromatosis
  Post-trauma
  Septo-optic dysplasia
  After meningitis/encephalitis

Exogenous sources of steroid. There have a been few reports of sexual precocity due to absorption of topical steroid creams. There is no epidemiological evidence to suggest that environmental oestrogens or hormones used in farming are responsible for sexual precocity. Prepubertal girls who take contraceptive pills on one occasion can provoke vaginal bleeding but not pubertal development.

The clinical presentation of sexual precocity
(Figures 24.2 and 24.3).

The majority of patients with sexual precocity are girls, partly because of the difference in activity of the hypothalamic–pituitary–gonadal axis between males and females. Clinical assessment will suggest the

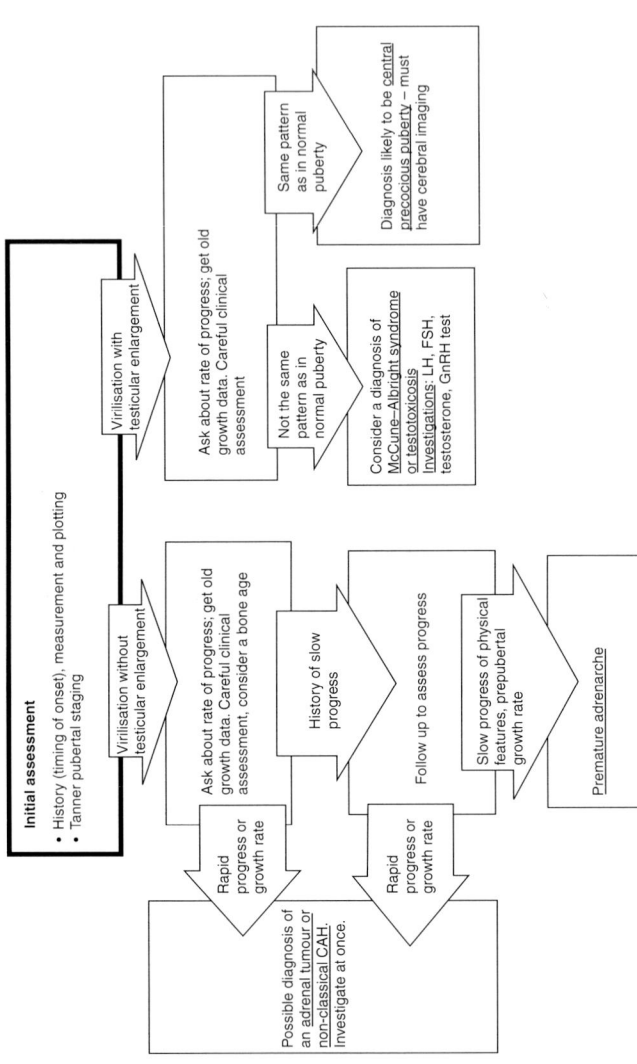

Figure 24.2 The diagnosis of sexual precocity in males. CAH = congenital adrenal hyperplasia; FSH = follicle-stimulating hormone; GnRH = gonadotrophin-releasing hormone; LH = luteinising hormone.

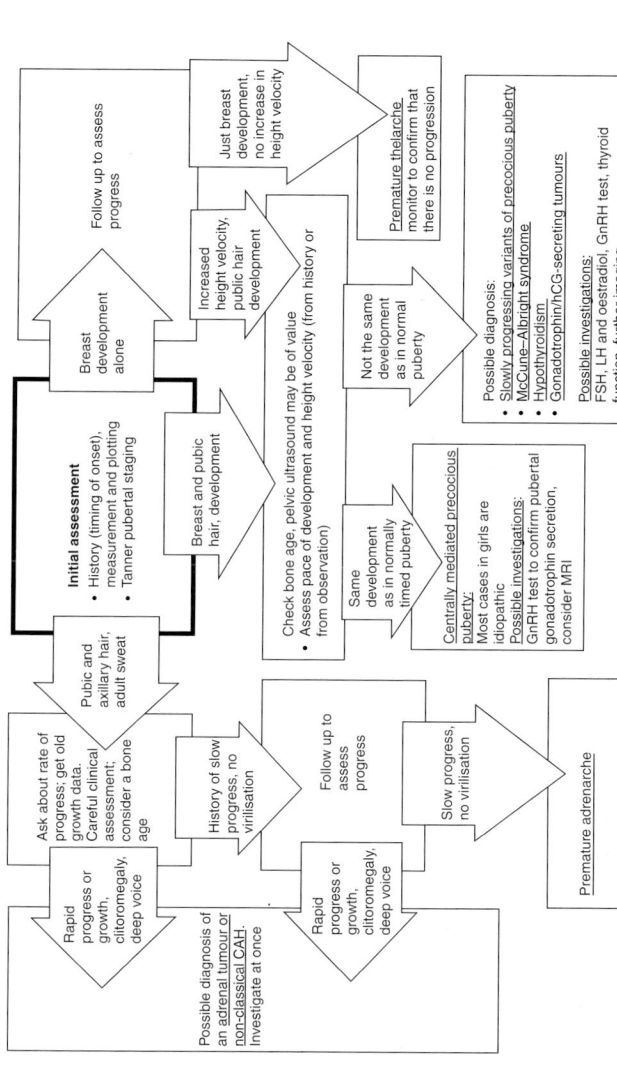

Figure 24.3 The diagnosis of sexual precocity in females. CAH = congenital adrenal hyperplasia; FSH = follicle-stimulating hormone; GnRH = gonadotrophin-releasing hormone; hCG = human chorionic gonadotrophin; LH = luteinising hormone; MRI = magnetic resonance imaging.

likely source of steroid secretion. There are a number of different clinical presentations:

Sexual precocity secondary to gonadal steroids

Gonadotrophin-mediated development in females – premature the-larche, thelarche variant, slowly progressing central precocious puberty and central precocious puberty. Premature thelarche usually presents in the first few years of life with breast develop-ment, which may be one sided or cyclical. There are no other signs of puberty and no increase in growth rate or progress in puberty. Final height is normal. Ultrasound may demonstrate small ovarian cysts. Sampling studies have demonstrated FSH pulsatility, which is thought to stimulate low levels of oestrogen secretion.

In central precocious puberty the pattern of endocrine changes and the pattern of physical events is the same as in normally timed puberty. The endocrine picture is the same as normal puberty with predominantly LH pulsatility occurring mainly at night. Most cases of central precocious puberty in girls are idiopathic with no lesion on MRI scanning. There is no sex difference in the incidence of secondary central precocious puberty caused by cerebral lesions and, because idiopathic central precocious puberty is very rare in boys (and may not exist at all), this means that the majority of cases of central precocious puberty occur in girls. A number of intracra-nial tumours or lesions can provoke central precocious puberty (see Box 24.1). Increased intracranial pressure may be an important factor. Central precocious puberty in children with shunts for hydrocephalus is related to a history of increased intracranial pres-sure in the neonatal period.

Central precocious puberty occurs much more commonly in girls adopted in early childhood from developing countries. Elevated sex steroid levels in prepuberty appear to mature the hypothalamus and can result in central precocious puberty in both sexes; e.g. when there has been a period of inadequate treatment in CAH.

In females there is a clinical spectrum between premature thelarche and central precocious puberty. The endocrine pattern follows a spectrum between predominantly FSH pulsatility in pre-mature thelarche and predominantly LH in central precocious puberty. These variations are labelled as thelarche variant or slowly progressing variations of precocious puberty. Some girls with central precocious puberty will turn out to progress very slowly, and some who seem to have premature thelarche will turn out to progress a little. Assessment of the pace of progress is important in determining the need for treatment in central precocious puberty.

Gonadotrophin-mediated development in males – central precocious puberty. There appears to be no equivalent of premature thelarche in boys, and central precocious puberty normally progresses at the same pace as normally timed puberty. Central precocious puberty in males is rare and must be investigated to look for a central lesion. There have been very few reports of idiopathic central precocious puberty in males, so great caution should be exercised in making this diagnosis.

Gonadotrophin-independent sex steroid secretion – males and females. In this group of disorders there is secretion of sex steroids without gonadotrophin stimulation. Gonadotrophin levels are low and the gonadotrophin response to GnRH stimulation is suppressed, whereas sex steroid concentrations are high. Physical development does not necessarily follow the same pattern as normal puberty. In girls high oestrogen concentrations can result in menstruation before breast development has reached Tanner stage 4.

In McCune Albright syndrome there is a defect in the G protein associated with the LH receptor, resulting in continued receptor activation without LH binding. The G protein is shared with a number of other hormone receptors, and autonomous secretion of other hormones has been reported (Cushing's thyrotoxicosis, gigantism). The defect is a somatic cell line mutation and occurs in both sexes. Presentation is highly variable and depends on which cells carry the mutation. There may be associated pigmented skin lesions and bony abnormalities (polyostostic fibrous dysplasia).

In testotoxicosis there is a dominantly inherited defect of the LH receptor. A number of mutations of the transmembrane domain of the receptor have been described that result in continuing G-protein activation and autonomous testosterone secretion. Females who carry the mutation appear unaffected.

Hypothyroidism

In untreated hypothyroidism there is a rise in FSH as well as TSH. Elevated FSH can result in breast development or presentation with vaginal bleeding with insufficient breast development. FSH falls with thyroxine treatment.

Sexual precocity secondary to adrenal steroids – premature adrenarche (also known as premature pubarche)

Most children do not have any physical changes at the time of adrenarche, but a few develop growth of pubic or axillary hair and adult-smelling sweat. There may be a small increase in height velocity at the time of adrenarche. Genetic factors are very important – premature adrenarche is more common in children with origins in the Middle East, the Indian subcontinent and some parts of Africa. Children of African origin can present with a much more marked growth spurt and significant bone age advance. True central puberty starts at a normal age in these children and final height is within the target range for parents.

Congenital adrenal hyperplasia

Boys with non-salt-losing 21-hydroxylase deficiency who have not had salt losing may present in the first few years of life with virilisation (genital growth, pubic hair but no testicular enlargement, increased muscle bulk). There is tall stature with significant bone age advancement, resulting in impaired adult height.

Adrenal tumours

An adrenal tumour should be considered if there is rapid growth or progressive virilisation, acne, cushingoid appearance, development of a deep voice or clitoromegaly. Most larger tumours (over 5 cm) are malignant.

Assessment and investigation of sexual precocity

All children should have height and weight measured and Tanner pubertal stages recorded. The history may give information on the rate of development, although parents occasionally fail to notice the development of secondary sexual characteristics.

Clinical assessment should suggest the likely source of sex steroids. In most cases the most important investigation is to follow the pace of growth and development. If the likely source of the steroids is adrenal, clinical assessment will indicate those who may not have premature adrenarche and these need further investigation.

The following investigations may be useful:

Bone age.   Pubertal levels of sex steroids result in bone age advance into the pubertal range.

Pelvic ultrasound (see above).   In central precocious puberty, changes in uterine shape occur at the same time as physical development. In premature thelarche, the uterus does not change shape and there is no endometrium. In slowly progressing variants of central precocious puberty, uterine growth mirrors pubertal development.

MRI scan of the hypothalamus and pituitary.   This scan must be done in every boy with central precocious puberty. The chances of detecting a lesion in girls with central precocious puberty are small. Younger girls are more likely to have an abnormality. Most clinicians scan younger girls, although practice varies as to the cut-off age.

Gonadotrophin response to GnRH.   One-off measurement of gonadotrophins may not be helpful. A pubertal response to GnRH stimulation suggests that an individual is in centrally mediated puberty. In McCune–Albright syndrome, the gonadotrophin response to GnRH is suppressed.

Urine steroid profile, serum adrenal androgens.   These are the initial tests for a possible adrenal tumour.

Bone scan.   To look for fibrous dysplasia in McCune–Albright syndrome.

Assessing the need for treatment

Treatment to hold up development should be considered in central precocious puberty or gonadotrophin-independent sexual precocity. The following problems might be reasons to start treatment:

Loss of adult height.   The height gained in the pubertal growth spurt is normal but growth starts when there has been insufficient childhood growth. The bone age rapidly advances into the range appropriate for puberty with a loss of height prediction and reduced adult height. However, most children with central precocious puberty have an adult height within the normal range.

Social problems.   Children appear much older than they are and this can cause difficulties socially and at school.

Behaviour problems.   Pubertal levels of sex steroids can produce mood swings and difficult behaviour.

Early menarche.   Periods in very young girls may present a practical problem.

Which patients require treatment?

Potential benefits should be weighed against the burden of regular injections and hospital visits. The small proportion of very young children who present with progressive central precocious puberty obviously need treatment for social and psychological reasons, whatever their final height. For older patients, the benefits may be more marginal – adult height potential may be normal (even if less than expected for their parents). Behavioural and social problems are often not resolved with treatment. Many quite young girls can cope extremely well with periods. Monitoring to determine the pace of progress will find a proportion of girls who have slowly progressing variants of precocious puberty and will not need treatment. Holding up puberty within the normal age range does not improve final height.

Currently used treatments are given below.

GnRH analogues.   GnRH analogues suppress gonadotrophin secretion and halt development with, in some cases, regression of secondary sexual characteristics. Monthly or 3-monthly depot injections are the most convenient formulation. GnRH analogues are more effective and have less side effects than cyproterone acetate, and are the primary treatment for central precocious puberty. Suppression of sex steroid secretion results in a slowing of growth, which is most marked in those with an advanced bone age. Most studies have reported a small increase in final height over height prediction at the start of treatment.

Cyproterone acetate.   Cyproterone acetate remains the main treatment option in gonadotrophin-independent sexual precocity and is second choice for central precocious puberty. It is less effective in suppressing pubertal development and there is no evidence of benefit in terms of final height. Treatment frequently results in tiredness and can cause significant adrenal suppression. Cyproterone is useful in suppressing the temporary increase in pubertal progress that occurs at the start of treatment with GnRH analogues.

Testolactone, spironolactone and ketoconazole.   These compounds have all been used in trials of treatment for gonadotrophin-independent precocity: there are limited long-term data.

Long-term outcome in sexual precocity

There is no consensus about when to stop treatment, but there is no evidence of benefit in continuing beyond the normal age of pubertal onset. A proportion of pubertal growth will have already occurred, and pubertal growth after the treatment has worn off will be limited, particularly in those with advanced bone age. Subsequent development and fertility is normal, except in gonadotrophin-independent precocious puberty, where the abnormal pattern of activation continues and can result in impaired fertility. Some studies suggest an increased risk of poly-cystic ovarian disease following premature adrenarche and central precocious puberty.

Calcium Disorders in Infants and Children

Nutritional rickets in infants and young children

Prolonged exclusive breast-feeding, pigmented skin, lack of sun-shine exposure in child and mother, failure to give supplements and limited diets are all risk factors for nutritional rickets, which may present in the following ways:

- The typical thickened epiphyses are noticed. These are most obvious around the wrists and ankles and as the 'ricketty rosary', which is the thickened costochondral junction. Epiphyseal cupping may be noted on an X-ray taken for other reasons.
- Infants can present with bowing of the legs when they start to walk. These infants typically have muscle weakness and may be reluctant to weight bear because of pain.
- The first presentation may be symptoms of hypocalcaemia such as tetany or fits.
- In children with severe rickets, craniotabes – the ability to dent the skull slightly under pressure.

Growth may be completely normal. A child who has a risk factor and typical radiological findings does not need extensive investiga-tion – check serum calcium, phosphate, albumin and urea and elec-trolytes. Alkaline phosphatase measurement provides a useful way of monitoring treatment. Consider further investigations if there seems to be no risk factors, biochemical or radiological investigations are not typical or there is alopecia (associated with about 50% of cases of vitamin D receptor abnormality). Rickets is associated with a generalised aminoaciduria, which resolves with treatment. A falling alkaline phosphatase is a sign of adequate treatment, whereas improvement on X-ray may take months. Even quite bowed legs can straighten as bone remodelling occurs, and few need surgical treatment. Failure to resolve on treatment may be caused by inherited forms of rickets, but in practice is more often due to poor compliance. It may be helpful to look at the vitamin D status of the mother and siblings.

Further Reading

Brunner HG, Otten BJ. Precocious puberty in boys. *N Engl J Med* 1999;**34**:1763–5.

Carel JC, Roger M, Ispas S *et al*. Final height after long term treatment with triptorelin slow release for central precocious puberty: importance of statural growth after interruption of treatment. *J Clin Endocrinol Metab* 1999;**84**:1973–8.

Donaldson MD, Thomas PH, Love JG, Murray GD, McNinch AW, Savage DC. Presentation acute illness and learning difficulties in salt wasting 21 hydroxylase deficiency. *Arch Dis Child* 1994;**70**:214–18.

Downie BA, Mulligan J, Stratford RJ, Betts PR, Voss LD. Are short children at a disadvantage? The Wessex growth study. *Br Med J* 1997;**314**:97–100.

Guyda HJ. Four decades of growth hormone therapy for short children: what have we achieved? *J Clin Endocrinol Metab* 1999;**84**:4307–15.

Hulse JA, Grant DB, Jackson D, Clayton BE. Growth development and reassessment of hypothyroid infants diagnosed by screening. *Br Med J* 1982;**284**:1435–7.

Kaplowicz PB, Oberfeld SE. Re-examination of the age limit for defining when puberty is precocious in girls in the United States: implications for evaluation and treatment. *Pediatrics* 1999;**104**(1): 936–41.

Karlberg J, Albertsson Wickland K. Growth in full term small for gestational age infants: from birth to final height. *J Pediatr* 1995;**38**:733–9.

Klein KO. Editorial: precocious puberty: Who has it? Who should be treated? *J Clin Endocrinol Metab* 1999;**84**:411–14.

Klein KO, Mericq V, Brown-Dawson J, Larmore K, Cabenzas P, Cortinez A. Estrogen levels in girls with premature thelarche compared with normal prepubertal girls as determined by an ultrasensitive recombinant cell bioassay. *J Pediatr* 1999;**134**:190–2.

Palmert MR, Malin HV, Boepple PA. Unsustained or slowly progressive puberty in young girls: initial presentation and long term follow up of 20 untreated patients. *J Clin Endocrinol Metab* 1999;**84**:415–23.

Saenger P. Growth promoting strategies in Turner's syndrome. *J Clin Endocrinol Metab* 1999;**84**:4345–8.

Wolthers O, Cameron FJ, Scheimberg I *et al.* Androgen secreting adreno-cortical tumours. *Arch Dis Child* 1999;**80**:46-50.

25

Paget's Disease of the Bone

Anne Marie McLaughlin and Donal O'Shea

Introduction

Paget's disease was first described by Sir James Paget in 1877. It is a chronic skeletal disorder characterised by increased bone remodelling that results in abnormal bone architecture. Paget's disease affects up to 10% of the elderly, although only 5% of these are symptomatic. It is more common in males with a ratio of 3 : 1. In Paget's disease there are increased numbers of osteoclasts and osteoblasts, resulting in overproduction of poor quality bone.

Various aetiological factors have been implicated, including measles, respiratory syncytial virus and canine distemper. More recently, cytokines, in particular interleukin-6 (IL-6), have been implicated in the pathogenesis of Paget's disease of the bone. IL-6 is produced by pagetic patients' osteoclasts, which also express IL-6 receptors. Increased levels of IL-6 are found in the marrow and serum of patients with Paget's disease. In addition, RANK ligand (RANKL) (receptor activator of NF-Kappa B), a member of the tumour necrosis factor (TNF) family, has recently been identified as a critical osteoclastogenic factor. The osteoclasts in Paget's disease demonstrate increased responsiveness to RANKL; this is thought to be in part due to IL-6. These factors may contribute to the increased numbers of osteoclasts in pagetic lesions.

Clinical Features

1. Bone pain is the most common symptom. The pain is typically present at rest and is dull and aching in nature. Skeletal deformities may occur in patients with long-standing Paget's disease; these deformities include bowing deformity of long bones, acetabular protrusion of the hips, skull enlargement, frontal bossing, kyphosis or scoliosis. Pathological fractures may occur, most commonly of the femur or tibia.

2. Neurological symptoms are rare; however, involvement of the skull may result in mixed sensory and conductive hearing loss and, less commonly, cranial nerve palsies. Patients may develop progressive sensory and motor symptoms due to pagetic stenosis of the spine. Basilar invagination may result in entrapment of lower cranial nerves, vertebrobasilar insufficiency and obstructive hydrocephalus.

3. Malignant degeneration in Paget's disease occurs in < 1%; the most common sites for neoplastic transformation are the femur, pelvis and humerus.

4. Cardiac failure due to high output may occur as a result of increased blood flow through the involved area of bone. In addition, there is cutaneous vasodilation causing hyperthermia of overlying skin. This combination of increased blood flow through the bone and decreased peripheral vascular resistance results in high cardiac output, which may lead to cardiomegaly or left ventricular hypertrophy and, eventually, to congestive heart failure.

5. Hypercalcaemia is an infrequent complication, but may occur in situations of immobilisation, e.g. following a fracture.

Diagnosis

A diagnosis of Paget's disease should be considered in a patient giving a history of bone pain, particularly if the pain is periarticular. Affected patients complain of a dull ache, which is aggravated by weight-bearing activities. These symptoms are also common in degenerative joint disease, which may produce a diagnostic dilemma.

Radiographs of affected bones are usually diagnostic, with areas of lysis due to increased osteoclastic resorption and sclerosis due to osteoblastic bone formation. Scintigraphy is a sensitive but nonspecific procedure for the diagnosis of Paget's disease and is mainly used to assess the distribution of Paget's disease.

Table 25.1   Biochemical markers of Paget's disease

MARKERS OF BONE FORMATION

Amino terminal propeptide of type 1 pro-collagen (PINP)	This protein is a product of the process whereby procollagen becomes collagen It is a marker of the synthesis stage of bone formation Measured from serum samples
Bone specific alkaline phosphatase (BAP)	This is a glycoprotein found on the cell surface of osteoblasts It is a marker of the maturation stage of bone formation Measured from serum samples
Osteocalcin	Synthesised by osteoblasts and incorporated into the bone matrix. Osteocalcin binds calcium; its main function is in matrix mineralisation Measured from serum samples

MARKERS OF BONE RESORPTION

Deoxypyridinoline (D-PYR)	This protein is a product of bone resorption. Type 1 collagen molecules in bone matrix are linked by pyridinoline crosslinks (pyridinoline or deoxypyridinoline). During osteoclastic bone resorption pyridinoline crosslinks are released into the circulation. Urine samples are required for D-PYR measurement
N-terminal telopeptide	In the circulation the pyridinoline crosslinks may be attached to fragments of C-terminal or N-terminal of the type 1 collagen molecule. Urinary measurement of these are also used as markers of bone resorption

Paget's disease is associated with normal serum concentrations of calcium, phosphate and parathyroid hormone despite an increase in bone turnover. A number of biochemical markers are used to assist in the diagnosis and to monitor response to treatment (Table 25.1). A raised alkaline phosphatase on biochemical screening may be the only abnormality.

Management

Asymptomatic patients or those with mild joint pain may be treated with nonsteroidal anti-inflammatory drugs (NSAIDs); however, their biochemical markers should be monitored for evidence of increased disease activity.

Bisphosphonates are the most important drug in the management of Paget's disease. They are analogues of inorganic pyrophosphate. Bisphosphonates inhibit bone resorption by being selectively taken up by and binding to the mineral surface of bone, where they interfere with the action of osteoclasts. It is thought that bisphosphonates are internalised by the osteoclasts and interfere with their biochemical processes, resulting in their apoptosis. In Paget's disease there are increased numbers of osteoclasts and increased osteoclast activity; this is thought to occur because they do not undergo apoptosis in the normal way. If this is true, then bisphosphonates may be viewed as a drug that specifically targets the cause of the disease.

Etidronate, pamidronate and tiludronate are currently licensed for the management of Paget's disease in the United Kingdom. Etidronate is given orally at a dose of 400 mg daily for 6 months and will reduce bone turnover by 50%. The dose and duration of the drug are limited by the development of defective mineralisation with high dosage. Its main side effects are abdominal cramps and diarrhoea, which at the indicated dose should occur in > 20%. Pamidronate is administered intravenously 30 mg weekly or 60 mg in alternate weeks. Bone turnover is reduced by 70%. Transient pyrexia, myalgia and lymphopenia are seen in 20% during the first infusion. Calcium and vitamin D supplements are given to prevent the hypocalcaemia and hypophosphataemia which may occur. Tiludronate is given as a 400 mg daily dose for 3 months and will reduce bone turnover by 50%. In clinical trials gastrointestinal side effects were no more common than placebo and bone biopsy showed no evidence of defective mineralisation.

Calcitonin has been largely superseded by the bisphosphonates. It acts via specific receptors to inhibit osteoclast differentiation and activity, resulting in decreased bone turnover. It also reduces bone vascularity and is occasionally used to reduce bone blood flow before surgery. Calcitonin has to be administered subcutaneously or by intranasal insufflation. Transient flushing, nausea and diarrhoea occur in 15–20% of patients.

There is no evidence that any therapy alters outcome in terms of fracture or malignancy; currently, treatment is therefore symptomatic.

Further Reading

Alvarez L, Guanebens N, Peris P *et al.* Discriminative value of biochemical markers of bone turnover in assessing the activity of Paget's disease. *J Bone Miner Res* 1995;**10**:458–65.

Barker DJP, Chamberlain AT, Guyer PB, Gardner MJ. Paget's disease of the bone: the Lancashire focus. *Br Med J* 1980;**280**:1105–7.

Compston JE. The therapeutic use of bisphosphonates. *Br Med J* 1994;**309**:711–15.

Delmas PD, Meunier PJ. The management of Paget's disease of the bone. *New Eng J Med* 1997;**336**:558–65.

Franck WA, Bress NM, Singer FR, Krane SM. Rheumatic manifestations of Paget's disease of the bone. *Am J Med* 1974;**56**:592–603.

Greditzer HG, Mcleod RA, Unni K, Beabout JW. Bone sarcomas in Paget's disease. *Radiology* 1983;**146**:327–33.

Hosking DJ. Advances in the management of Paget's disease of the bone. *Drugs* 1990;**40**(6):829–40.

Lorenzo J. Interactions between immune and bone cells: new insights with many remaining questions. *J Clin Invest* 2000;**106**:749–52.

Mee AP. Paramyxoviruses and Paget's disease; the affirmative view. *Bone* 1999;**24**:195–215.

Menaa C, Reddy S, Kurihara N *et al*. Enhanced RANK ligand expression and responsivity of bone marrow cells in Paget's disease of the bone. *J Clin Invest* 2000;**105**:1833–8.

Roux C, Gennari C, Farrerons J *et al*. Comparative prospective, double blind, multicentre study of the efficacy of tiludronate and etidronate in the treatment of Paget's disease of the bone. *Arthritis Rheum* 1995;**38**:851–8.

Protocols

Protocols:
1. Insulin tolerance test (ITT)
2. Glucagon stimulation test
3. Arginine stimulation test
4. Water deprivation test
5. Overnight dexamethasone suppression test (ODST)
6. Low-dose dexamethasone suppression test (LDDST)
7. High-dose dexamethasone suppression test (HDDST)
8. Petrosal venous sampling
9. Peripheral venous sampling
10. Glucose tolerance test
11. Adrenal aldosterone sampling
12. Short Synacthen test
13. Long Synacthen test
14. Insulinoma fast
15. Pentolinium suppression test
16. Clonidine suppression test

Protocol 1: Insulin Tolerance Test (ITT)

Indications

Assessment of ACTH/cortisol and GH reserve

Contraindications

Documented or suspected ischaemic heart disease
History of seizures

Protocol

An experienced practitioner should remain with the patient for the duration of the test

- Fast from midnight.

- In peripubertal children (bone age > 10 years) priming is needed:
  $\Rightarrow$M: 100 mg testosterone IM 3 days before testing
  $\Rightarrow$F: 100 µg ethinyloestradiol p.o. each for 3 days before the
  test.
- Check weight, ECG and plasma potassium concentration.
- Omit hydrocortisone or cortisone acetate on the morning of test
  (at least 12 hours elapse from last dose).
- 8.30 am insert IV cannula.
- 9.00 am take basal blood samples for glucose, cortisol, GH.
- Administer IV bolus insulin (soluble). Consideration should be
  given to using a higher dose of insulin in patients in whom
  insulin resistance is suspected:
  $\Rightarrow$ Normal pituitary function 0.15 U/kg
  $\Rightarrow$ Hypopituitary 0.10 U/kg
  $\Rightarrow$ Acromegaly, diabetes, Cushing's 0.2–0.3 U/kg.
- Monitor for hypoglycaemia (expected at approximately 20–40
  min).
- Tachycardia and sweating are common and patients frequently
  become drowsy.
- Capillary glucose may be used to monitor the development of
  hypoglycaemia; however, they are not very accurate and are
  only a guide. If there is no clinical evidence of hypoglycaemia
  by 45 min, give further 0.1 U/kg of insulin IV. It will then be
  necessary to extend the period of sampling by 1 hour.
- After hypoglycaemia has been confirmed (clinically and with
  BM stix) the patient should be given a sweet drink and snack. If
  severe or persistent hypoglycaemia occurs, IV dextrose should
  be administered.
- Samples for serum glucose, cortisol and GH taken at 30, 60, 90
  and 120 min. An additional sample should be taken for glucose
  when the patient is hypoglycaemic.
- The patient should be given a meal and observed for 2 hours
  after the end of the test.

Problems in insulin stress test and their management

Severe hypoglycaemia

Adult:

- Dextrose 50%, 1 ml/kg IV
- If patient remains unconscious, give hydrocortisone 100 mg IV

Children:

- Dextrose 10%, 2 ml/kg IV over 3 min. Continue with infusion at 0.1 ml/kg/min IV.
- If patient remains unconscious, give hydrocortisone 100 mg IV.
- Aim for glucose concentrations 5–8 mmol/l.
- Higher values may precipitate cerebral oedema. Complications in ITT have been related to overzealous treatment of hypoglycaemia rather than the hypoglycaemia itself.

Interpretation

- The test cannot be interpreted unless hypoglycaemia (≤2.2 mmol/l) is achieved.
- Adequate cortisol response is defined as a rise of greater than 170 nmol/l to above 500 nmol/l (these numbers will depend on local laboratory). Patients with slightly impaired cortisol responses may only need steroid cover for major illnesses or stresses. They will need instruction about this and should carry a steroid card.
- In Cushing's syndrome there will be a rise of less than 170 nmol/l above the fluctuations of basal levels of cortisol.
- Adequate GH response is a rise to > 20 mU/l. In adults this may be a sensitive indicator of hypopituitarism but its principal role is in children who may require GH treatment. In children a rise to greater than 39 mU/l (15 ng/ml) is considered normal (2.59 mU/l = 1 ng/ml). Appropriate priming is very important if they are peri-pubertal. Before treatment with growth hormone children should have two stimulatory tests.

Sensitivity and specificity

If there is adequate hypoglycaemia and the patient is not hypothyroid then cortisol response is a good test of ACTH/adrenal reserve: 5–15% of normals will show a suboptimal response as defined by these two criteria.

Protocol 2: Glucagon Stimulation Test

Indications

- Assessment of ACTH/cortisol and GH reserve
- Used in patients in whom an ITT is contraindicated

- Often useful in diabetic patients in whom predictable hypogly-caemia is difficult to achieve with the ITT

Protocol

- Fast from midnight
- Omit hydrocortisone or cortisone acetate on the morning of test (at least 12 hours elapse from last dose)
- 8.30 am insert IV cannula
- 9.00 am take basal blood samples for glucose, cortisol, GH
- Administer 1mg IM glucagon
- Note: In children or individuals > 90 kg, consideration should be given to modifying the dose of glucagon used
- Samples for blood glucose, cortisol, GH taken at 30, 60, 90, 120, 150 and 180 min.
- It is essential that the test be continued for 180 min as the peak GH/cortisol response to glucagon is often seen at this time
- The patient should be given a meal after the end of the test.

Side effects

Side effects are unusual, but occasional patients experience nausea and may vomit.

Note

The peak cortisol response to glucagon stimulation is lower than that seen to the ITT. A normal response is therefore >400 nmol/l.

Protocol 3: Arginine Stimulation Test

Indications

Assessment of GH reserve

Protocol

- Fast from midnight
- 8.30 am insert IV cannula
- 9.00 am
    Take basal blood sample for GH
    Administer IV infusion arginine into the other cannula over 30 min
    Dose: (related to body surface area) 20 g/m^2

- Samples for GH taken at 30, 60, 90, 120 and 150 min
- The patient should be given a meal after the end of the test.

Side effects

- Side effects are unusual
- Occasional flushing, light headedness, hypotension, nausea and vomiting
- Hypoglycaemia secondary to stimulation of insulin release is a possibility which is theoretical rather than real.

Note

In normal individuals, arginine is a less profound or reliable stimulus of GH release than the ITT. Failure to reach a value > 5 mU/l is consistent with severe GH deficiency, but interpretation should take into account the clinical picture.

Protocol 4: Water Deprivation Test

Indications

Differential diagnosis of polyuria.

Cautions

Thyroid and adrenal status should be normal.

Protocol

- The patient should receive food and especially fluid (except tea and coffee) up to 0800 h on the morning of the test.
- The patient should not smoke before or during the test.
- The last dose of DDAVP should be given 24 hours before the start of the test.
- Begin test 0800–0830 h: the full test takes 10 hours.
- Weigh the patient.
- Insert IV cannula in antecubital vein.
- At the start of the test and at hourly intervals throughout the test the patient should empty their bladder and the urine volume is recorded. A 10-ml aliquot is retained for osmolality. The weight of the patient should also be recorded.
- At 30 min, $3\frac{1}{2}$, $6\frac{1}{2}$, $7\frac{1}{2}$ and 10 hours throughout the test blood samples should be taken for U&E's and serum osmolality.

- At 8 hours, a test dose of DDAVP (2 μg IM) is given to determine whether there is then an improvement in urine concentration. The weight of the patient need not be recorded after this and he/she may eat and drink normally.
- Further urine and blood specimens are taken for 2 hours to determine the response to DDAVP in order to distinguish between cranial and nephrogenic diabetes insipidus.

Problems and their management

The patient should be reviewed by the supervising physician if:

- Cumulative weight loss > 3% of initial value: check serum osmolality urgently and if > 305 mosmol/kg give DDAVP.
- Cumulative urine output > 5 litres in the absence of any significant weight loss (strongly suggests surreptitious drinking).

Protocol 5: Overnight Dexamethasone Suppression Test

Indication

Initial screening test for Cushing's syndrome in a patient with a low clinical suspicion of Cushing's. If you have a high index of suspicion of Cushing's, omit this test and go directly to the LDDST.

Contraindications

- Patients on enzyme-inducing drugs, e.g. anticonvulsants, may rapidly metabolise dexamethasone.
- Oestrogens (e.g. pregnancy, HRT or COC) may induce cortisol-binding protein and artefactually increase total cortisol levels.
- Urine collection for 24-hour urinary free cortisol must not occur during this test.

Preparation

Outpatient test with no particular patient preparation.

Method

1. The patient takes 1 mg dexamethasone p.o. at 2300 h and the 0900 h cortisol is measured the next morning (7 ml clotted blood, in red top Vacutainer).

2. If the patient is collecting a 24-hour urine sample for urinary free cortisol this should be completed before taking the dexamethasone.

Interpretation

If the 0900 h cortisol value is less than 35 nmol/l the patient has shown suppression. Failure to suppress is seen in the autonomous secretion of cortisol found in Cushing's syndrome. With this cutoff, there will be a high false-positive rate.

Sensitivity and specificity

Suppression in patients with Cushing's syndrome is rare with this test (2%).

The reported cases metabolise dexamethasone slowly and so achieve higher circulating levels than expected. If there is strong clinical or biochemical evidence for Cushing's syndrome this test should be repeated or a formal low-dose dexamethasone test performed.

Normal subjects rarely (2%) fail to suppress with overnight dexamethasone unless they are depressed (10–50%), obese (10%) or systemically unwell (10–20%). The formal low-dose dexamethasone test is more specific.

This is a good screening test, especially if combined with urinary free cortisol.

Protocol 6: Low-Dose Dexamethasone Suppression Test (LDDST)

Indication

Screening test for Cushing's syndrome, especially if the result of the overnight suppression test contradicts other investigations. In women with a high testosterone this test may be used to differentiate PCO and partial hydroxylase deficiencies (CAH) from autonomous androgen-secreting tumours.

Contraindications

- Patients on enzyme-inducing drugs, e.g. anticonvulsants, may rapidly metabolise dexamethasone.

- Oestrogens (e.g. pregnancy, HRT or COC) may induce cortisol-binding protein and artificially increase total cortisol levels.
- *Care in diabetes mellitus and patients who are psychologically unstable.*

Preparation

This is usually an inpatient test with no particular patient preparation.

Stop all oral oestrogen therapy 6 weeks prior to test. Patients on sex steroid implants might generate results that are difficult to interpret. Measuring SHBG and CBG might be helpful in this circumstance.

Method

1. The patient takes 0.5 mg dexamethasone orally at *strict* 6-hour intervals (i.e. 0900 h, 1500 h, 2100 h and 0300 h) for 48 hours.
2. The cortisol is measured at 0900 h (before the first dose) on the first day ('2 + 0') of the test and 48 hours later (6 hours after the last dose) ('2 + 48'); samples are taken in red top Vacutainers (serum). The same sample can be used to measure SHBG and CBG if needed.

Interpretation

If the 0900 h cortisol value is less than 38 nmol/l the patient has shown suppression. Failure to suppress is seen in the autonomous secretion of cortisol found in Cushing's syndrome. In virilisation from PCO or partial hydroxylation deficiencies there will be suppression of testosterone. This is not seen in ovarian or adrenal tumours.

Sensitivity and specificity

Suppression in patients with Cushing's syndrome is rare (2–5%). Some reported cases metabolise dexamethasone slowly and so achieve higher circulating levels than expected. This test is more specific than the overnight suppression test with a lower false-positive rate. Failure of suppression in patients is rarely seen in patients with systemic illness, endogenous depression, or on enzyme-inducing drugs, e.g. phenytoin or rifampicin. In virilisation, some cases of PCO do not show suppression so imaging and venous sampling is required to exclude ovarian or adrenal tumours.

Protocol 7: High-Dose Dexamethasone Suppression Test

Indication

Patients with definite Cushing's syndrome of unknown aetiology.

Contraindications and preparation

As low-dose dexamethasone.

Method

- This test often follows the LDDST. The final sample from the LDDST (2 + 48) can often be used as the basal sample for this test. Basal 0900 h cortisol (red top Vacutainer) and ACTH (purple tops Vacutainers on ice) are measured ('8 + 0').
- During the test the patient takes 2 mg dexamethasone p.o. at *strict* 6-hour intervals (i.e. 0900 h, 1500 h, 2100 h and 0300 h) for 48 hours.
- The cortisol and ACTH are measured at 0900 h on the first day of the test and 48 hours later ('8 + 48'). In some patients the dexamethasone may be continued for 72 hours, in which case an additional 0900 h serum cortisol and ACTH are taken ('8 + 72').

Interpretation

If the 0900 h cortisol is less than 50% of the basal value after 48 hours of dexamethasone, this is classified as showing suppression. Suppression with high-dose dexamethasone is usually seen in Cushing's disease but not in ectopic ACTH production or adrenal tumours.

Sensitivity and specificity

The high-dose dexamethasone test is useful but not totally reliable in the differential diagnosis of Cushing's syndrome as it is neither very sensitive nor specific. Suppression occurs in 75% of patients with Cushing's disease, 10–25% of patients with ectopic ACTH and 0–6% of patients with adrenal tumours.

Patients with ectopic ACTH who show suppression tend to have occult and relatively benign tumours with lower levels of ACTH and cortisol. These patients are very hard to differentiate from Cushing's disease.

The 0900 h cortisol after 48 hours is considered to be the best parameter to use to discriminate between Cushing's disease and ectopic ACTH. The criterion of 50% suppression at 48 hours should not be applied too rigidly, as many cases of Cushing's disease will suppress by 40 or 45% or suppress after 72 hours. In difficult cases it is advisable to repeat the test as no patients with an adrenal tumour have been shown to have reproducible suppression and cases of Cushing's syndrome may show cyclical variation.

Protocol 8: Bilateral Simultaneous Inferior Petrosal Sinus Sampling (IPSS) with CRF

Indication

Patients with Cushing's syndrome and high ACTH levels in whom there is not a clinically definite pituitary source. The aim of this test is to differentiate pituitary from a non-pituitary source of ACTH and to lateralise a corticotroph adenoma.

Contraindications

- Allergy to contrast dye
- Ischaemic heart disease
- Orthopnoea
- Bleeding tendencies (severe).

Preparation

- Discuss with radiology
- Metyrapone and ketoconazole need to be stopped 1 week before IPSS
- Order synthetic *human or ovine* corticotrophin releasing factor (CRF) in advance from Pharmacy
- Warn endocrinology lab (34681) 48 hours in advance
- Consent patient (risks of bleeding from cannula sites, CVA, dye allergy, pulmonary embolus)
- Fast for at least 4 hours
- Two people to attend to assist sample processing
- Syringes for sampling and flushing cannulae with ice
- Discuss with laboratory the arrangements to transfer for immediate centrifugation.

Side effects

CRF can cause flushing and hypotension, but this is rare with 100 µg. No complications of IPS sampling have been reported in over 50 patients reported in the literature, but we have had one patient who had a pulmonary embolus following the procedure and one who became asystolic during the procedure but recovered when the procedure was abandoned.

Method

1. One catheter is placed in each inferior petrosal sinus (IPS) and their position confirmed on screening. A third catheter is placed peripherally (P) in the arm.
2. Two baseline samples are taken at approximately -5 and 0 min. Ask the radiologist for 10 ml from each site: one purple for ACTH and one red Vacutainer at each site. At $T = 0$ the CRF is injected as a bolus over 1 min peripherally. For adults the dose is 100 µg or 60 µg per square meter body surface in children.
3. Simultaneous samples from the 3 sampling sites are taken at $T = 2$, 5 and 10 min. At the same time as one of the sets of basal samples an arterial sample may be taken from the femoral artery if a pulmonary source of ACTH is possible, and peripheral samples may be taken at $T = 60$ and 90 min (see below). Only samples taken for ACTH should be stored in ice and spun within 15 min.
4. ACTH is measured in all samples. Cortisol is measured in the basal samples from all sites and in all the peripheral samples. Prolactin is measured in both IPS series.

Interpretation

- A basal IPS:P ratio > 2.0 indicates a pituitary source with 95% sensitivity and 100% specificity. A CRH stimulated ratio > 3.0 increases the sensitivity to 100%, the 2- and 5-min samples usually being sufficient. Pituitary ACTHomas are usually paramedian or lateral and there is suppression of the normal corticotrophs on the contralateral side.
- If, in addition, the basal or stimulated ACTH level for one IPS sample is 1.5 times as high as the simultaneous contralateral side, this localises the pituitary tumour to the ipsilateral side with a sensitivity of 99% and a specificity of 82%. It has also

been reported that prolactin and GH are often raised on the side of the tumour and that this is augmented by CRF.

- In IPS sampling the principal difficulty arises from the positioning of the sampling catheter. Jugular venous samples do not consistently show lateralisation. The measurement of prolactin can be used as a marker of proximity to the pituitary.

- Using the peripheral samples it is possible to look at the response to CRF of venous levels of cortisol. The interpretation of this response is difficult, but in general patients with Cushing's disease tend to have an exaggerated response (> 850 nmol/l) and ectopic ACTH sources have a reduced response. The interpretation of the CRF test at present is uncertain as the reported series use different end points, varying doses of CRF and small numbers of patients. Until there is more local experience of this test it should not be used to differentiate sources of ACTH.

- It appears that in ectopic ACTH production a cortisol response greater than normal has not been described. It is not a sensitive test, as approximately 25% of Cushing's disease do not respond to CRF with cortisol responses greater than normals.

Protocol 9: Peripheral Venous Sampling for Sources of Ectopic ACTH

Indication

Patients with Cushing's syndrome with high ACTH in whom there is strong evidence for an ectopic source and no evidence, including inferior petrosal sampling, to support a pituitary source. Sampling should be preceded by fine cut CT scanning of the chest and abdomen.

Contraindications

As for IPS.

Preparation

As for IPS.

Side effects

- Rarely, local bleeding
- Very rare, adrenal infarction.

Method

1. One large catheter (14–16 g) is placed peripherally to take a background venous level simultaneously with each selective site.
2. Sites will include adrenal veins, high IVC, hepatic vein, azygos and hemiazygos veins, Rt atrium, Rt & Lt innominate and thymic vein, both jugular and both superior and middle thyroid veins.
3. An arterial sample is needed as a difference between arterial and venous levels may be seen in a pulmonary source.
4. If CT scanning or tumour markers have shown a possible tumour site then super selective samples will be taken from the venous drainage.
5. Samples for ACTH should be stored in ice and spun within 15 min.
6. ACTH is measured in all samples. Cortisol is measured in the adrenal, IVC and Rt atrium samples. Prolactin is measured in the high jugular and IVC samples.

Interpretation

Local and reported experience with this technique have been disappointing with difficulties arising due to the pulsatile secretion of ACTH and wide variations in venous drainage. Results can either be expressed as a ratio of the simultaneous background ACTH or considered positive when the selective sample exceeds the maximum level recorded in the background samples.

Sensitivity and specificity

The largest and most successful study was reported from Bart's.[1] In this study high levels were found appropriately in 6 of 16 sources of ectopic ACTH; however, in only 4 cases was this the major evidence for the source. Often the level found was only slightly higher than background and in 4 of the 5 patients whose source remains undiagnosed there were levels recorded higher than the background samples and these did not help localisation. CT and tumour markers were more helpful.

Protocol 10: Glucose Tolerance Test

Indications

- Suspected diabetes mellitus. An oral glucose tolerance test is not required if the diagnosis of diabetes is not in doubt or if a fasting venous plasma glucose is greater than 7.0 mmol/l (twice if there are no symptoms) or a random venous plasma glucose is greater than 11.1 mmol/l.
- In acromegaly, to establish the diagnosis and assess patients after treatments.
- Suspected reactive hypoglycaemia when the test is prolonged to 3 hours.

Contraindications

None.

Side effects

Nausea and occasional vomiting.

Preparation

- The subject should have been on a diet containing an adequate amount of carbohydrate (250 g/day) for at least 3 days before the test
- Overnight fast
- 75 g anhydrous glucose
- Fluoride oxalate tubes × 3 (grey top Vacutainers)
- Plain tubes × 3 (red top Vacutainers) – if acromegaly
- 19 g cannula
- Saline flush
- Syringes × 3.

Method

- *Diabetes:*
  insert cannula
  take a baseline glucose at time 0
  give oral glucose load (75 g anhydrous glucose in 250–350 ml water)
  repeat blood samples at 60 and 120 min after glucose load.
- *Acromegaly:*
  insert cannula

take a baseline glucose and GH at time 0

give glucose load (75 g anhydrous glucose in 250–350 ml water)

repeat blood samples for glucose and GH at 30, 60, 90 and 120 min.

• *Reactive hypoglycaemia:*
take blood glucose at -30, 0, 30, 60, 90, 120, 150 and 180 min.

Interpretation

The WHO criteria for diabetes and impaired glucose tolerance are given in Table A1.

Acromegaly

In normal people GH will suppress to < 2 mU/l with a glucose load. Failure to suppress also occurs in chronic liver disease, renal impairment and poorly controlled diabetes.

Sensitivity and specificity

Macrovascular risk is a continuum increasing through normal and impaired glucose tolerance to diabetes.

Microvascular risk is absent in normal subjects and increases with a fasting plasma glucose >6.9 mmol/l or 2 hour glucose >11.1 mmol/l.

These criteria were revised by the WHO in 1997 and remain arbitrary.

Remember that acute illness (e.g. myocardial infarction) and drugs may affect glucose tolerance.

In acromegaly it is very rare for GH to suppress to the normal range with a glucose load. In fact there is often a paradoxical rise in

Table A1. WHO criteria for diabetes and impaired glucose tolerance

Condition	Plasma glucose (mmol/l)	
	Fasting	2 hours after glucose load
Diabetes mellitus	>6.9	>11.1
Impaired glucose tolerance		>7.8–11.0
Impaired fasting glucose	>6.0–6.9	
Normal	≤6.0	≤7.8

GH. Some normals, especially if stressed, do not suppress. The definition of 'cure' in acromegaly is very difficult. Patients may show dramatic clinical improvement but not suppress with glucose.

Protocol 11: Adrenal Venous Sampling for Aldosterone

Indication

Differential diagnosis of primary hyperaldosteronism, between aldosterone-producing adenoma and idiopathic hyperaldosteronism where CT has demonstrated no definite tumour and when the results of selenium cholesterol scanning are ambiguous.

Contraindications

Discuss with radiologist:
- bleeding tendency
- accelerated hypertension
- allergy to contrast
- significant ischaemic heart disease.

Side effects

- Bleeding
- Adrenal infarction, rarely.

Preparation

- Remember liquorice ingestion and carbenoxolone may mimic hyperaldosteronism.
- Discontinue drugs:
  $\Rightarrow$ spironolactone, oestrogens 6 weeks
  $\Rightarrow$ diuretics 4 weeks
  $\Rightarrow$ ACE inhibitors 2 weeks
  $\Rightarrow$ NSAIDs 2 weeks
  $\Rightarrow$ calcium antagonists 1 week
  $\Rightarrow$ sympathomimetics 1 week
  $\Rightarrow$ beta-blockers 1 week.
- If antihypertensive therapy needs to be continued then prazosin, doxazosin or bethanidine may be used.
- Patient should be on unrestricted sodium intake before admission.
- Consent (risks of bleeding from sheath sites, venous thrombosis).
- Fast overnight.

- Tetracosactrin 250 µg (Synacthen).
- Arrangements for immediate transfer of samples to laboratory. Two assistants required for this.

Method

Catheter inserted via femoral vein and adrenal veins selectively cannulated under X-ray control. Bolus of Synachten may be given 20 min prior to sampling. Samples taken simultaneously for cortisol, DHEAS, androstenedione and aldosterone.

Interpretation

Normal adrenal vein aldosterone 100–400 ng/dl. In aldosterone-producing adenoma the ipsilateral value is 1000–10,000 ng/dl. Ratio of >10:1 between sides is considered diagnostic.

Confirm that adrenal veins have been cannulated by comparing cortisol and adrenal androgen levels on the two sides.

Sensitivity and specificity

The main problem with this procedure is difficulty in catheterising the right adrenal vein; this is because it enters the inferior vena cava at an acute angle and may be multiple. Even in the best hands cannulation is not possible in 26% of patients.

In patients in whom both adrenal veins are successfully cannulated (as demonstrated by a symmetrical cortisol response to ACTH) this procedure is 90–95% successful in correctly distinguishing between idiopathic hyperaldosteronism and aldosterone-producing adenoma by demonstrating a unilateral increase in aldosterone secretion.

Protocol 12: Short Synacthen Test

Indication

- Used in the diagnosis of hypoadrenalism as a screening test
- It is an increasingly used alternative to the insulin tolerance test to diagnose secondary hypoadrenalism due to pituitary hypofunction
- May also be used to ascertain that the adrenals are functioning normally after a prolonged course of corticosteroids
- Diagnosis and characterisation of 21-hydroxylase deficiency and other causes of adrenal hyperplasia.

Contraindications

- Not needed for hypoadrenalism if random cortisol > 580 nmol/l
- Allergy to egg albumin.

Side effects

None.

Preparation

- If on steroids, ensure that none is taken the night prior to the test. The final dose should be at 0900 h, 24 hours prior to the test.
- Admission is required if there is a risk of addisonian crisis (virtually never).
- 1 ampoule of 250 μg tetracosactrin (Synacthen).

Method

1. 0900 h: take 7 ml blood for cortisol and discuss with laboratory.
2. Give 250 μg tetracosactrin IM (ideally) or IV.
3. 0930 h: Take 7 ml blood for cortisol.
4. 1000 h: Take 7 ml blood for cortisol.
5. For the diagnosis of congenital adrenal hyperplasia the samples taken for cortisol are also analysed for 17-OH progesterone to exclude 21-hydroxylase deficiency. In some cases 17-OH pregnenolone is measured to differentiate between 21-OH and 3β-HSD deficiency.

Interpretation

- Normal response if test done at 0900 h (considerable diurnal variation):
    - basal plasma cortisol >170 nmol/l
    - stimulated plasma cortisol > 580 nmol/l (may be 500–600 depending on local laboratory)
    - incremental rise of at least 190 nmol/l.
- If impaired cortisol response, and ACTH > 200 ng/l then diagnosis is primary adrenal failure.
- If ACTH <10 ng/l, then diagnosis is secondary adrenal failure.
- Response of 17-OH progesterone in suspected 21-hydroxylase deficiency (cryptic): marked rise after ACTH stimulation, which varies according to whether the patient is homozygous or heterozygous.

Sensitivity and specificity

A normal cortisol response does not exclude adrenal failure, since impending adrenal failure might be associated with a much greater loss of zona glomerulosa function. The latter would be suggested by an elevated plasma renin activity.

If equivocal result and no urgency, repeat test after a few weeks.

An abnormal response is consistent with primary or secondary adrenal failure, and should be investigated further. Consider long Synacthen test or pituitary function testing.

Protocol 13: Long Synacthen Test

Indication

- Confirmation of diagnosis of hypoadrenalism.
- Differentiating primary and secondary hypoadrenalism (note that measurement of basal 0900 h ACTH levels is far more sensitive than cortisol response in the long Synacthen test).
- The first three samples should give the same result as the short Synacthen test.

Contraindications

None.

Side effects

None.

Preparation

- Patients who have already been taking corticosteroids should have been on these for less than 2 weeks and should be switched to dexamethasone 24 hours before the test.
- 1 mg tetracosactrin (depot preparation). This is not the same as ordinary Synacthen!

Method

0900 h: insert cannula and flush; take blood for baseline cortisol and ACTH; give 1 mg depot Synacthen IM

0930 h, 1000 h, 1100 h, 1300 h, 1700 h, 0900 h: take blood for cortisol measurement (i.e. additional 2, 4, 8 and 24 hours)

Interpretation

- *Normal response*: baseline cortisol >170 nmol/l with rise to >900 nmol/l (peak)
- *Primary adrenal insufficiency*: little or no response
- *Secondary adrenal insufficiency*: some patients may show a rise in cortisol, which may be delayed (but a subnormal response does not exclude this – measure ACTH levels).

Sensitivity and specificity

More sensitive than short Synacthen test for primary adrenal insufficiency (for nomogram, see Burke.[2]).

Protocol 14: Prolonged Supervised Fast for Insulinoma

Indication

Used to demonstrate fasting hypoglycaemia and diagnose insulinoma if not shown spontaneously or after an overnight fast.

Preparation

- Screen with three fasting plasma glucose, diagnose with this test
- Admit to perform test under close supervision with glucose (p.o./IV) available
- Leave a copy of this protocol sheet in the nurse's notes and a copy above the patient's bed.

Method

- Cannulate patient and commence 72-hour fast.
- Water/non-caloric beverages allowed. Patient should be active during waking hours.
- Blood glucoses should be done at regular (4–6 hours) intervals and whenever the patient has symptoms suggestive of hypoglycaemia. Decrease to 2-hour intervals if the patient consistently has glucoses <3.0 mmol/l.
- If blood glucoses are ≤ 2.2 mmol/l or symptoms are convincing:
  Bleep endocrine SHO urgently.
  Take blood for glucose, insulin and C peptide in a plain clotted tube (7 ml) and a fluoride oxalate tube.
  Take blood and spot urine for sulphonylurea screen in a plain clotted tube (7 ml) and a Sterilin universal container.

Take to chemistry labs to be separated and frozen within 30 min. Ring Biochemistry up for an urgent glucose.

Do not reverse hypoglycaemia until the lab confirms hypoglycaemia, or unless the patient becomes unconscious or fits.

- If no symptoms during the fast, finish with 15–30 min exercise, e.g. a brisk walk around the hospital.
- Take final samples for glucose, insulin and C peptide, sulphonylurea screen.

Interpretation

- Normals do not become hypoglycaemic, although young women can run glucoses in the region of 2.2–3.0 mmol/l without symptoms.
- True hypoglycaemia must be demonstrated (glucose ≤ 2–2.2 mmol/l) before we are able to either interpret insulin results or consider insulinoma.
- If hypoglycaemia with raised insulin but low C peptide, consider self-administration of insulin.
- If hypoglycaemia with raised insulin, and raised C peptide, make sure sulphonylurea screen is negative!
- With hypoglycaemia, insulin and endogenous insulin production (estimated by C peptide) should be undetectable:

Insulin >6 mU/l (>50 pmol/l); C peptide >300 pmol/l = insulinoma

Insulin >3–6 mU/l (25–50 pmol/l); C peptide 100–300 pmol/l = possible insulinoma but needs further tests

Insulin <3 mU/l (<25 pmol/l); C peptide <75 pmol/l = normal response.

- Ketones should be suppressed with insulinoma even though patient is fasting because of the excess insulin.

Sensitivity and specificity

By 24 hours, 66% insulinomas develop hypoglycaemia and by 48 hours, >95% insulinomas can be diagnosed. After 72 hours fast plus exercise, if no hypoglycaemia, insulinoma is very unlikely.

Protocol 15: Pentolinium Suppression Test

Indication

To try and exclude the diagnosis of phaeochromocytoma in patients with hypertension and borderline changes in plasma catecholamines or 24-hour urinary catecholamines.

Contraindications

No absolute contraindications, but beware frail patient and patients with severe coronary or carotid vascular disease.

Side effects

May cause severe transient hypotension.

Preparation

- Order the pentolinium from Pharmacy (difficult to obtain). It comes as 10 mg/ml
- Stop hypotensive treatment for at least 24 hours before the test (especially centrally acting drugs such as methyldopa)
- Fast overnight
- Quiet environment
- Sphygmomanometer or electronic BP monitor
- Cannula, 19 g
- Ice and lithium heparin tubes
- Contact biochemistry laboratory, who measure catecholamines before doing the test; enquire how they would like the samples taken and arrange for their delivery.

Method

1. Rest for 1/2 hour.
2. Monitor BP and pulse at onset and every time blood taken.
3. Take two baseline samples at 5-min intervals for catecholamines. Blood needs to be taken into lithium heparin, kept on ice, spun at 4°C and frozen until assay.
4. At time 0, give 2.5 mg pentolinium IV.
5. Take blood at 1 hour.

Interpretation

Pentolinium is a sympathetic ganglion blocker. Normal subjects may show an initially elevated plasma adrenaline and noradrenaline, but these will fall to within the normal plasma range with pentolinium. In contrast, the autonomous secretion of a phaeochromocytoma will not suppress.

Sensitivity and specificity

This test has a low false-positive and false-negative rate as determined in series of known phaeochromocytomas and normals but published information is very scanty. The most likely theoretical problem is a fall in plasma catecholamine levels in a phaeochromocytoma patient whose tumour is only secreting episodically.

Protocol 16: Clonidine Suppression Test

Indication

To try and exclude the diagnosis of phaeochromocytoma in patients with hypertension and borderline changes in plasma catecholamines or urinary catecholamine metabolites.

Contraindications

Frail patient with a history of hypotensive episodes or severe coronary or carotid disease.

Side effects

Hypotension and sedation.

Preparation

- Order the clonidine from Pharmacy (readily obtainable)
- Stop hypotensive treatment for at least 24 hours before the test if possible
- Fast overnight
- Quiet environment
- Sphygmomanometer
- Contact biochemistry laboratory, who measure catecholamines before doing the test; enquire how they would like the samples taken and arrange for their delivery.

Method

1. Insert cannula
2. Rest for 1/2 hour
3. Monitor BP and pulse at onset and every time blood taken
4. Take two baseline samples at 5-min intervals
5. Give, at time 0, 0.3 mg clonidine hydrochloride orally
6. Take blood at hourly intervals for 3 hours.

Interpretation

Clonidine acts via the alpha preganglionic receptors to reduce catecholamine secretion.

In normals, even if they are anxious, the plasma catecholamines will suppress into the normal range 3 hours after clonidine (noradrenaline 0.2–0.8 ng/ml, adrenaline 0.04–2 ng/ml). Phaeochromocytoma patients should not.

Sensitivity and specificity

This test gives similar information as the pentolinium test; there have been no formal comparisons of the two tests. Case reports[3] have illustrated false negatives. The 24-hour urinary metanephrines/catecholamines have replaced VMA (vanillylmandelic acid) as the cornerstone of screening for phaeochromocytoma. If a dopamine-secreting phaeochromocytoma is suspected on the basis of normo- or hypotension, then urinary dopamine and its metabolites should be assayed.

References

1. Besser M, Trainer PJ (eds). *The Barts Endocrine Protocols.* London: Churchill Livingstone, 1995.

2. Burke CW. Adrenocortical insufficiency. *Clin Endocrinol Metab* 1985;**14**:947–76.

3. Clonidine-suppression test for diagnosis of pheochromacytoma. *N Engl Med J* 1982;**306**:49-50.

Further Reading

Abdu TA, Elhadd TA, Neary R, Clayton RN. Comparison of the low dose short synacthen test (1 microg), the conventional dose short synacthen test (250 microg), and the insulin tolerance test for assessment of the hypothalamic-pituitary-axis in patients with pituitary disease. *J Clin Endocrinol Metab* 1999;**84**:838–43.

Bravo EL, Tarazi RC, Fouad FM, Vidt DG, Gifford RW Jr. Clonidine-suppression test: a useful aid in the diagnosis of pheochromocytoma. *N Engl J Med* 1981;**305**:623–6.

Brown MJ, Allison DJ, Jenner DA, Lewis PJ, Dollery CT. Increased sensitivity and accuracy of phaeochromocytoma diagnosis achieved by use of plasma-adrenaline estimations and a pentolinium-suppression test. *Lancet* 1981;**1**:174–7.

Clayton RN. Diagnosis of adrenal insufficiency. *BMJ* 1989;**298**:271–2.

Crapo A. Cushing's syndrome: a review of diagnostic tests. *Metabolism* 1979;**28**:955–77.

Friesen SR. Update on the diagnosis and treatment of rare neuroendocrine tumours. *Surg Clin North Am* 1987;**67**:379–93.

Greenwood FC, Landon J, Stamp TC. The plasma sugar, free fatty acid, cortisol, and growth hormone response to insulin. I. In control subjects. *J Clin Invest* 1966;**45**:429–36.

Landon J, Greenwood FC, Stamp TC, Wynn V. The plasma sugar, free fatty acid, cortisol, and growth hormone response to insulin, and the comparison of this procedure with other tests of pituitary and adrenal function. II. In patients with hypothalamic or pituitary dysfunction or anorexia nervosa. *J Clin Invest* 1966;**45**:437–49.

Melby JC. Diagnosis and treatment of primary aldosteronism and isolated hypoaldosteronism. *Clin Endocrinol Metab* 1985;**14**:977–95.

New MI, Lorenzen F, Lerner AJ et al. Genotyping steroid 21-hydroxylase deficiency: hormonal reference data. *J Clin Endocrinol Metab* 1983;**57**:320–6.

Oldfield EH, Doppman JL, Nieman LK et al. Petrosal sinus sampling with and without corticotropin-releasing hormone for the differential diagnosis of Cushing's syndrome. *N Engl J Med* 1991;**325**:897–905.

Rao RH, Spathis GS. Intramuscular glucagon as a provocative stimulus for the assessment of pituitary function: growth hormone and cortisol responses. *Metabolism* 1987;**36**(7):658–63.

Savage MO. Congenital adrenal hyperplasia. *Clin Endocrinol Metab* 1985;**14**:893–909.

Young WF, Klee GG. Primary aldosteronism. Diagnostic evaluation. *Endocrinol Metab Clin North Am* 1988;**17**:367–95.

Useful Addresses

Patient groups

Addison's Disease Self-Help Group
21 George Road
Guildford
Surrey
GU1 4NP
Tel: 01483 830 673
E-mail: deana@adshg.freeserve.co.uk
http://www.surreyweb.net\adshg

The National Association for the Relief of Paget's Disease
323 Manchester Road
Walkden
Worsley
Manchester
M28 3HH
Tel: 0161 799 4646
E-mail: NARPD@aol.com
http://www.paget.org.uk

Thyroid Federation International
Headquarters
96 Mack Street
Kingston
ON
Canada K7L 5J7
Tel: 613 544 8364
E-mail: tfi@kos.net
http://www.thyroid-fed.org

Thyroid Foundation
PO Box 97
Clifford
Wetherby
W Yorks
LS23 6XD
Tel: 0113 292 4600
http://www.british-thyroid-association.org

Thyroid Eye Disease Association
Head Office
Solstice
Sea Road
Winchelsea Beach
East Sussex
TN36 4LH
Tel: 01797 222338
E-mail: tedassn@eclipse.co.uk

The Pituitary Foundation
PO Box 1944
Bristol
BS99 2UB
Tel: 0117 927 3355
E-mail: helpline@pituitary.org.uk
http://www.pituitary.org.uk

Weight Watchers
Weight Watchers UK Ltd
Ludlow Road
Maidenhead
Berkshire
SL6 2SL
Tel: 08457 123000
http://www.weightwatchers.co.uk

Professional groups

Association of the Study of Obesity
20 Brook Meadow Close
Woodford Green
Essex
IG8 9NR
Tel: 020 8503 2042
http://www.aso.org.uk

Society for Endocrinology
17/18 The Courtyard
Woodlands
Bradley Stoke
Bristol BS32 4NQ
Tel: 01454 642200
E-mail: info@endocrinology.org
http://www.endocrinology.org

Index

Page numbers in *italics* refer to illustrations, tables or boxes.